VOLUME EIGHTY TWO

ADVANCES IN PHARMACOLOGY

VOLUME EIGHTY TWO

ADVANCES IN PHARMACOLOGY

Apprentices to Genius: A tribute to Solomon H. Snyder

Edited by

GAVRIL W. PASTERNAK
Memorial Sloan Kettering Cancer Center, New York, NY, United States

JOSEPH T. COYLE
Harvard Medical School, Boston; McLean Hospital, Belmont, MA, United States

Serial Editor

S.J. ENNA
University of Kansas Medical Center, Kansas City, KS, United States

Managing Editor

LYNN LECOUNT
University of Kansas Medical Center, School of Medicine, Kansas City, KS, United States

ELSEVIER

ACADEMIC PRESS
An imprint of Elsevier

Academic Press is an imprint of Elsevier
50 Hampshire Street, 5th Floor, Cambridge, MA 02139, United States
525 B Street, Suite 1800, San Diego, CA 92101-4495, United States
The Boulevard, Langford Lane, Kidlington, Oxford OX5 1GB, United Kingdom
125 London Wall, London, EC2Y 5AS, United Kingdom

First edition 2018

Notices
Knowledge and best practice in this field are constantly changing. As new research and experience broaden our understanding, changes in research methods, professional practices, or medical treatment may become necessary.

Practitioners and researchers must always rely on their own experience and knowledge in evaluating and using any information, methods, compounds, or experiments described herein. In using such information or methods they should be mindful of their own safety and the safety of others, including parties for whom they have a professional responsibility.

To the fullest extent of the law, neither the Publisher nor the authors, contributors, or editors, assume any liability for any injury and/or damage to persons or property as a matter of products liability, negligence or otherwise, or from any use or operation of any methods, products, instructions, or ideas contained in the material herein.

ISBN: 978-0-12-814087-1
ISSN: 1054-3589

For information on all Academic Press publications
visit our website at https://www.elsevier.com/books-and-journals

Publisher: Zoe Kruze
Acquisition Editor: Zoe Kruze
Editorial Project Manager: Shellie Bryant
Production Project Manager: Vignesh Tamil
Cover Designer: Victoria Pearson

Typeset by SPi Global, India

CONTENTS

CONTRIBUTORS

Darrick T. Balu
Harvard Medical School, Boston; McLean Hospital, Belmont, MA, United States

Jay M. Baraban
Johns Hopkins School of Medicine, Baltimore, MD, United States

A. Harrison Brody
Program in Cellular Neuroscience, Neurodegeneration & Repair, Yale University School of Medicine; Yale University, New Haven, CT, United States

David B. Bylund
University of Nebraska Medical Center, Omaha, NE, United States

Joseph T. Coyle
Harvard Medical School, Boston; McLean Hospital, Belmont, MA, United States

Ted M. Dawson
Neuroregeneration and Stem Cell Programs, Institute for Cell Engineering, Johns Hopkins University School of Medicine, Baltimore, MD; Adrienne Helis Malvin Medical Research Foundation; Diana Helis Henry Medical Research Foundation, New Orleans, LA, United States

Valina L. Dawson
Neuroregeneration and Stem Cell Programs, Institute for Cell Engineering, Johns Hopkins University School of Medicine, Baltimore, MD; Adrienne Helis Malvin Medical Research Foundation; Diana Helis Henry Medical Research Foundation, New Orleans, LA, United States

Yi Na Dong
Children's Hospital of Philadelphia, Philadelphia, PA, United States

S.J. Enna
University of Kansas Medical Center, Kansas City, KS, United States

Lloyd D. Fricker
Albert Einstein College of Medicine, Bronx, NY, United States

Xiuping Fu
Johns Hopkins School of Medicine, Baltimore, MD, United States

Moshe Gavish
Faculty of Medicine, Rappaport Institute, Technion—Israel Institute of Technology, Haifa, Israel

Amy J. Gleichman
Perelman School of Medicine, University of Pennsylvania, Philadelphia, PA, United States

Alan I. Green
Geisel School of Medicine at Dartmouth; Dartmouth Clinical and Translational Science Institute, Dartmouth College, Hanover, NH, United States

Angela M. Henricks
Geisel School of Medicine at Dartmouth; Dartmouth Clinical and Translational Science Institute, Dartmouth College, Hanover, NH, United States

Ioline D. Henter
Molecular Imaging Branch, National Institute of Mental Health, Bethesda, MD, United States

Robert B. Innis
Molecular Imaging Branch, National Institute of Mental Health, Bethesda, MD, United States

Samie R. Jaffrey
Weill Medical College, Cornell University, New York, NY, United States

Jonathan A. Javitch
College of Physicians & Surgeons, Columbia University; Division of Molecular Therapeutics, New York State Psychiatric Institute, New York, NY, United States

Caline S. Karam
College of Physicians & Surgeons, Columbia University; Division of Molecular Therapeutics, New York State Psychiatric Institute, New York, NY, United States

Jibran Y. Khokhar
Geisel School of Medicine at Dartmouth; Dartmouth Clinical and Translational Science Institute, Dartmouth College, Hanover, NH, United States

William C. Kreisl
Taub Institute, Columbia University Medical Center, New York, NY, United States

David R. Lynch
Children's Hospital of Philadelphia; Perelman School of Medicine, University of Pennsylvania, Philadelphia, PA, United States

Jessica A. Panzer
Children's Hospital of Philadelphia; Perelman School of Medicine, University of Pennsylvania, Philadelphia, PA, United States

Gavril W. Pasternak
Memorial Sloan Kettering Cancer Center, New York, NY, United States

Amy Rattelle
Children's Hospital of Philadelphia, Philadelphia, PA, United States

Kylie Roslin
Children's Hospital of Philadelphia, Philadelphia, PA, United States

Aparna Shah
Johns Hopkins School of Medicine, Baltimore, MD, United States

Stephen M. Strittmatter
Program in Cellular Neuroscience, Neurodegeneration & Repair, Yale University School of Medicine; Yale University, New Haven, CT, United States

Emily D.K. Sullivan
Geisel School of Medicine at Dartmouth; Dartmouth Clinical and Translational Science Institute, Dartmouth College, Hanover, NH, United States

Leo Veenman
Faculty of Medicine, Rappaport Institute, Technion—Israel Institute of Technology, Haifa, Israel

Herman Wolosker
Rappaport Faculty of Medicine and Research Institute, Technion—Israel Institute of Technology, Haifa, Israel

PREFACE

The molecular biology revolution and technological advances over the past few decades have transformed biomedical science, enabling us to view biology at the atomic level—a far cry from the descriptive biology of the last century. Yet, some things have not changed. The academic preparation of today's future scientists is outstanding, but their training as investigators remains heavily dependent upon a close mentoring relationship—much like an apprentice of old. Mentors teach how to approach problems and solve them, but most critically, to determine which questions are the most important to address.

Mentors and students develop strong bonds, with mentors commonly referred to as "scientific mothers or fathers," going back to scientific grandparents and even great-grandparents. Two decades ago, Robert Kanigel, in his book *Apprentice to Genius*, explored the generational transfer of mentorship from Bernard Brodie to Julius Axelrod and from him to Solomon Snyder, likening it to a family tree. The tree has continued to grow tall, with branches spreading out into many different areas of neuroscience.

This volume is dedicated to Solomon Snyder. Sol is an extraordinary scientist, winner of the Lasker Award and the Wolfe Prize among others. However, he considers his greatest accomplishment the cadre of scientists he has trained over the years—his "children" and even "grandchildren." This volume is an acknowledgment by some of the "kids" of his profound impact on their science, their careers, and their lives. The chapters are from a representative sample of his trainees. With several hundred trainees, it would be impossible to include them all, but everyone is one family.

The book encompasses a wide range of topics. Assay development was an integral component of the Axelrod laboratory, carried forward by Snyder and more recently with the development of RNA-based fluorescent biosensors. The explosion in receptor biology started with the development of receptor binding assays in the 1970s, as described by Bylund and Enna. The early work from the Snyder laboratory on opioid receptors that led to his Lasker Award is described and extended in another chapter, while the continuation of his early investigations on enkephalins carried forward with the identification of a range of novel neuropeptides. Other chapters expand on nitric oxide and the "peripheral benzodiazepine receptor" and explore a range of neurologic and psychiatric entities, including anti-NMDA receptor encephalitis and degenerative diseases. The extended range of topics in this volume illustrates the broad impact of Sol and his trainees in neuroscience, neurology, and psychiatry.

His students and fellows have described his laboratory as "transformative" and "infected by the excitement of discovery research." The laboratory was filled with "counter watchers"—those unable to wait until the next day to find out the results of their experiments. Many recollect writing a manuscript over lunch in his office—something few of us have been able to accomplish since. His wife, Elaine, played the role of our "mother," inviting us to dinners, lab parties, and other celebrations, which often ended with Sol playing classical guitar music. Most of all, we remember his warmth, generosity of spirit (and ideas), and the feeling of belonging to a wonderful family.

Gavril W. Pasternak
Joseph T. Coyle
S.J. Enna
October 30, 2017

APPENDIX

Soloman H. Snyder, M.D.	
Trainees as of November 1, 2017	
Bahman Aghdasi	William Logan
Ishrat Ahmed	Hongbo Luo
Lauren Albacarys	David Lynch
Robert Anholt	Ernie Lyons
Hasti Atashi Shirazi	Martin Ma
BI Bae	Ting Martin Ma
Jay Baraban	David Maag
David Baranano	Mathew MacCumber
Roxanne Barrow	Adarsha Malla
Marie Bell	Micah Maxwell
James Bennett	Maureen McEnery

Soloman H. Snyder, M.D.	
Trainees as of November 1, 2017	
Isaac Bernstein	Susan McTeer
Rashna Bhandari	Robbie Mealer
Deeya Bhattacharya	Jordana Meisel
Seth Blackshaw	James Meyerhoff
Darren Boehning	Ginny Miller
Felice Borisy-Rudin	Jack Moriarty
Jimo Borjigin	Jean-Pierre Mothet
Karen Braas	Weitong Mu
David Bredt	Alexandra Murray
Robert Bruns	Asif Mustafa
Patrick Burnett	Eiichiro Nagata
David Burt	Latika Nagpal
David Bylund	Jeffrey Nye
Andrew Cameron	Gavril Pasternak
Jiyoung Cha	Randen Patterson
Anutosh Chakraborty	Bindu Paul
Michael Charness	Stephen Peroutka
Jaime Cheah	David Perry
Stephen Childers	Jonathan Pevsner
Alfred Chin	Andrew Pieper
Sayan Chowdhury	Joe Pietropaoli
Noam Cohen	Feng Rao
Marisol Cortes	Luke Reilly
Pedro Cortes	Adam Resnick
Joseph Coyle	Ian Reynolds
Ian Creese	Cristina Ricco
Robert D'Amato	Elliott Richelson

Continued

Soloman H. Snyder, M.D.

Trainees as of November 1, 2017

Sonye Danoff	Terry Rogers
Ted Dawson	Tomas Rojas
Jay Dinerman	Gabriele Ronnett
Dawn Dodson	Christopher Ross
Sylvain Dore	Robin Roychaudhuri
Jeffrey Ehmsen	Martial Ruat
Mikael Eliasson	David Sabatini
Salvatore Enna	Adolfo Saiardi
Ming Fang	Masoumeh Saleh
Christopher Ferris	Akira Sawa
Majid Fotuhi	Juan Sbodio
Jonathan Freedman	Michael Schell
Lloyd Fricker	Paul Scherer
Chenglai Fu	Tom Sedlak
Moataz Gadalla	Balakrishnan Selvakumar
Moshe Gavish	Evan Semenza
Charles Glatt	Nilkantha Sen
Robert Goodman	Alan Sharp
Robert Gould	Rabi Simantov
Alan Green	Kate Sixt
David Greenberg	Pamela Sklar
Prasun Guha	Pam Smith
Andrew Gundlach	Adele Snowman
Makoto Hara	Joe Steiner
Maged Harraz	Stephen Strittmatter
Edith Hendley	Srinivasa Subramaniam
Lynda Hester	Surachai Supattapone
Daniel Higginson	Ken Taylor

Soloman H. Snyder, M.D.

Trainees as of November 1, 2017	
David Hirsch	Anne Theibert
Evelyn Ho	Jing Tian
Gary Ho	Robert Tokhunts
Alex Huang	Lawrence Toll
Yunfei Huang	Isaac Treisman
K. Joe Hurt	Rosario Trifiletti
Patrick Hussman	Richa Tyagi
Paul Hwang	George Uhl
Robert Innis	David U'Prichard
Samie Jaffrey	Ted Usdin
Jonathan Javitch	Damien van Rossum
Krishna Juluri	Scott Vandiver
Mitchell Jung	Chirag Vasavda
Bingnan Kang	Ajay Verma
Josh Kang	Susan Voglmaier
Michael Kapiloff	John Wagner
Adam Kaplin	Loren Walensky
Jefferson Katims	Crystal Watkins
Adil Khan	Kent Werner
David Kim	Urbain Weyemi
Paul Kim	Herman Wolosker
Sangwon Kim	Paul Worley
Seyun Kim	Jing Xu
Michael Koldobskiy	Risheng Xu
Michael Kornberg	Keqiang Ye
Ruchita Kothari	Anne Young
Michael Kuhar	Nicholas Zaccor

Continued

Soloman H. Snyder, M.D.	
Trainees as of November 1, 2017	
Michael Lai	Jie Zhang
Chi Ming Lee	Barbara Ziegler
Xiadong Li	Stephen Zukin
Xiao-Jiang Li	

FOREWORD

It is a pleasure and an honor to contribute to this volume celebrating Sol Snyder's 50 years of research at Johns Hopkins and his impending 80th birthday. I have known Sol as a friend and colleague for more than 50 years, beginning with our time together as young scientists at the NIH working with Julie Axelrod. Julie inspired us and others in the frantic pace of work at the time as molecular studies of the brain were just exploding. I went on from the NIH to a year at Harvard Medical School to work with Stephen Kuffler and Ed Kravitz, two other world leaders in this expanding field. Following my stint at Harvard I returned to Cambridge, England. Until Julie's death in 2004, Sol remained his close friend as he considered Julie his first, and most important, scientific mentor.

Spontaneity was a key component of Julie's research style. Julie remained constantly open to new challenges, avenues of research and ideas, with a talent for always finding ingenious ways of testing them in the laboratory. In many ways Sol has emulated the Axelrod's approach. His oeuvre is characterized by a broad range of research projects with many notable successes. His research pioneered the development of molecular approaches for defining central nervous system function. In particular, he focused on projects that might ultimately provide new therapies for complex psychiatric disorders, such as schizophrenia. As a psychiatrist, Sol's knowledge of the clinical characteristics of these disorders gives him particularly keen insights and perspectives in designing and interpreting experiments in this field.

His first notable discovery came in the early 1970s with his finding that opiate receptors could be studied, and their molecular properties defined, in vitro using radioligand binding. Up to that time the existence of these receptors could only be inferred by the characteristic physiological responses elicited by drugs such as morphine. The use of Sol's radioligand binding technique for identifying brain neurotransmitter and hormone receptors quickly became a vital tool for biochemical pharmacologists in both academia and industry. Sol's work on radioligand binding to dopamine receptors identified directly the site and mechanism of action of antipsychotic drugs as dopamine D2 receptor antagonists. This finding encouraged others to undertake new approaches for designing and developing agents for this important drug class. Over the years Sol's research on receptor identification and mechanisms included studies on nitric oxide, the modulation of glutamate NMDA receptor function by serine transport, GABA, glycine, serotonin, acetylcholine, and noradrenaline receptors, among others. His work is described in hundreds of research, review, and monograph articles, as well as books he has authored for both lay and scientific audiences.

The breadth of the research performed by Sol and his students and colleagues is well represented in this volume. Much of it is aimed at identifying the molecular mechanisms of CNS disorders. The studies range from the genetics of schizophrenia, to the role of RNA metabolism, and the identification of novel substances that may serve as biomarkers or potential therapeutic targets. (At this stage I confess that GOOGLE had to be asked to translate some of the acronyms!)

Probably the most important of Sol's contributions was the training of so many successful scientists, many of whom contributed to this volume. Just as Sol and I were inspired by Julie Axelrod, Sol has inspired dozens of students and postdoctoral fellows with his "Axelrod-like" enthusiasm for science. Thus, besides his research accomplishments, Sol has played a major role in populating the current generation of research-oriented neuroscientists and clinicians, ensuring his legacy in the field.

Long may he continue!

Les Iversen
29 May 2017

CHAPTER ONE

Multiple Pathways Mediate MicroRNA Degradation: Focus on the Translin/Trax RNase Complex

Jay M. Baraban[1], Aparna Shah, Xiuping Fu
Johns Hopkins School of Medicine, Baltimore, MD, United States
[1]Corresponding author: e-mail address: jay.baraban@gmail.com

Contents

Abstract

The discovery of the microRNA system has revolutionized our understanding of translational control. Furthermore, growing appreciation of the pivotal role that de novo translation plays in activity-dependent synaptic plasticity has fueled interest among neuroscientists in deciphering how the microRNA system impacts neuronal signaling and the pathophysiology of neuropsychiatric disorders. Although we have a general understanding of how the microRNA system operates, many key questions remain. In particular, the biosynthesis of microRNAs and their role in translational silencing are fairly well understood. However, much less is known about

Advances in Pharmacology, Volume 82
ISSN 1054-3589
https://doi.org/10.1016/bs.apha.2017.08.003

how microRNAs are degraded and silencing is reversed, crucial aspects of microRNA signaling. In contrast to microRNA synthesis which is mediated almost exclusively by a single pathway that culminates in Dicer, recent studies indicate that there are multiple pathways of microRNA degradation that target different subpopulations of microRNAs. While the Lin-28 pathway of microRNA degradation has been investigated extensively, the translin/trax RNase complex has emerged recently as another pathway mediating microRNA degradation. Accordingly, we summarize herein key features of the translin/trax RNase complex as well as important gaps in our understanding of its regulation and function that are the focus of ongoing studies.

ABBREVIATIONS

BDNF brain-derived neurotrophic factor
ERE Egr response element
NGF nerve growth factor
PLCbeta phospholipase C beta
pre-miRNAs precursor microRNAs
pri-miRNAs primary transcripts of microRNAs
RISC RNA-induced silencing complex
SSRIs selective serotonin reuptake inhibitors

1. INTRODUCTION

Sol has infected generations of students with his contagious enthusiasm for "figuring out" how things work, the creative urge at the heart of science. In tribute to Sol's extraordinary mentorship, we present an overview of progress in "figuring out" the function of the translin/trax RNase complex, which plays a key role in regulating the microRNA system. To place these studies in context, we will first provide a brief overview of the microRNA system and its role in neuronal signaling.

2. CANONICAL VIEW OF MicroRNA SYNTHESIS AND MicroRNA-MEDIATED SILENCING

The discovery of the microRNA system has revolutionized our understanding of translational control (Bartel, 2004, 2009). Every cell generates hundreds of microRNAs, small, ~22-nucleotide RNA species, that can each silence dozens of mRNA transcripts. At first glance, this system appears to be impossibly chaotic. While each cell transcribes thousands of mRNAs destined for translation, it simultaneously generates hundreds of different microRNA species charged with intercepting these mRNAs before they undergo translation. However, a closer look reveals that this elaborate choreography of mRNAs and microRNAs is not designed to suppress translation indiscriminately, but to provide an elegant means of fine-tuning which mRNAs are translated at any given time in response to dynamic changes in cellular demands. While this system plays a ubiquitous role in regulating translation throughout the body, neuroscientists are particularly eager to understand its impact on neuronal signaling, in light of growing evidence that many forms of neuronal plasticity are mediated by de novo translation (Mayford, Siegelbaum, & Kandel, 2012).

Following the discovery of the microRNA system (Fire et al., 1998; Ruvkun, 2008), attention focused on deciphering how these tiny RNA species are generated (Bartel, 2004). Rapid progress in this area revealed that primary transcripts containing microRNAs (pri-miRNAs) are transcribed in a pol II-dependent fashion and then processed by the Drosha complex to stem-loop structures, referred to as precursor microRNAs (pre-miRNAs). After export from the nucleus, pre-miRNAs are acted on by Dicer to generate mature microRNAs, short, double-stranded RNA oligos with overhangs. Mature microRNAs are then separated into "guide" and "passenger" strands, with the guide strand loaded onto the RNA-induced silencing complex (RISC) which enables it to bind to a complementary sequence in the 3′UTR of a target mRNA (Fig. 1). While the steps in processing microRNAs from initial transcription of pri-miRNAs to association with RISC are reasonably well worked out, the exact mechanism mediating silencing of translation remains unclear and is under active investigation (Chapat et al., 2017; Filipowicz & Sonenberg, 2015).

A major function of silencing is to restrain translation of targeted mRNAs *temporarily* so that it can proceed rapidly in response to cellular demands. Therefore, an important challenge facing this field is to define the mechanisms controlling rapid reversal of silencing. From this perspective, the microRNA system can be viewed as a second messenger system that triggers translation by reversing silencing of selected mRNAs in response to extracellular signals (Fu et al., 2016). Accordingly, these findings have focused attention on identifying the pathways mediating degradation of microRNAs and how they are regulated.

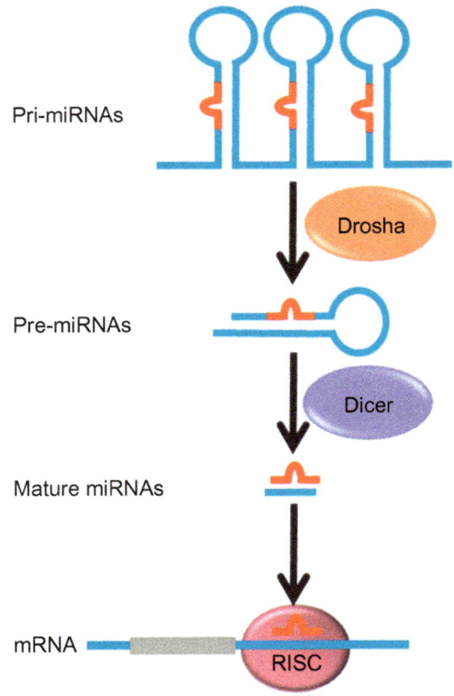

Fig. 1 Overview of microRNA biogenesis. Generation of mature microRNAs is mediated almost exclusively via sequential conversion of the primary microRNA transcripts (pri-miRNAs) by Drosha to hairpin structures, called precursor-microRNAs (pre-miRNAs), which are then cleaved by Dicer to form double-stranded mature microRNAs (mature miRNAs). At this point, the guide strand, *shown in red*, is separated from its complementary passenger strand, *shown in blue*, prior to being loaded onto the RNA-induced silencing complex (RISC). Once loaded onto RISC, the guide strand directs RISC to cognate binding sites in the 3′UTR of target mRNAs to suppress their translation. *Figure modified from Fu, X., Shah, A., & Baraban, J. M. (2016). Rapid reversal of translational silencing: Emerging role of microRNA degradation pathways in neuronal plasticity* Neurobiology of Learning and Memory, 133, *225–232.*

3. FOCUS ON MicroRNA DEGRADATION

The initial discovery of the microRNA system emerged from efforts aimed at understanding the interplay of let-7 and Lin-28 in *C. elegans* which display complementary patterns of expression (Ruvkun, 2008). These observations led to the discovery that Lin-28 triggers degradation of the let-7 family of microRNAs (Rybak et al., 2008; Viswanathan, Daley, & Gregory, 2008). In this pathway (Fig. 2), Lin-28 recognizes a sequence motif

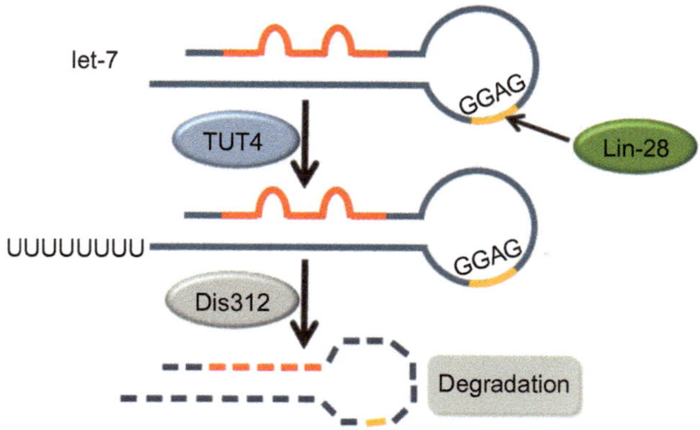

Fig. 2 Lin-28 microRNA degradation pathway. Nearly all let-7 family members contain a Lin-28 binding motif, GGAG, located toward the 3′ end of the pre-microRNA loop (*top panel*). Binding of Lin-28 to let-7 pre-microRNA recruits TUT4, an enzyme that adds a poly U tract to the 3′ end of the pre-microRNA (*middle panel*). The polyuridylated form is then degraded by Dis132 (*bottom panel*).

in the loop of pre-let-7 microRNAs (Heo et al., 2008), which leads to polyuridylation of pre-let-7 microRNAs by TUT4 (Hagan, Piskounova, & Gregory, 2009; Heo et al., 2009). After polyuridylation, pre-let-7 is cleaved by an exonuclease, Dis312 (Chang, Triboulet, Thornton, & Gregory, 2013).

Recent studies have identified a central role of Lin-28 in mediating the rapid translational response to brain-derived neurotrophic factor (BDNF) and other growth factors (Amen et al., 2017; Huang, Ruiz, Eyler, Lin, & Meffert, 2012). Stimulation of primary hippocampal neurons with BDNF triggers simultaneous activation of Dicer and Lin-28 (Fig. 3). This two-pronged response elicits a global increase in microRNA synthesis via activation of Dicer, as well as selective degradation of let-7 microRNAs via activation of Lin-28. Thus, BDNF stimulation produces a generalized suppression of translation while at the same time selectively blocking silencing of let-7 targets. In this way, BDNF achieves selective translation of let-7 targets which include several prominent plasticity-related transcripts, such as Arc. As these findings have established that neuronal stimuli can trigger rapid reversal of silencing, they have heightened interest in deciphering the role of the microRNA system in neuronal signaling and plasticity. The selectivity of Lin-28 for let-7 family members suggests that there might be additional pathways of microRNA degradation to target other subpopulations of microRNAs. Consistent with this prediction, recent studies have led to the identification of the translin/trax RNase complex as another pathway of microRNA degradation.

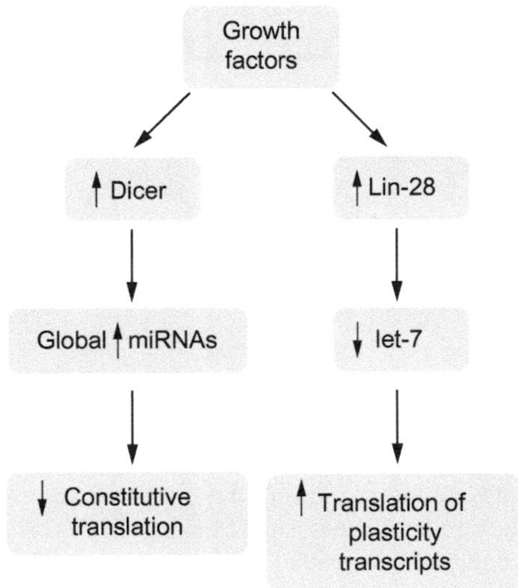

Fig. 3 Growth factor-induced activation of Dicer and Lin-28. Growth factors, such as BDNF, trigger coordinated activation of both Dicer and Lin-28. Dicer activation elicits a global increase in most microRNAs; activation of Lin-28 drives degradation of let-7 family pre-miRNAs. This combination of actions leads to a generalized decrease in constitutive translation, while relieving silencing of transcripts targeted by let-7 family members. *Figure modified from Fu, X., Shah, A., & Baraban, J. M. (2016). Rapid reversal of translational silencing: Emerging role of microRNA degradation pathways in neuronal plasticity* Neurobiology of Learning and Memory, 133, *225–232.*

4. IDENTIFICATION OF THE TRANSLIN/TRAX COMPLEX

The Baraban lab initially became interested in studying this complex as an offshoot of studies investigating the rapid activation of immediate early genes by neuronal stimulation. This line of research demonstrated that Egr1, a transcription factor, was rapidly and robustly induced in dentate granule cells by brief tetanic stimulation of the perforant path input in an NMDA receptor-dependent fashion (Cole, Saffen, Baraban, & Worley, 1989). As these studies assayed Egr1 activation by in situ hybridization, we proceeded to confirm that Egr1 protein was also induced as expected. Furthermore, we wanted to check if this protein was able to bind to the previously defined Egr response element (ERE), a short sequence of double-stranded DNA, targeted by all four members of the Egr family. To this end, we conducted gel-shift or electrophoretic mobility shift assays with a double-stranded radiolabeled probe containing the ERE sequence.

Surprisingly, incubation of hippocampal extracts with this probe yielded multiple bands that displayed sequence-specific binding to the ERE. In addition to Egr1, the other prominent bands were identified as isoforms of Egr3 that were generated by utilization of multiple translation start sites (O'Donovan & Baraban, 1999).

In an effort to identify all the factors in the hippocampus that were able to bind to ERE sites, we explored the possibility that the double-stranded ERE might "melt" to expose binding sites for factors that bind to single-stranded DNA. Accordingly, to look for such hypothetical factors, we conducted gel-shift studies with probes made up of individual strands of the ERE rather than the standard double-stranded form. Remarkably, one of these strands yielded a robust binding complex, while the complementary strand did not (Taira & Baraban, 1997).

Having found an unexpected ssDNA binding factor, we considered whether it was worthwhile "figuring out" what it was. To help make an informed decision, we examined the tissue distribution of this complex which revealed that it was enriched in brain. Furthermore, it seemed unlikely that this new factor was related to the Egr family since it bound with high affinity to mutant ERE sequences that abolish Egr family member binding (Taira & Baraban, 1997). Based on these limited data, we decided to undertake identification of this factor. However, we still needed to decide the best strategy for cloning it. One important consideration that had to be taken into account was whether the factor might be composed of multiple proteins that are needed to confer binding activity. If so, then conventional expression cloning would not be suitable. To address this question, we exposed the factor-probe complex to UV irradiation and found that two proteins were cross-linked to the probe, suggesting that both may be needed to confer binding activity. Accordingly, we decided to employ a classical biochemical purification of this factor followed by microsequencing of peptides generated by cleavage of its constituent proteins.

Employing this approach led to the identification of the two proteins that were cross-linked to the probe as translin and trax (Finkenstadt, Jeon, & Baraban, 2002; Taira, Finkenstadt, & Baraban, 1998). Translin had been identified as a ssDNA binding protein implicated in mediating chromosomal translocations, such as those linked to malignant transformations (Aoki et al., 1995), while trax had been identified in a yeast two-hybrid assay as a translin interactor (Aoki, Ishida, & Kasai, 1997). Thus, our study provided confirmation that endogenous translin and trax participate in a heteromeric complex, as predicted by yeast two-hybrid studies (Fig. 4).

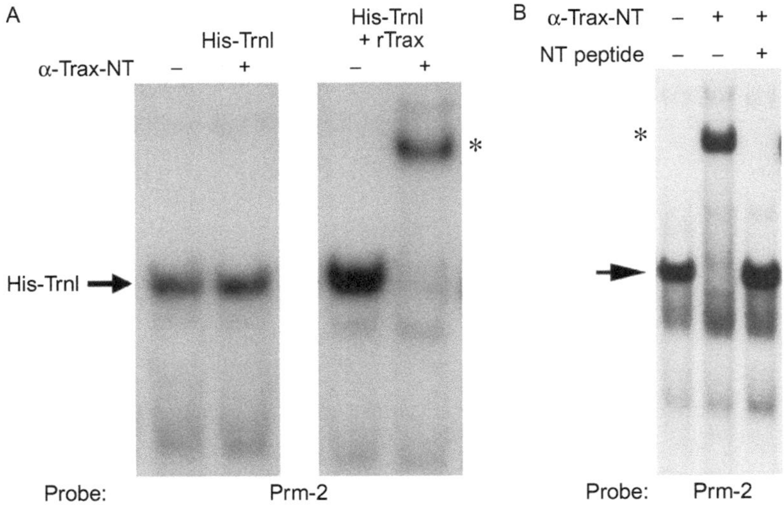

Fig. 4 Translin/trax gel-shift complex. (A) The *left panel* illustrates the robust gel-shift complex formed by overexpression of His-tagged translin (His-Trnl). The *right panel* shows that coexpression of His-translin and trax leads to formation of a gel-shift complex that migrates with similar mobility. Incorporation of trax in this complex was confirmed by demonstrating that its mobility is further slowed (*asterisk on right edge*) by preincubation with trax antibodies (α-Trax-NT). (B) The native gel-shift complex detected in mouse cerebellar extracts also contains trax as it is completely supershifted (*asterisk on left edge*) by incubation with trax antibodies. This supershift is blocked by preincubation of the antibody with the epitope peptide (NT peptide), confirming its specificity. Gel-shift studies were conducted using a fragment of protamine-2 3′UTR (Prm-2) as described in Li, Wu, and Baraban (2008). *Figure modified from Li, Z., Wu, Y., & Baraban, J. M. (2008). The translin/trax RNA binding complex: Clues to function in the nervous system.* Biochimica et Biophysica Acta, 1779, *479–485.*

5. DOES THE TRANSLIN/TRAX COMPLEX MEDIATE DENDRITIC TRAFFICKING OF mRNAs?

As the translin/trax complex was able to bind to single-stranded RNA and localized to dendrites, our working hypothesis was that it was involved in dendritic trafficking of mRNAs, such as BDNF mRNA (Wu et al., 2011). Support for this view came from studies demonstrating that siRNA-mediated knockdown of translin in primary hippocampal neurons inhibited the ability of KCl-induced depolarization to trigger dendritic translocation of BDNF transcripts (Chiaruttini et al., 2009). However, it is unclear if this effect is mediated by direct interaction of translin/trax with BDNF mRNA or via an indirect effect of translin knockdown on signaling pathways linking

KCl-induced depolarization to dendritic trafficking. Furthermore, examination of BDNF mRNA translocation induced by pilocarpine in vivo revealed a complex picture (Wu et al., 2011). In translin KO mice, the basal level of BDNF mRNA translocation into dendrites was reduced; however, the ability of pilocarpine to trigger BDNF mRNA translocation into dendrites was not impaired. Thus, these studies indicate that translin deletion decreases basal level of dendritic BDNF mRNA but that translin/trax is not necessary for activity-induced dendritic translocation of BDNF mRNA in vivo.

6. SURPRISING DISCOVERY OF TRANSLIN/TRAX RNase ACTIVITY

To help clarify the role of the translin/trax complex in dendritic trafficking of mRNAs, we had made several attempts to identify the RNA species bound to the translin/trax complex using a variety of cross-linking methods. However, as these were unsuccessful, we were about to put the translin/trax project on hold, when the Liu laboratory published their unexpected finding that the translin/trax complex possesses RNase activity (Liu et al., 2009). This breakthrough caught the field by surprise for two reasons. First, since many RNase enzymes are dependent on divalent ions such as Mg^{2+} or Ca^{2+}, the standard buffer for conducting gel-shift studies with RNA probes includes EDTA, a divalent ion chelator, to minimize digestion of the RNA probe by RNase activity inevitably present in tissue homogenates. As a result, the RNase activity of the translin/trax complex, which is Mg^{2+} dependent, was suppressed during gel-shift assays. Second, neither translin nor trax, which are highly homologous proteins, contains domains with homology to RNase enzymes. Accordingly, there was no reason to suspect that they might contain RNase activity. However, in retrospect, it makes perfect sense that our attempts to "pull down" RNA targets bound to the translin/trax complex were unsuccessful as these hypothetical target RNAs would be rapidly cleaved by the intrinsic RNase activity of the translin/trax complex.

The line of research that uncovered the RNase activity of the translin/trax complex emerged from studies trying to figure out how translational silencing works in Drosophila. Researchers attempting to reconstitute this process using recombinant factors noted that they could not match the efficiency of the silencing process displayed by native Drosophila cell extracts. Accordingly, they postulated that this discrepancy was due to the absence of a key component. Therefore, the Liu laboratory undertook a classic biochemical purification approach to search for fractions that contained this missing component. This approach yielded identification of both translin and trax in highly purified active fractions. Accordingly, these investigators proceeded to confirm that inclusion of recombinant translin/trax mimicked the ability of the active fractions to improve the efficiency of the reconstituted silencing process. Detailed analysis of the key step that was catalyzed by recombinant translin/trax indicated that this complex facilitated separation of the guide and passenger strands so that the guide strand could be loaded more efficiently onto the RISC. In particular, these studies suggested that translin/trax facilitated degradation of the passenger strand after it had been nicked by Ago, a key component of the RISC (Fig. 5B).

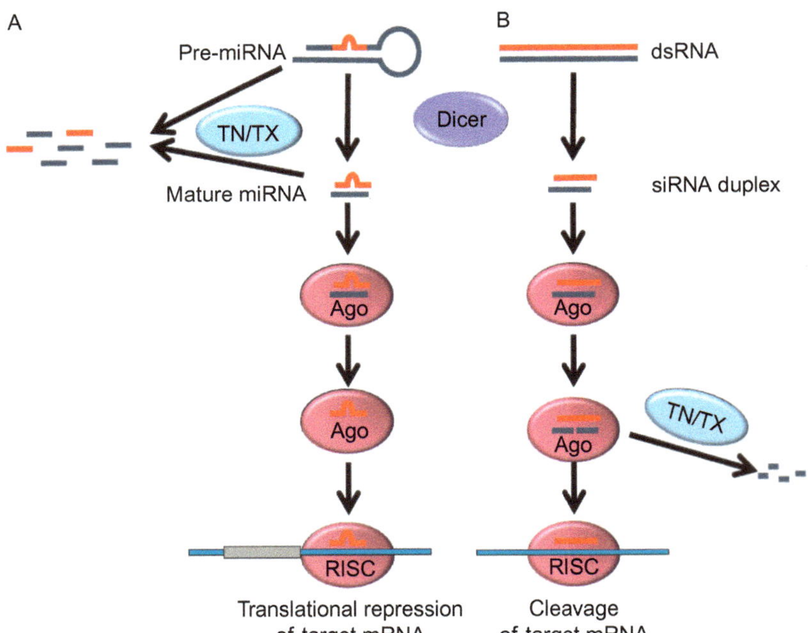

Fig. 5 Differential effects of translin/trax on siRNA- and miRNA-mediated silencing. As depicted in panel (A), the translin/trax complex is able to cleave the double-stranded stem of pre-microRNAs, as well as mature microRNAs, containing mismatches. Therefore, it inhibits or reverses microRNA-mediated silencing. In contrast, as shown in panel (B), the translin/trax complex potentiates siRNA-mediated silencing by catalyzing degradation of the passenger strand after it is nicked by Ago. In this way, translin/trax speeds association of the guide strand with the RISC to facilitate siRNA-mediated silencing.

With this new information in hand, examination of structural models of translin and trax suggested that this complex possesses RNase activity, a hypothesis that was readily corroborated with recombinant translin/trax generated in bacteria. Furthermore, these studies established that translin homomeric complexes do not display RNase activity and that mutation of key glutamate residues in trax, thought to form the catalytic pocket, abolished the RNase activity of the translin/trax complex.

These new findings provided a strong impetus to conduct crystallographic studies to define the organization of the complex (Ye et al., 2011). These revealed that the holo-complex is an octamer composed of four dimers. Two of these are translin homodimers, while the other two are translin/trax heterodimers. Thus, altogether, the octamer is composed of six copies of translin and two of trax, with the active catalytic pockets formed by the translin/trax dimers, while the translin homodimers provide scaffolding.

7. TRANSLIN/TRAX MEDIATES MicroRNA DEGRADATION

This Drosophila-based study inferred that the translin/trax complex plays a key role in facilitating silencing by degrading the passenger strand, thereby expediting association of the guide strand with the RISC. However, attempts by our lab and others to confirm this model of translin/trax action in the context of microRNA signaling in mammalian cells were unsuccessful. These unexpected results forced us to reconsider this model of translin/trax action and led to the realization that the translin/trax RNase has the opposite effect in the mammalian microRNA system, i.e., it acts to degrade microRNAs and to suppress translational silencing (Asada et al., 2014).

The Paroo laboratory embarked on an unbiased biochemical search for identifying RNases capable of degrading pre-microRNAs. Using a synthetic pre-miRNA as a substrate, they identified fractions that were able to degrade this substrate. Using this approach, they identified the active factor as the translin/trax complex. In vitro, this complex competed with Dicer for access to pre-miRNA substrates to produce opposite outcomes (Fig. 5A). Cleavage of pre-miRNAs with Dicer yielded mature double-stranded microRNAs that were then passed on to Ago. In contrast, cleavage with translin/trax yields inactive fragments. Thus, these findings suggest that the translin/trax RNase complex provides a mechanism for suppressing silencing, comparable to the role played by the Lin-28 pathway (Huang et al., 2012).

To assess whether translin/trax is able to act in competition with Dicer in vivo, Asada et al. (2014) assessed the effect of translin deletion on microRNA levels in vivo or in cell lines expressing shRNAs targeting translin or trax. Interestingly, they found that only a small subset of microRNAs showed elevated levels, suggesting that under basal conditions, Dicer may outcompete translin/trax for access to most pre-miRNA substrates. This appears to be the case, since suppression of Dicer expression increases the impact of translin knockdown. Cells expressing a hypomorphic allele of Dicer display 50% reduction in Dicer protein levels with a commensurate decrease in global microRNA levels, consistent with Dicer being the rate-limiting step in microRNA synthesis. However, under these conditions, suppression of translin or trax expression triggered a more robust effect, as the majority of microRNAs show increased levels. Thus, these findings support the view that reduced expression of Dicer leads to decreased microRNA levels via two mechanisms: decreased generation of microRNAs due to decreased Dicer levels, as well as increased degradation of microRNAs by the translin/trax complex. As decreased Dicer levels have been implicated in the pathophysiology of a broad range of diseases (Dias et al., 2014; Herav-Moussavi et al., 2012; Kumar et al., 2009; Mori et al., 2012; Schneeberger et al., 2012), inhibition of the translin/trax RNase may have therapeutic applications since it might be able to help restore microRNA levels toward normal levels (Asada et al., 2014). To this end, Asada, Canestrari, and Paroo (2016) have also demonstrated that this complex is druggable and have identified lead compounds that inhibit recombinant translin/trax RNase selectively, as they are inactive at suppressing Dicer RNase activity.

8. LIN-28 AND TRANSLIN/TRAX PATHWAYS TARGET DIFFERENT FEATURES OF PRE-miRNAs

Detailed analysis of the initial cleavage sites produced by translin/trax in pre-microRNA substrates revealed that it acts on the stem at "mismatch" sites. In contrast, mutant versions of pre-microRNAs lacking these mismatches in the stem are poor substrates for translin/trax. At present, the sequence or structural features of pre-miRNAs that render them sensitive to cleavage by translin/trax have not been defined. However, pilot studies conducted with double-stranded mature microRNAs that lack a loop indicate that the presence of a few mismatches in the stem is not sufficient to render these microRNA analogs sensitive to cleavage by recombinant translin/trax (Baraban, unpublished data). Accordingly, an important goal of future studies will be to define the subset of microRNAs that are substrates for translin/trax. From the observation that translin or trax knockdown in Dicer hypomorph cells causes a widespread increase in microRNAs, it seems likely that translin/trax can cleave a wide range of microRNAs and that its specificity is not as restricted as that displayed by the Lin-28 pathway. Nevertheless, the ability of Dicer to outcompete translin/trax for access to pre-miRNAs under normal conditions appears to limit the impact of translin deletion to producing elevations in a highly restricted subset of microRNAs. Perhaps, these microRNAs are present in microdomains that are enriched with translin/trax relative to Dicer and are therefore more sensitive to loss of translin/trax. Taken together, these studies indicate that the translin/trax complex represents a second degradation pathway for microRNAs and that further studies are needed to define the subpopulation of microRNAs that are targeted by this complex.

9. CRITICAL DIFFERENCES BETWEEN siRNA AND miRNA SILENCING PATHWAYS

Both the initial Drosophila-based study and the subsequent examination of the role of translin/trax in mammalian cells demonstrated that this complex plays a key role in RNA-mediated silencing pathways. However, it appeared to have opposite effects in these systems; in Drosophila it potentiated silencing, while in mammalian cells it inhibited silencing. In retrospect, this discrepancy may reflect fundamental differences between the organization of RNA-mediated silencing pathways in these organisms. It is well established that Drosophila possess two quite distinct silencing pathways, referred to as siRNA and microRNA pathways, respectively (He & Hannon, 2004; Liu & Paroo, 2010). The siRNA pathway appears to be designed primarily for host defense and uses RNA oligos that are perfectly complementary to foreign RNAs to target them for degradation. In contrast, the microRNA pathway appears to be designed to use genomically encoded microRNAs to reversibly regulate translation of endogenous mRNAs. In Drosophila these pathways are biochemically and genetically distinct, while in mammalian systems, they have merged into a single system. This distinction is important in trying to understand the different functional role assigned to translin/trax based on Drosophila and mammalian studies.

The Drosophila studies were done using the siRNA pathway, and therefore addressed how translin/trax could facilitate processing of double-stranded RNA oligos that are perfectly complementary. As subsequent studies indicate that translin/trax cannot cleave most double-stranded siRNAs, translin/trax did not affect siRNA stability until a nick was introduced into the passenger strand by Ago. Once this nick is present, then translin/trax can rapidly cleave the passenger strand, while the guide strand is presumably protected from cleavage. In contrast, in mammalian systems, pre-microRNAs with mismatches in their stem would be subject to cleavage by translin/trax which has the effect of suppressing microRNA signaling (Fig. 5).

Of note, studies in mammalian systems suggest that translin/trax may also facilitate siRNA-mediated silencing as reported in Drosophila. In particular, Sahu, Philip, and Scarlata (2014) reported that siRNA-mediated knockdown of GAPDH is potentiated by translin/trax, while siRNAs targeting Hsp70 are not. Thus, these findings suggest that translin/trax may exert contrasting effects on microRNA- and siRNA-mediated silencing.

10. MULTIPLE PATHWAYS OF MicroRNA DEGRADATION CONFER VERSATILITY

In addition to translin/trax and Lin-28 pathways of microRNA degradation, recent studies also suggest that MCPIP1 provides a third pathway of microRNA degradation (Suzuki et al., 2011). As Dicer mediates synthesis of nearly all mature microRNAs, modulation of its activity would be expected to produce global alterations in microRNA levels. Thus, this arrangement does not provide a mechanism for differential processing of distinct subsets of microRNAs. In contrast, the availability of multiple pathways of microRNA degradation seems advantageous for differentially altering microRNA profiles that would allow cells to fine-tune silencing of selected classes of transcripts. As described above, BDNF and other growth factors utilize this versatility to selectively suppress silencing mediated by let-7 family members, which triggers translation of key plasticity transcripts. Thus, it will be important to define which cell signaling pathways regulate the activity of translin/trax or MCPIP1 and whether selective activation of these microRNA degradation pathways triggers translation of a distinct cohort of mRNAs (Fig. 6). Furthermore, it will be interesting to determine whether there are additional pathways of microRNA degradation remaining to be discovered.

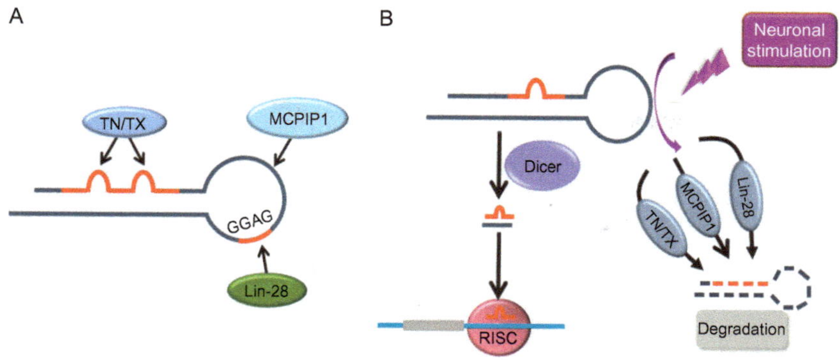

Fig. 6 Multiple pathways of microRNA degradation. (A) Distinct substrate selectivites. The three identified microRNA degradation pathways target different features of substrate pre-microRNAs. Lin-28 binds to a consensus sequence, GGAG, in the portion of the loop close to the 3′ stem present in nearly all let-7 family members. Translin/trax targets mismatches in the stem. MCPIP1 targets the loop; however, the nature of its binding site has not been defined. (B) Differential activation of microRNA degradation pathways. Based on the ability of BDNF and other growth factors to stimulate activation of the Lin-28 pathway of microRNA degradation, we hypothesize that the translin/trax and MCPIP1 pathways may also be activated rapidly by extracellular stimuli to trigger degradation of their substrate microRNAs leading to rapid reversal of silencing of their target transcripts. The presence of three distinct pathways of microRNA degradation that target distinct subpopulations of microRNAs enables the cell to reverse silencing selectively and fine-tune translation in response to extracellular signals. *Figure reproduced from Fu, X., Shah, A., & Baraban, J. M. (2016). Rapid reversal of translational silencing: Emerging role of microRNA degradation pathways in neuronal plasticity* Neurobiology of Learning and Memory, 133, *225–232.*

11. CLUES TO REGULATION OF TRANSLIN/TRAX

The identification of the translin/trax RNase complex as playing a key role in regulating microRNA degradation has heightened interest in understanding how its activity might be regulated. From this perspective, the observation that translin/trax interacts with phospholipase C beta (PLCbeta) has provided an interesting lead (Aisiku et al., 2010; Philip et al., 2012; Sahu et al., 2014). This line of research indicates that PLCbeta interacts with the translin/trax complex by binding to trax and, thereby, inhibits its RNase activity. These investigators have found evidence that translin/trax can potentiate siRNA-mediated knockdown for selected siRNAs and have found that conditions that promote association of PLCbeta with translin/trax block siRNA-mediated knockdown of GAPDH. Furthermore, recent studies indicate that this mechanism may play a key role in nerve growth factor (NGF)'s ability to drive neuronal differentiation of PC12 cells (Garwain & Scarlata, 2016). Knockdown of either trax or PLCbeta1 blocks NGF-induced differentiation in this system. Furthermore, NGF stimulation elicits a transient increase in association of PLCbeta1 with trax as monitored by FRET at 24 h following NGF stimulation. However, at 48 h, increased expression of Gαq enables it to recapture PLCbeta1 blocking its interaction with the translin/trax complex. Thus, NGF is thought to transiently inhibit translin/trax activity. Further studies are needed to determine how PLCbeta1 and trax are critical in the differentiation process, as it is unclear whether it is the transient suppression of translin/trax activity that is critical. In addition, although these investigators focus on translin/trax's role in potentiating siRNA-induced silencing, a reasonable alternative scenario is that translin/trax may act to degrade microRNA and thereby block silencing in this system. Accordingly, further studies aimed at identifying the dynamics of microRNAs and endogenous siRNAs during NGF-induced differentiation may be useful in distinguishing between these options.

12. RNase-INDEPENDENT FUNCTIONS OF TRAX

Using yeast two-hybrid studies, Chern and colleagues identified trax as a protein that binds to the C-terminal segment of the A2a adenosine receptor (Sun et al., 2006). Furthermore, they have shown that trax plays a key role in activating ATM, a central component of a DNA repair pathway activated by double-strand breaks (Wang, Chen, Sun, Chien, & Chern, 2016). Of note, they did not detect translin in the ATM/trax complex. Furthermore, a point mutant in trax that abolishes the RNase activity of translin/trax complex does not inhibit trax's ability to stimulate ATM activation. Thus, these findings lead to two unexpected conclusions. First, these studies indicate that trax has cellular functions that are independent of its RNase activity. Second, they suggest that trax may interact with other protein partners besides translin. This inference is paradoxical in light of compelling evidence that trax protein is degraded in translin KO mice (Chennathukuzhi et al., 2003; Yang et al., 2004). Based on this striking observation, it had been assumed that trax's interaction with translin is necessary for its stability and, therefore, that it formed a complex exclusively with translin. However, this inference needs to be reevaluated. Conceivably, the absence of translin may activate a cellular pathway that targets trax for degradation. However, if translin is present, then trax may be able to form complexes with other partners. Further studies are clearly needed to resolve this paradox.

13. CONCLUSION

Emerging evidence implicating defects in the microRNA system in the pathophysiology of a wide variety of disease states, including neuropsychiatric illnesses, provide an important impetus to "figure out" how this system works and to identify potential targets for drugs that may be useful in combatting these illnesses. It is well established that the rate-limiting steps in turning off biological signals can be powerful points of intervention. For example, blockade of the serotonin plasma membrane transporter, the rate-limiting step in inactivating serotonin signaling, is the basis for selective serotonin reuptake inhibitors (SSRIs), one of the most widely used class of drugs. Accordingly, ongoing efforts to identify the pathways that mediate reversal of microRNA-mediated silencing may also represent a fertile area of research for identifying useful targets to manipulate microRNA signaling.

Although the translin/trax RNase complex has been identified as mediating microRNA degradation, further studies are needed to understand how its activity is regulated in brain. As PLC beta1 has been found to interact with the complex and inhibit its activity, this represents an important starting point. Accordingly, it will be interesting to assess whether activation of receptors linked to PLCbeta1 either with pharmacological agents or by synaptic stimulation are able to inhibit TN/TX activity in brain neurons.

Recent studies indicate that trax may possess cellular functions that are independent of its association with translin. Although these findings appear to be inconsistent with the observation that the stability of trax protein depends on its interaction with translin, this assumption needs to be reevaluated. Thus, "figuring out" the cellular functions of translin and trax remains an active area of investigation that promises to shed light on the role of the microRNA signaling system in neuronal function and the pathophysiology of neuropsychiatric disorders.

CONFLICT OF INTEREST

The authors have no conflicts of interest to declare.

REFERENCES

Aisiku, O. R., Runnels, L. W., & Scarlata, S. (2010). Identification of a novel binding partner of phospholipase cβ1: Translin-associated factor X. *PLoS One*, *5*, e15001.

Amen, A. M., Ruiz-Garzon, C. R., Shi, J., Subramanian, M., Pham, D. L., & Meffert, M. K. (2017). A rapid induction mechanism for Lin28a in trophic responses. *Molecular Cell*, *65*, 490–503.

Aoki, K., Ishida, R., & Kasai, M. (1997). Isolation and characterization of a cDNA encoding a translin-like protein, TRAX. *FEBS Letters*, *401*, 109–112.

Aoki, K., Suzuki, K., Sugano, T., Tasaka, T., Nakahara, K., Kuge, O., et al. (1995). A novel gene, translin, encodes a recombination hotspot binding protein associated with chromosomal translocations. *Nature Genetics*, *10*, 167–174.

Asada, K., Canestrari, E., Fu, X., Li, Z., Makowski, E., YC, W., et al. (2014). Rescuing dicer defects via inhibition of an anti-dicing nuclease. *Cell Reports*, *9*, 1471–1481.

Asada, K., Canestrari, E., & Paroo, Z. (2016). A druggable target for rescuing microRNA defects. *Bioorganic & Medicinal Chemistry Letters*, *26*, 4942–4946.

Bartel, D. P. (2004). MicroRNAs: Genomics, biogenesis, mechanism and function. *Cell*, *116*, 281–297.

Bartel, D. P. (2009). MicroRNAs: Target recognition and regulatory functions. *Cell*, *136*, 281–297.

Chang, H. M., Triboulet, R., Thornton, J. E., & Gregory, R. I. (2013). A role for the Perlman syndrome exonuclease Dis3l2 in the Lin28-let-7 pathway. *Nature*, *497*, 244–248.

Chapat, C., Jafarnejad, S. M., Matta-Camacho, E., Hesketh, G. G., Gelbart, I. A., Attig, J., et al. (2017). Cap-binding protein 4EHP effects translation silencing by microRNAs. *Proceedings of the National Academy of Sciences of the United States of America*, *114*, 5425–5430.

Chennathukuzhi, V., Stein, J. M., Abel, T., Donlon, S., Yang, S., Miller, J. P., et al. (2003). Mice deficient for testis-brain RNA-binding protein exhibit a coordinate loss of TRAX, reduced fertility, altered gene expression in the brain, and behavioral changes. *Molecular and Cellular Biology*, *23*, 6419–6434.

Chiaruttini, C., Vicario, A., Li, Z., Baj, G., Braiuca, P., Wu, Y., et al. (2009). Dendritic trafficking of BDNF mRNA is mediated by translin and blocked by the G196A (Val66Met) mutation. *Proceedings of the National Academy of Sciences of the United States of America*, *106*, 16481–16486.

Cole, A. J., Saffen, D. W., Baraban, J. M., & Worley, P. F. (1989). Rapid increase of an immediate early gene messenger RNA in hippocampal neurons by synaptic NMDA receptor activation. *Nature*, *340*, 474–476.

Dias, C., Feng, J., Sun, H., Shao, N. Y., Mazei-Robison, M. S., Damez-Werno, D., et al. (2014). β-catenin mediates stress resilience through Dicer1/microRNA regulation. *Nature*, *516*, 51–55.

Filipowicz, W., & Sonenberg, N. (2015). The long unfinished march towards understanding microRNA-mediated repression. *RNA*, *21*, 519–524.

Finkenstadt, P. M., Jeon, M., & Baraban, J. M. (2002). Trax is a component of the translin-containing RNA binding complex. *Journal of Neurochemistry*, *83*, 202–210.

Fire, A., Xu, S., Montgomery, M. K., Kostas, S. A., Driver, S. E., & Mello, C. C. (1998). Potent and specific genetic interference by double-stranded RNA in C. elegans. *Nature*, *391*, 806–811.

Fu, X., Shah, A., & Baraban, J. M. (2016). Rapid reversal of translational silencing: Emerging role of microRNA degradation pathways in neuronal plasticity. *Neurobiology of Learning and Memory*, *133*, 225–232.

Garwain, O., & Scarlata, S. (2016). Phospholipase Cβ-TRAX association is required for PC12 cell differentiation. *The Journal of Biological Chemistry*, *291*, 22970–22976.

Hagan, J., Piskounova, E., & Gregory, R. (2009). Lin28 recruits the Tutase Zcchc11 to inhibit let-7 maturation in mouse embryonic stem cells. *Nature Structural & Molecular Biology, 16*, 1021–1025.

He, L., & Hannon, G. J. (2004). MicroRNAs: Small RNAs with a big role in gene regulation. *Nature Reviews. Genetics, 5*, 522–531.

Heo, I., Joo, C., Cho, J., Ha, M., Han, J., & Kim, V. (2008). Lin28 mediates the terminal uridylation of let-7 precursor microRNA. *Molecular Cell, 32*, 276–284.

Heo, I., Joo, C., Kim, Y., Ha, M., Yoon, M., Cho, J., et al. (2009). TUT4 in concert with Lin28 suppresses microRNA biogenesis through pre-microRNA uridylation. *Cell, 138*, 696–708.

Herav-Moussavi, A., Anglesio, M. S., Cheng, S. W., Senz, J., Yang, W., Prentice, L., et al. (2012). Recurrent somatic DICER1 mutations in nonepithelial ovarian cancers. *The New England Journal of Medicine, 366*, 234–242.

Huang, Y. W., Ruiz, C. R., Eyler, E. C., Lin, K., & Meffert, M. K. (2012). Dual regulation of miRNA biogenesis generates target specificity in neurotrophin-induced protein synthesis. *Cell, 148*, 933–946.

Kumar, M. S., Pester, R. E., Chen, C. Y., Lane, K., Chin, C., Lu, J., et al. (2009). Dicer1 functions as a haploinsufficient tumor suppressor. *Genes & Development, 23*, 2700–2704.

Li, Z., Wu, Y., & Baraban, J. M. (2008). The translin/trax RNA binding complex: Clues to function in the nervous system. *Biochimica et Biophysica Acta, 1779*, 479–485.

Liu, Q., & Paroo, Z. (2010). Biochemical principles of small RNA pathways. *Annual Review of Biochemistry, 79*, 295–319.

Liu, Y., Ye, X., Jiang, F., Liang, C., Chen, D., Peng, J., et al. (2009). C3PO, an endoribonuclease that promotes RNAi by facilitating RISC activation. *Science, 325*, 750–753.

Mayford, M., Siegelbaum, S., & Kandel, E. R. (2012). Synapses and memory storage. *Cold Spring Harbor Perspectives in Biology, 4*.

Mori, M. A., Raghavan, P., Thomou, T., Boucher, J., Robida-Stubbs, S., Macotela, Y., et al. (2012). Role of microRNA processing in adipose tissue in stress defense and longevity. *Cell Metabolism, 16*, 336–347.

O'Donovan, K. J., & Baraban, J. M. (1999). Major Egr3 isoforms are generated via alternate translation start sites and differ in their abilities to activate transcription. *Molecular and Cellular Biology, 19*, 4711–4718.

Philip, F., Guo, Y., Aisiku, O., & Scarlata, S. (2012). Phospholipase Cβ1 is linked to RNA interference of specific genes through translin-associated factor X. *The FASEB Journal, 26*, 4903–4913.

Ruvkun, G. (2008). The perfect storm of tiny RNAs. *Nature Medicine, 14*, 1041–1045.

Rybak, A., Fuchs, H., Smirnova, L., Brandt, C., Pohl, E., Nitsch, R., et al. (2008). A feedback loop comprising lin-28 and let-7 controls pre-let-7 maturation during neural stem cell commitment. *Nature Cell Biology, 10*, 987–993.

Sahu, S., Philip, F., & Scarlata, S. (2014). Hydrolysis rates of different small interfering RNAs (siRNAs) by the RNA silencing promoter complex, C3PO, determines their regulation by phospholipase Cβ. *The Journal of Biological Chemistry, 289*, 5134–5144.

Schneeberger, M., Altirriba, J., García, A., Esteban, Y., Castaño, C., García-Lavandeira, M., et al. (2012). Deletion of miRNA processing enzyme Dicer in POMC-expressing cells leads to pituitary dysfunction, neurodegeneration and development of obesity. *Molecular Metabolism, 2*, 74–85.

Sun, C. N., Cheng, H. C., Chou, J. L., Lee, S. Y., Lin, Y. W., Lai, H. L., et al. (2006). Rescue of p53 blockage by the A(2A) adenosine receptor via a novel interacting protein, translin-associated protein X. *Molecular Pharmacology, 70*, 454–466.

Suzuki, H., Arase, M., Matsuyama, H., Choi, Y., Ueno, T., Mano, H., et al. (2011). MCPIP1 ribonuclease antagonizes Dicer and terminates microRNA biogenesis through precursor microRNA degradation. *Molecular Cell*, *44*, 424–436.
Taira, E., & Baraban, J. M. (1997). Identification of a strand-specific Egr response element binding complex enriched in rat brain. *Journal of Neurochemistry*, *68*, 2255–2262.
Taira, E., Finkenstadt, P. M., & Baraban, J. M. (1998). Identification of translin and trax as components of the GS1 strand-specific DNA binding complex enriched in brain. *Journal of Neurochemistry*, *71*, 471–477.
Viswanathan, S., Daley, G., & Gregory, R. (2008). Selective blockade of microRNA processing by Lin28. *Science*, *320*, 97–100.
Wang, J. Y., Chen, S. Y., Sun, C. N., Chien, T., & Chern, Y. (2016). A central role of TRAX in the ATM-mediated DNA repair. *Oncogene*, *35*, 1657–1670.
Yang, S., Cho, Y. S., Chennathukuzhi, V. M., Underkoffler, L. A., Loomes, K., & Hecht, N. B. (2004). Translin-associated factor X is post-transcriptionally regulated by its partner protein TB-RBP, and both are essential for normal cell proliferation. *The Journal of Biological Chemistry*, *279*, 12605–12614.
Wu, Y. C., Williamson, R., Li, Z., Vicario, A., Xu, J., Kasai, M., et al. (2011). Dendritic trafficking of brain-derived neurotrophic factor mRNA: Regulation by translin-dependent and -independent mechanisms. *Journal of Neurochemistry*, *116*, 1112–1121.
Ye, X., Huang, N., Liu, Y., Paroo, Z., Huerta, C., Li, P., et al. (2011). Structure of C3PO and mechanism of human RISC activation. *Nature Structural & Molecular Biology*, *18*, 650–657.

CHAPTER TWO

Receptor Binding Assays and Drug Discovery

David B. Bylund*[,1], S.J. Enna[†]
*University of Nebraska Medical Center, Omaha, NE, United States
[†]University of Kansas Medical Center, Kansas City, KS, United States
[1]Corresponding author: e-mail address: dbylund@unmc.edu

Contents

Abstract

Although Solomon Snyder authored hundreds of research reports and several books covering a broad range of topics in the neurosciences, he is best known by many as the person who developed neurotransmitter receptor radioligand binding assays. By demonstrating the utility of this approach for studying transmitter receptors in brain, Dr. Snyder provided the scientific community with a powerful new tool for identifying and characterizing these sites, for defining their relationship to neurological and psychiatric disorders, and their involvement in mediating the actions of psychotherapeutics. Although it was hoped the receptor binding technique could also be used as a primary screen to speed and simplify the identification of novel drug candidates, experience has taught that ligand binding is most useful for drug discovery when it is used in conjunction with functional, phenotypic assays. The incorporation of ligand binding assays into the drug discovery process played a significant role in altering the search for new therapeutics from solely an empirical undertaking to a mechanistic and hypothesis-driven enterprise. This illustrates the impact of Dr. Snyder's work, not only on neuroscience research but on the discovery, development, and characterization of drugs for treating a variety of medical conditions.

Advances in Pharmacology, Volume 82
ISSN 1054-3589
https://doi.org/10.1016/bs.apha.2017.08.007

ABBREVIATIONS

EC_{50} the concentration of an agent that induces 50% of the maximal effect
K_D the equilibrium disassociation constant for a ligand and a receptor binding site

1. INTRODUCTION

1.1 The Snyder Approach to the Development of Neurotransmitter Receptor Binding Assays

The decade of the 1970s was an exciting time for those engaged in neuroscience research. It began with the 1970 Nobel Prize in Physiology or Medicine being awarded to Bernard Katz, Ulf von Euler, and Julius Axelrod for their seminal work on chemical neurotransmission. The Society for Neuroscience held its first annual meeting in 1971. In 1970, Dr. Solomon Snyder, who earlier was a Research Associate with Dr. Axelrod and later became President of the Society of Neuroscience, was promoted to Professor of Pharmacology and Psychiatry at Johns Hopkins University School of Medicine. This elevation came just 4 years after his initial appointment as an Assistant Professor. It was no accident that his meteoric rise in rank coincided with the dramatic advances in the neurosciences given his many contributions to the field. Among these was the development of a rapid, simple, and inexpensive ligand binding procedure for characterizing the biochemical, molecular, and pharmacological properties of neurotransmitter receptors.

Some of the earliest studies utilizing a radioligand binding technique were aimed at characterizing the estrogen receptor (Gorski, Taft, Shyomala, Smith, & Notides, 1968; Jensen & Jacobson, 1962). For this work the investigators had to synthesize their own [^{3}H]estradiol to achieve a specific activity sufficient for detection of the extremely low quantities of specifically bound radioligand. Using [^{3}H]atropine, Paton and Rang (1965) were among the first to attempt to label a neurotransmitter receptor with a radioactive substance. However, the low specific activity of the radioligand resulted in a high nonspecific/specific binding ratio, making it inadequate for characterizing this site. The subsequent use of alkylating agents, such as benzilylcholine mustards (Gill & Rang, 1966) and the snake venom α-bungarotoxin (Meunier et al., 1972), made it possible to more selectively label muscarinic and nicotinic cholinergic receptors, respectively. Because such ligands bind irreversibly, or nearly so, to the receptor, they were useful for the autoradiographic visualization and biochemical purification of these sites. However, they were of limited value in examining other receptor properties, such as kinetics, allosteric interactions, and pharmacological selectivity. Others identified binding sites in vivo by administering a radiolabeled drug and mapping the distribution of the selectively labeled, pharmacologically relevant targets (Bylund, Charness, & Snyder, 1977; Enna, DaPrada, & Pletscher, 1974; Enna & Shore, 1971; Murrin, Enna, & Kuhar, 1977). While useful for identifying the tissue, cellular, and subcellular localization of a drug target under biological conditions, this method is costly and cumbersome, with pharmacokinetics and the in vivo metabolic stability of the labeling agent sometimes limiting the interpretation of results.

Among the many insights Dr. Snyder gained while working with Dr. Axelrod is the value of developing simple laboratory techniques for asking questions in new ways. Novel assays virtually assure the generation of novel insights. Also, the person who develops a new assay can exploit its use before others. During his training, Dr. Snyder also came to appreciate the value of radiolabeled chemicals for defining the biochemical properties of neuronal systems. Dr. Axelrod employed such substances extensively in the studies that earned him the Nobel Prize. A third characteristic of Dr. Snyder's approach to research is his habit of following developments in fields outside his main interests, not only because of his native curiosity but also on the chance he might discover a new technique or a technology that could be adapted to his own work. These three factors were crucial in the development of neurotransmitter receptor binding assays.

From his knowledge of the literature, and his conversations with Dr. Pedro Cuatrecasas, a faculty colleague at Johns Hopkins, Dr. Snyder became intrigued by the possibility of labeling neurotransmitter receptors which, at that time, were enigmatic and, in the minds of some, purely theoretical entities (Kobinger, 1986). Dr. Cuatrecasas (1971), as well as others (Freychet, Roth, & Neville, 1971), had developed a simple assay system for studying insulin receptor binding in adipose tissue and liver plasma membranes. To this end they had to prepare a radioligand with a high specific activity, in this case ^{125}I-insulin, and to develop a procedure capable of rapidly rinsing the tissue and incubation vessel to quickly separate the unbound ligand from that attached to the target site. A custom-designed filtration apparatus achieved this goal and allowed for the simultaneous analysis of dozens of samples. This met all of Dr. Snyder's criteria for an innovative, simple, and rapid procedure that had the potential to yield new insights into synaptic transmission in general and neurotransmitter receptors in particular. What needed to be determined was whether the assay would work with synaptic membranes, and whether the available neurotransmitter receptor radioligands had the specific activity needed to detect the small quantities bound to receptor sites. It was also crucial that these radioactive compounds have the affinity and selectivity for the target site required to clearly distinguish specific receptor binding from nonspecific attachment to other tissue components.

The utility of this new approach for studying neurotransmitter and hormone receptor sites was first demonstrated with publications by Dr. Snyder and his group characterizing the binding of nerve growth factor in sympathetic ganglia and of opiates in rat brain (Banerjee, Snyder, Cuatrecasas, & Greene, 1973; Pert & Snyder, 1973). Although others had attempted previously to achieve this goal with opiates (Goldstein, Lowney, & Pal, 1971), the results were inconclusive because of the small percentage of detectable ligand that attached to a possible receptor. The rapid washing and filtering approach adopted by Dr. Snyder proved to be the technical advance needed to demonstrate conclusively the existence of specific receptors for opiates in the central nervous system. Given its implications for defining drug mechanisms of action, for discovering new therapeutics, and for understanding the relationship between receptors and mental illness, the Pert and Snyder work was publicized widely in both the scientific and lay press. Others quickly adopted this protocol for their studies.

1.2 Applications

Following publication of the opiate and nerve growth factor binding assay, studies were quickly undertaken by Dr. Snyder and other investigators to determine the general utility of this technique. Given the breadth of his interests and expertise, Dr. Snyder set out to develop ligand binding assays for all of the major neurotransmitter receptors in brain. To this end, each graduate student and postdoctoral fellow in his laboratory was assigned a receptor target for study. This was not a trivial undertaking for those receiving these assignments because the optimal conditions for detecting specific binding differ somewhat among receptors. The first step in developing a neurotransmitter receptor binding assay is to purchase or prepare and purify an appropriate radioligand having the requisite specific activity. This is followed by analyses of its binding in brain tissue using various buffers at different temperatures and pH (Enna & Snyder, 1977). The chemical stability of the radiolabel under the incubation conditions needs to be demonstrated, as does the incubation time required for the binding to reach a steady state, and the time needed for the radioligand to bind to (on rate) and vacate (off rate) the site. Such information is required to ensure the use of assay conditions that will yield consistent and reliable results. Once these technical details are known, the number of projects that can be undertaken using the binding assay were seemingly endless, with the time necessary to complete each being generally brief. In the early days, a study initiated on a Monday was often completed during the same week, with the manuscript written and submitted a few days thereafter. It was not unusual for those working with Dr. Snyder to publish a dozen or more high impact articles over a 2-year period, illustrating the importance and value of new technology for the advancement of science.

Many of those trained in Dr. Snyder's laboratory during this period went on to distinguished careers as neuroscientists and pharmacologists. Members of this group, and the receptors they were assigned during their time with Dr. Snyder include Gavril Pasternak (opiates), David Bylund (β-adrenergic), David Burt (dopamine), Henry Yamamura (cholinergic muscarinic), S.J. Enna (GABA), Ian Creese (dopamine), James Bennett (serotonin), David U'Prichard (α-adrenergic), and Anne Young (glycine), to name a few. Assistant Professors in the unit at that time were Joseph Coyle, Elliott Richelson, and Michael Kuhar. While establishing their own independent laboratories, they took full advantage of the information and new technologies generated by the Snyder group. This contributed to Coyle's identification and characterization of glutamate receptors, Richelson's work on cholinergic muscarinic receptors, and Kuhar's development of autoradiographic techniques for mapping the distribution of neurotransmitter and drug binding sites in the central nervous system. As orchestrated by Dr. Snyder, the receptor binding program led to collaborations and cross-fertilization of ideas among this enthusiastic and creative group of young scientists. The research and training environment he fostered had a lasting impact on their careers and the field.

This work identified the many ways this new methodology could be employed to address issues of importance to neuroscientists and pharmacologists. This included its use for the isolation and characterization of receptor sites (Hollenberg, 1990), for identifying changes in neurotransmitter receptors associated with brain development, drug treatment, and neurological and psychiatric disorders (Enna, 1978; Enna et al., 1976; Reisine et al., 1977), for use as an analytical procedure for quantifying drug and neurotransmitter levels in biological tissues and fluids (Creese & Snyder, 1977;

Enna & Snyder, 1976), for defining drug mechanisms of action (Creese, Burt, & Snyder, 1976), for discovering new receptor subtypes (Bylund, 1988), and as a screening technique for identifying new chemical entities that may have therapeutic potential (Creese, 1985).

2. RECEPTOR BINDING ASSAYS AND DRUG DISCOVERY

2.1 Compound Screening

Historically, initial analysis of a drug candidate involved the determination of a biological response in isolated organ systems or animal models of the targeted condition. Such tests are limited as primary screens because of the quantity of test agent required, the costs associated with such assays, and the time and expertise needed for their establishment, execution, and interpretation of the findings. Also, with these assays the turnaround time between the synthesis of a chemical agent and preliminary biological data is slow, often requiring months or years of testing chemical analogs to identify the active pharmacophore, for optimizing the pharmacological response and minimizing untoward effects. As receptor binding assays make it possible to examine rapidly the selectivity and affinity of a test agent at a receptor target, they greatly shorten the time needed to refine a chemical structure to generate a lead compound. Moreover, because receptor binding assays make possible the screening of hundreds of chemical candidates in a day, investigators can examine at the target site the interaction of large numbers of structurally unrelated agents with the aim of discovering novel drug candidates and to guide the synthesis of innovative products.

The use of receptor binding assays as a primary screen for new therapeutics was also fostered by the growing interest in first identifying such agents on the basis of their interaction with a particular target, such as an enzyme or receptor site, rather than on a pharmacological effect (phenotypic response) for which the mechanism of action was unknown. With the traditional approach, drugs, especially those for treating central nervous system disorders, were discovered empirically in laboratory animal studies or in the clinic, while the agent was used for other purposes (Coyle & Enna, 1998). Once proven to be therapeutically useful, such therapeutics were then examined using biochemical assays to define their mechanism and site of action. With the growing number of biological targets known to be affected by, or to contribute to, disease processes, many investigators became convinced that drug development could be streamlined significantly by focusing discovery efforts on the identification or design of compounds that interact selectively with a target molecule after which its pharmacological effects would be defined in more complex systems and in intact animals. Spurred by this notion, receptor binding facilities, many of them highly automated, were established in both the pharmaceutical industry and academia. Millions of chemicals were screened, with thousands identified as interacting with neuronal targets, such as transmitter uptake and receptor sites. While some of these discoveries ultimately resulted in the development of a useful drug, most did not, even after refinement of the chemical structure and enhancement of target selectivity. Overall, during the past 40 years use of receptor binding assays as a primary screening technique has been more successful in generating new ligands as research tools than as pharmaceuticals. Although receptor binding assays are still widely used in drug discovery, it is now appreciated that the predictive value of such data alone is limited with regard to clinical utility.

2.2 Limitations of Ligand Binding Assays in Drug Discovery

There are many reasons why receptor binding assays are limited as a primary drug-screening technique (Enna & Williams, 2009a, 2009b). Included is the fact that while binding assays are useful for identifying compounds that interact with a particular receptor site, they reveal nothing about the pharmacokinetics of the compound and provide only limited information about off-target actions that may cause significant side effects or toxicities. Pharmacokinetic issues and toxicity are two of the more common reasons for the failure of drug candidates. Also, from a simple receptor binding screen alone, it is difficult to know whether a test agent interacts with the receptor as a full, partial, inverse, or biased agonist or antagonist. Moreover, particularly for agonists, there is often little relationship between the binding affinity (K_D) of the ligand for the site and its potency (EC_{50}) and efficacy (maximal effect) in generating a biological response (e.g., change in the production of cyclic AMP or inositol phosphate, Ca^{2+} mobilization, channel opening). A major reason for this is that the functional potency of an agonist is dependent not only on its receptor binding affinity but also on its ability to activate the coupling of the appropriate receptor component to the biochemical effector system. This complicates studies on the relationship between chemical structure and biological activity. Thus, not only can there be a large separation between K_D and EC_{50} values for a particular compound, the potency of an agent can vary among different biochemical and physiological assay systems. These factors limit the conclusions that may be drawn concerning potential biological activity, let alone therapeutic utility, based solely on receptor binding data.

To increase the speed, efficiency, and reproducibility of receptor binding assays for compound screening, the receptor of interest is often expressed in cell culture. This makes it possible to generate a uniform system with a sufficient number of receptors for easy detection. While this approach enhances the throughput of compound screening and reduces cost, it confounds further the interpretation of binding data. Chief among the problems with expression systems is the possibility of posttranslational changes in the receptor molecule that have no counterpart in human tissue. This could lead to the identification of a ligand that is selective for the receptor expressed in this particular cell, but not in other tissues, such as human brain. This is especially true when a nonhuman cell line is employed for expression of the target site.

Another limitation of the binding assay as a primary drug-screening technique is the fact that many pharmacologically active agents allosterically modify receptor function by acting on a component of the receptor that is remote from the ligand binding recognition site (Berizzi et al., 2016; Changeux & Christopoulos, 2016; Zhang & Kavana, 2015). Indeed, the benzodiazepines, barbiturates, and many other sedative/hypnotics and general anesthetics would not have been identified as having therapeutic potential if screened solely in a receptor binding assay because they do not attach with a high affinity to any known neurotransmitter receptor recognition site.

Binding data are of limited value for predicting clinical activity because of a lack of knowledge at the systems level about the physiological responses following activation or inhibition of the target site. This is especially true for central nervous system receptors. In addition, it is likely that for some drugs to be effective, they must interact at multiple receptors, perhaps as an agonist at one and as a partial agonist or antagonist at another. This appears to be particularly true for drugs used to treat central nervous system disorders. As the optimal multitarget profile is unknown, binding assays, even when conducted over a large number of receptors, cannot by themselves be used to drive a drug design and discovery program in these cases. In fact, it is possible that the lack of success in using receptor binding data to identify novel psychotherapeutics is due in large measure to the focus on identifying agents that act selectively at a single site when in fact many clinically effective agents in this drug class are known to attach to multiple receptors in brain (Enna, 2014).

2.3 Functional, Phenotypic Screening

There have been several publications detailing reasons for the decline in recent years in the discovery and approval of novel therapeutics (Enna & Williams, 2009b; Swinney & Anthony, 2011). Among the factors cited is the increasingly reductionistic approach taken for drug discovery. For millennia drug candidates were first identified empirically in intact animals, often humans, or by screening chemicals in isolated organ systems. These functional, or phenotypic, assays were discarded as initial drug screens as biochemical and molecular methodologies, including receptor binding assays, evolved because the latter allow for a less expensive and more rapid analysis of chemical libraries. This represented a shift from pursuing the refinement and development of an agent with known biological, and therefore potentially pharmacological, activity but an unknown mechanism of action, to first proposing a mechanism, such as blockade or activation of a particular receptor, then identifying an active compound using a ligand binding assay. Only after a chemical lead was identified as a high affinity and selective ligand for the receptor of interest was it tested in more complex systems to assess its therapeutic potential. While many drug candidates were identified using this approach, the vast majority were ultimately found to be of no clinical value. This failure rate is generally attributed to the fact that, as opposed to many phenotypic screens, conventional ligand binding assays provide no information on the pharmacokinetics and metabolism of a chemical lead, and only limited information on potential side effects and toxicities. Moreover, unless the physiological and functional relationship between the targeted site and the organ system of interest is well defined in humans, it is impossible to predict with any precision the ultimate biological response to a receptor ligand in a complex organism. This is especially true for agents that interact with sites within the central nervous system. In fact, the lack of progress made in discovering new, centrally active therapeutics using the reductionistic approach is, in part, the reason why many pharmaceutical firms have abandoned, or greatly reduced, drug discovery efforts in this area (Schoepp, 2011).

As the limitations of receptor ligand binding as a primary screen in a drug discovery program became apparent, efforts turned toward developing high-throughput phenotypic assays capable of detecting relevant biological responses to test agents (Swinney, 2013; Wagner, 2016). Such assays range from in vitro whole cell techniques (Grundmann, 2017; Parker et al., 2017; Werley et al., 2017) to automated screens of animal behavior (Kafkafi,

Yekutieli, & Elmer, 2009; Tecott & Nestler, 2004). The information generated by these methods yields important hints about therapeutic utility beyond that provided by a receptor binding assay. Because of the functional endpoint, phenotypic assays are more useful than ligand binding analysis for structure–activity studies in the search for the most selective and active compound. In addition, phenotypic assays are more likely to identify a novel therapeutic lead that interacts with a site or biological system not detected or examined in a ligand binding screen. Although the mechanism of action may not be apparent from such a hit, the functional readout could indicate the serendipitous discovery of a new drug class. Ligand binding assays can then be employed to identify the site of action of the novel, pharmacologically active, agent.

As with ligand binding assays, phenotypic assays have limitations as primary drug screens. The precise relationship between the functional response measured and the desired pharmacological response in humans is, in most cases, unknown. This is especially true when working with isolated cells and tissue in vitro. Also, as with ligand binding assays, in vitro phenotypic analysis provides no information on the pharmacokinetics and potential toxicities of the test agent. While in vivo phenotypic testing, the most costly and labor-intensive form of preliminary screening, provides the greatest information on the pharmacological response, pharmacokinetics, and safety profile of a test substance, its predictive value for identifying therapeutics is positively related to the relevance of the selected end-point to the target disorder. This is a particular problem for conditions for which the underlying biological abnormality is unknown, such as schizophrenia and major depression (Markou, Chiamulera, Geyer, Tricklebank, & Steckler, 2009). At best the animal models recapitulate only some of the symptoms of these disorders, limiting drug discovery to the identification of agents that may palliate, but not cure, the condition. Nonetheless, the generation of functional data in a primary drug-screening program provides greater insight into therapeutic possibilities than receptor binding alone.

The growing popularity in high-throughput phenotypic screens is not a wholesale indictment of the radioligand binding assay as a tool for drug discovery. Rather, it is an acknowledgment that by delaying to late in the discovery process the determination of whether a chemical candidate has relevant pharmacological activity, the reductionistic approach has encouraged the pursuit of too many false leads. This underscores the fact that much remains to be learned about the response to activation and inhibition of receptor systems in a complex, diseased organism. Today, a well-balanced primary screening program includes both ligand binding and high-throughput phenotypic assays: the former for the initial analysis of large compound libraries over selected receptor targets, and the latter for testing a more limited number of compounds to define their effect on cell and organ function and to perhaps identify empirically active compounds that fail to test positive in the ligand binding assay. For the foreseeable future, receptor ligand binding, as pioneered by Dr. Snyder, will remain an indispensable tool for drug discovery, and for characterizing the site and mechanism of action of established therapeutics.

3. CONCLUSION

Like Henry Ford, Solomon Snyder was not the first to recognize the value of a new technology or to attempt its design and implementation. Rather, as Ford did with the automobile, Dr. Snyder refined, simplified, and adapted a technology that was initially created by others. His efforts dramatically increased the popularity and use of this technique, with transformative effects on research in the neurosciences and on drug discovery. The results of his accomplishment remain in evidence today.

The impact of receptor binding assays on characterizing transmitter receptors, in identifying drug mechanisms of action, and in the identification of novel drug candidates is an excellent illustration of how methods development plays a crucial role in the advancement of science. It is remarkable the impact that such a simple, inexpensive procedure has had on the neurosciences in general and drug discovery in particular. While more sophisticated and informative in vitro screening techniques have been developed since Dr. Snyder published the initial binding studies in 1973, the ligand binding assay that he perfected remains an invaluable tool for characterizing neurotransmitter and hormone receptors, and the interaction of drugs and drug candidates at these sites.

ACKNOWLEDGMENT

The authors thank Ms. Lynn LeCount for her outstanding editorial assistance.

CONFLICT OF INTEREST

The authors declare no conflict of interest pertaining to the material contained in this report.

REFERENCES

Banerjee, S. P., Snyder, S. H., Cuatrecasas, P., & Greene, L. A. (1973). Binding of nerve growth factor receptor in sympathetic ganglia. *Proceedings of the National Academy of Sciences of the United States of America, 70,* 2519–2523.

Berizzi, A. E., Gentry, P. R., Rueda, P., Den Hoedt, S., Sexton, P. M., Langmead, C. J., et al. (2016). Molecular mechanisms of action of M5 muscarinic acetylcholine receptor allosteric modulators. *Molecular Pharmacology, 90,* 427–436.

Bylund, D. B. (1988). Subtypes of α_2-adrenoceptors: Pharmacological and molecular biological evidence converge. *Trends in Pharmacological Sciences, 9,* 356–361.

Bylund, D. B., Charness, M. E., & Snyder, S. H. (1977). Beta adrenergic receptor labeling in intact animals with [^{125}I]-hydroxybenzylpindolol. *The Journal of Pharmacology and Experimental Therapeutics, 201,* 644–653.

Changeux, J. P., & Christopoulos, A. (2016). Allosteric modulation as a unifying mechanism for receptor function and regulation. *Cell, 166,* 1084–1102.

Coyle, J. T., & Enna, S. J. (1998). Overview of neuropsychopharmacology. In S. J. Enna & J. T. Coyle (Eds.), *Pharmacological management of neurological and psychiatric Disorders,* (pp. 1–26). New York: McGraw Hill.

Creese, I. (1985). Receptor binding as a primary drug screen. In H. I. Yamamura, S. J. Enna, & M. J. Kuhar (Eds.), *Neurotransmitter receptor binding (2nd Edition),* (pp. 189-233). New York: Raven Press.

Creese, I., Burt, D. R., & Snyder, S. H. (1976). Dopamine receptor binding predicts clinical and pharmacological potencies of antischizophrenic drugs. *Science, 192,* 481–483.

Creese, I., & Snyder, S. H. (1977). A novel, simple and sensitive radioreceptor assay for antischizophrenic drugs in blood. *Nature, 270,* 261–263.

Cuatrecasas, P. (1971). Insulin-receptor interaction in adipose tissue cells: Direct measurement and properties. *Proceedings of the National Academy of Sciences of the United States of America, 68,* 1264–1268.

Enna, S. J. (1978). The GABA receptor binding assay: Focus on human disorders. In F. - Fonnum (Ed.), *Amino acids as chemical transmitters* (pp. 445–456). New York: Plenum Press.

Enna, S. J. (2014). Phenotypic drug screening. *Journal of the Peripheral Nervous System, 19,* S4–S5.

Enna, S. J., Bird, E., Bennett, J. P., Bylund, D. B., Yamamura, H. I., Iversen, L. L., et al. (1976). Huntington's chorea: Changes in neurotransmitter receptors in brain. *New England Journal of Medicine, 294,* 1305–1309.

Enna, S. J., DaPrada, M., & Pletscher, A. (1974). Subcellular distribution of reserpine in blood platelets: Evidence for multiple pools. *The Journal of Pharmacology and Experimental Therapeutics, 191,* 164–168.

Enna, S. J., & Shore, P. A. (1971). Regional distribution of specifically bound reserpine in rat brain. *Biochemical Pharmacology, 20,* 1910–1912.

Enna, S. J., & Snyder, S. H. (1976). A simple, sensitive and specific radioreceptor assay for endogenous GABA in brain tissue. *Journal of Neurochemistry, 26,* 221–224.

Enna, S. J., & Snyder, S. H. (1977). Influences of ions, enzymes and detergents on GABA receptor binding in synaptic membranes of rat brain. *Molecular Pharmacology, 13,* 442–453.

Enna, S. J., & Williams, M. (2009a). Challenges in the search for drugs to treat central nervous system disorders. *The Journal of Pharmacology and Experimental Therapeutics, 329,* 404–411.

Enna, S. J., & Williams, M. (2009b). Defining the role of pharmacology in the emerging world of translational research. In S. J. Enna & M. Williams (Eds.), *Advances in pharmacology, Vol. 57.* pp. 1-30, New York: Academic Press.

Freychet, P., Roth, J., & Neville, D. M. (1971). Insulin receptor in the liver: Specific binding of ^{125}I-insulin to the plasma membrane and its relation to insulin bioactivity. *Proceedings of the National Academy of Sciences of the United States of America, 68*, 1833–1837.

Gill, E. W., & Rang, H. P. (1966). An alkylating relative to benzilycholine with specific and long-lasting parasympatholytic activity. *Molecular Pharmacology, 2*, 284–297.

Goldstein, A., Lowney, L. I., & Pal, B. K. (1971). Stereospecific and nonspecific interactions of the morphine congener levorphanol in subcellular fractions of mouse brain. *Proceedings of the National Academy of Science of the United States of America, 68*, 1742–1747.

Gorski, J., Taft, D., Shyomala, G., Smith, D., & Notides, A. (1968). Hormone receptors: Studies on the interaction of estrogen with the uterus. *Recent Progress in Hormone Research, 24*, 45–80.

Grundmann, M. (2017). Label-free dynamic mass redistribution and bio-impedance methods for drug discovery. *Current Protocols in Pharmacology, 77*, 9.24.1–9.24-21. https://doi.org/10.1002/cpph.24.

Hollenberg, M. D. (1990). Receptor solubilization, characterization, and isolation. In H. I. Yamamura, S. J. Enna, & M. J. Kuhar (Eds.), *Methods in neurotransmitter receptor analysis*, (pp. 111–145). New York: Raven Press.

Jensen, E. V., & Jacobson, H. I. (1962). Basic guides to the mechanism of estrogen action. *Recent Progress in Hormone Research, 18*, 387–414.

Kafkafi, N., Yekutieli, D., & Elmer, G. I. (2009). A data mining approach to the in vivo classification of psychopharmacological drugs. *Neuropsychopharmacology, 34*, 607–623.

Kobinger, W. (1986). Rudolf Buchheim Lecture. Drugs as tools in research on adrenoceptors. *Naunyn-Schmiedeberg's Archives of Pharmacology, 332*, 113–123.

Markou, A., Chiamulera, C., Geyer, M. A., Tricklebank, M., & Steckler, T. (2009). Removing obstacles in neuroscience drug discovery: The future path for animal models. *Neuropsychopharmacology, 34*, 74–89.

Meunier, J.-C., Olsen, R. W., Menez, A., Fromageot, P., Boquet, P., & Changeux, J.-P. (1972). Some physical properties of the cholinergic receptor protein from Electrophorus electricus revealed by a tritiated α-toxin form Naja nigricollis venom. *Biochemistry, 11*, 1200–1210.

Murrin, L., Enna, S. J., & Kuhar, M. J. (1977). Autoradiographic localization of ^{3}H-reserpine binding sites in rat brain. *The Journal of Pharmacology and Experimental Therapeutics, 203*, 564–574.

Parker, C. G., Galmozzi, A., Wang, Y., Correia, B. E., Sasaki, K., Joslyn, C. M., et al. (2017). Ligand and target discovery by fragment-based screening in human cells. *Cell, 168*, 527–541.

Paton, W. D. M., & Rang, H. P. (1965). The uptake of atropine and related drugs by intestinal smooth muscle of the guinea-pig in relation to acetylcholine receptors. *Proceedings of the Royal Society B, 163*, 1–44.

Pert, C., & Snyder, S. H. (1973). Opiate receptor: Demonstration in nervous tissue. *Science, 179*, 1011–1014.

Reisine, T. D., Fields, J. Z., Yamamura, H. I., Bird, E., Spokes, E., Schreiner, P. S., et al. (1977). Neurotransmitter receptor alterations in Parkinson's disease. *Life Sciences, 21*, 335–344.

Schoepp, D. D. (2011). Where will new neuroscience therapies come from? *Nature Reviews. Drug Discovery, 10*, 715–716.

Swinney, D. C. (2013). The contribution of mechanistic understanding to phenotypic screening for first-in-class medicines. *Journal of Biomolecular Screening, 18*, 1186–1192.

Swinney, D. C., & Anthony, J. (2011). How were new medicines discovered? *Nature Reviews. Drug Discovery, 10*, 507–519.

Tecott, L. H., & Nestler, E. J. (2004). Neurobehavioral assessment in the information age. *Nature Neuroscience*, 7, 462–466.

Wagner, B. K. (2016). The resurgence of phenotypic screening in drug discovery and development. *Expert Opinion on Drug Discovery*, 121–125.

Werley, C. A., Brookings, T., Upadhyay, H., Williams, L. A., McManus, O. B., & Demsey, G. T. (2017). All-optical electrophysiology for disease modeling and pharmacological characterization of neurons. *Current Protocols in Pharmacology*, *78*, 11.20.1–11.20.X (in press).

Zhang, R., & Kavana, M. (2015). Quantitative analysis of receptor allosterism and its implication for drug discovery. *Expert Opinion on Drug Discovery*, *10*, 763–780.

CHAPTER THREE

The Role of Serine Racemase in the Pathophysiology of Brain Disorders

Joseph T. Coyle[*,†,1], **Darrick T. Balu**[*,†]
[*]Harvard Medical School, Boston, MA, United States
[†]McLean Hospital, Belmont, MA, United States
[1]Corresponding author: e-mail address: joseph_coyle@hms.harvard.edu

Contents

Abstract

The *N*-methyl-D-aspartate receptor (NMDAR) is unique in requiring two agonists to bind simultaneously to open its cation channel: the neurotransmitter, glutamate, and the coagonists, glycine, or D-serine. The Snyder laboratory was the first to clone serine racemase (SR), the enzyme that synthesizes D-serine, and to localize it immunocytochemically. Our laboratory has focused on the role of D-serine in brain disorders. Silencing the expression of SR, a risk gene for schizophrenia (SCZ), in mice (SR −/−), results in a phenotype that closely resembles SCZ including: cortical atrophy, reduced dendritic spine density and complexity, downregulation of parvalbumin-positive cortical GABAergic neurons, and cognitive impairments. This pathology can be reversed by treatment of SR −/− mice with D-serine in adulthood. SR −/− mice also exhibit abnormal response toward abusable substances, such as stimulants. They show reduced behavioral sensitization to D-amphetamine, but fail to extinguish it. Place preference to cocaine is altered, and the hedonic response to it is profoundly impaired as assessed by intracranial self-stimulation. D-cycloserine, a partial agonist at the NMDAR glycine modulatory site, shows therapeutic benefit for treating pathologic anxiety in combination with behavioral therapies. Studies in vitro with cortical culture and in vivo with middle cerebral artery occlusion show that silencing SR provides substantial protection

Advances in Pharmacology, Volume 82
ISSN 1054-3589
https://doi.org/10.1016/bs.apha.2017.10.002

against ischemic neuronal death. Finally, the switch of SR expression from neurons to reactive astrocytes after closed head trauma accounts for the reduced in vivo neuroplasticity, electroencephalogram abnormalities, and cognitive impairments.

ABBREVIATIONS

Arc	activity-regulated cytoskeleton-associated protein
BDNF	brain-derived neurotrophic factor
CCI	controlled cortical impact
CPP	conditioned place preference
CS	conditioned stimulus
DAAO	D-amino acid oxidase
DCS	D-cycloserine
FOLH1	gene encoding folate hydrolase 1
GABAergic	ϒ-amino-butyric acidergic
GCPII	glutamate carboxypeptidase II
GlyT1	glycine transporter 1
GMS	glycine modulatory site
GRIA1	gene for glutamate ionotropic receptor AMPA type subunit 1
GRIN2A	gene for glutamate ionotropic receptor NMDA type subunit 2A
GRM3	gene for glutamate metabotropic receptor 3
GWAS	genome-wide association study
ICSS	intracranial self-stimulation
Kyna	kynurenic acid
LTP	long-term potentiation
mTOR	mammalian target of rapamycin
NAAG	*N*-acetyl-L-aspartyl-L-glutamate
NAc	nucleus accumbens
NAALADase	*N*-acetyl-L-aspartyl-L-glutamate peptidase
NMDAR	*N*-methyl-D-aspartate receptor
PSD-95	postsynaptic density with mass of 95 Da
SR	serine racemase
UC	unconditioned stimulus
VGluT1	vesicular glutamate transporter-1
WT	wild type

1. INTRODUCTION

The Nishikawa laboratory was the first to report the presence of D-serine in the brain, thus upending the shibboleth that vertebrates utilize only L-amino acids (Hashimoto et al., 1992). This discovery also resolved a quarter of a century conundrum about the reason for the expression of D-amino acid oxidase (DAAO) in brain (Neims, Zieverink, & Smilack,

1966). Johnson and Ascher (1987) showed that the *N*-methyl-D-aspartate receptor (NMDAR) had the unusual characteristic of requiring a second ligand, glycine, to be bound to the receptor for glutamate to open the cation channel. Notably, Kleckner and Dingledine (1988) implicated D-serine as a potential coagonist at the NMDAR. They found D-serine to be more potent than glycine itself in the *Xenopus* expression system, although D-serine's presence in the brain awaited the Hashimoto et al. (1992) discovery.

Sol Snyder has had a deep interest in unusual signaling pathways in the nervous system such as nitric oxide and carbon monoxide (Bredt & Synder, 1969; Verma, Hirsch, Glatt, Ronnett, & Snyder, 1993). This interest undoubtedly drew his attention to D-serine, which was known to be a potential coagonist at the NMDAR (Kleckner & Dingledine, 1988) and to be present in the brain (Hashimoto et al., 1992). Thus, his laboratory undertook the purification and characterization of serine racemase (SR), the enzyme that synthesizes D-serine, from rat brain (Wolosker, Blackshaw, & Snyder, 1999). They then cloned SR and showed that it was a member of the family of pyridoxal-5′-phosphate-dependent enzymes in eukaryotes (Wolosker, Sheth, et al., 1999). They also demonstrated that there was a close correspondence in the expression of SR, NMDARs, and D-serine levels in the forebrain of the rat (Schell, Molliver, & Snyder, 1995). They developed compelling evidence that endogenous D-serine in fact was a coagonist at synaptic receptors by showing loss of NMDAR activity when culture hippocampal neurons and hippocampal slice were perfused with purified DAAO to catabolize synaptic D-serine (Mothet et al., 2000). Finally, they showed that during development there was an inverse relationship between D-serine levels and DAAO expression in the cerebellum and hindbrain where glycine was found in high concentrations and was likely the coagonist. Thus, the Snyder laboratory laid the foundation by establishing D-serine as the coagonist at synaptic NMDARs in forebrain, which has been confirmed repeatedly since then (Li et al., 2013; Meunier et al., 2016).

This chapter will review research from the Coyle laboratory to define the potential role of D-serine in the pathophysiology of brain disorders. This effort was built upon the foundation laid by the Snyder laboratory on the role of D-serine as the forebrain coagonist at synaptic NMDARs.

2. SCHIZOPHRENIA

For over 40 years the "dopamine hypothesis" has dominated the thinking about the pathophysiology of schizophrenia due to the fact that antipsychotic drugs act at the dopamine D2 receptor (Snyder, 1976). Subsequent imaging research substantiated the relationship between excessive forebrain dopamine D2 receptor activation and psychosis in patients (Ginovart & Kapur, 2012). However, with the possible exception of clozapine, antipsychotic drugs have no effects on negative symptoms and cognitive impairments, the most robust predictors of disability in schizophrenia (Lim et al., 2016). Furthermore, cortical atrophy correlates with negative symptoms and cognitive impairments in chronic schizophrenia but not with the severity of psychosis (Davis et al., 1998; Johnstone et al., 1989). Thus, the core features of schizophrenia, which are primarily responsible for persistent disability, are linked to pervasive cortical pathology and are unlikely the consequence of simply dopamine dysfunction.

The implications of dysfunction of glutamatergic neurotransmission and specifically NMDAR function evolved primarily out of two research strategies: pharmacologic challenges and postmortem neurochemical studies (for review, Coyle, Basu, Benneyworth, Balu, & Konopaske, 2012). Since dissociative anesthetics were first introduced to clinical practice 50 years ago, they were known to cause a syndrome clinically indistinguishable from schizophrenia (Anis, Berry, Burton, & Lodge, 1983). The demonstration that ketamine and phencyclidine are noncompetitive antagonists raised the question whether NMDARs might play a role in the pathophysiology of schizophrenia (Javitt & Zukin, 1991). Objective clinical challenge studies with ketamine confirmed that low-dose ketamine administered to normal volunteers caused negative symptoms and cognitive impairments, hypofrontality and increased forebrain dopamine release similar to schizophrenia, while it exacerbated core symptoms in stabilized schizophrenic subjects (for review, Moghaddam & Krystal, 2012).

Our laboratory identified a neuropeptide, *N*-acetyl-L-aspartyl-L-glutamate (NAAG), which is concentrated in forebrain glutamatergic neurons but is also found in spinal motor neurons. We identified its catabolic enzyme, glutamate carboxypeptidase II (GCPII; also known as folate hydrolase I or *FOLH 1*, prostate-specific membrane antigen, and *N*-acetyl-L-aspartyl-L-glutamate peptidase or NAALADase) (for review, Bergeron & Coyle, 2012). NAAG has a dual role in inhibiting glutamatergic neurotransmission by activating metabotropic glutamate 3 receptors (mGluR3) that inhibit glutamate release (Jackson & Slusher, 2001) and by antagonizing NMDARs at the glycine modulatory site (GMS) (Bergeron, Coyle, Tsai, & Greene, 2005). We carried out a postmortem analysis of the levels of glutamate and NAAG, as well as the activity GCPII in the cortex and hippocampus in controls and in subjects with the diagnosis of schizophrenia, and found evidence for a significant increase in NAAG and reduced glutamate and GCPII activity. These findings were consistent with reduced glutamatergic neurotransmission, specifically through the NMDAR (Tsai et al., 1995).

Our hypothesis, which linked the observations from ketamine challenges and the postmortem findings on glutamatergic parameters in schizophrenia, proposed that the fundamental pathophysiology of schizophrenia resulted from NMDAR hypofunction in the cortex, causing the cognitive deficits and negative symptoms with psychosis being a downstream, subcortical complication (Coyle, 1996). The hypothesis was supported by the demonstration that both the GMS partial agonist, D-cycloserine (DCS); and GMS full agonist, D-serine, reduced negative symptoms, and enhanced cognition in schizophrenic patients stabilized on antipsychotic drugs (Goff, Tsai, Manoach, & Coyle, 1995; Tsai, Yang, Chung, Lange, & Coyle, 1998).

Although there were several pharmacologic models for the NMDAR hypofunction in schizophrenia (Bakshi & Geyer, 1995; Farber et al., 1995), we were concerned that they represented at best a transient receptor dysfunction, whereas schizophrenia likely resulted from a congenital impairment of NMDAR function since cognitive and behavioral abnormalities were often present in childhood long before the onset of psychosis (Erlenmeyer-Kimling et al., 2000). Therefore, based on the foundational research of the Snyder laboratory and evidence of reduced cerebrospinal fluid of D-serine in schizophrenia (Hashimoto et al., 2005), we decided to "knock-out" SR since a deficiency in D-serine would likely impair, but not totally block NMDAR function because of the presence of the other coagonist glycine (Basu et al., 2009). Excising the first expressed exon of SR blocked expression of SR and in the homozygote state (SR −/−), resulted in a >85% reduction of endogenous D-serine in cortex and hippocampus.

Extensive phenotyping of the SR −/− mice have revealed striking homologies between them and the neuropathologic, neurochemical, and cognitive deficits associated with schizophrenia. The two most reproduced neuropathologic features of schizophrenia are downregulation of the cortical parvalbumin-positive GABAergic interneurons (Lewis, 2014) and reduced spine density and dendritic complexity of cortical pyramidal neurons, surrogates of glutamatergic synapses (Moyer, Shelton, & Sweet, 2015). In this regard, Selemon and Goldman-Rakic (1999) proposed that loss of neuropil, not loss of neurons, accounts for the cortical atrophy and ventricular enlargement in schizophrenia (1999). An in vivo MRI study revealed a significant 4% loss of cortical volume and a 23% increase of ventricular volume in adult SR −/− mice, values similar to what has been reported in schizophrenia (Puhl et al., 2015). This loss of cortical gray matter in male SR −/− mice reflected a wide-spread loss of dendritic complexity and spine density on pyramidal neurons in frontal cortex (DeVito et al., 2011), in the primary sensory cortex (Balu, Basu, Corradi, Cacace, & Coyle, 2012) and on the granule cells in the dentate gyrus of the hippocampus (Balu et al., 2013). In aggregate, the total reduction of cortical glutamatergic synapses (spine density × total dendritic length) is in the order of 30%, similar to schizophrenia.

Steullet et al. (2017) have summarized the evidence that an important pathologic feature of schizophrenia is the downregulation of the presynaptic markers for the cortical fast-firing PV + GABAergic neurons, which provide recurrent inhibition to the pyramidal neurons. They mounted evidence that these deficits result from oxidative stress, which damages the perineuronal net. Examination of these parameters in the SR −/− mice revealed a 26% reduction in the number of PV+ neurons and a 35% reduction of PV + neurons surrounded by perineuronal nets. These changes were accompanied by a fourfold increase in 8-oxo-2′-deoxyguanosine, a marker of oxidative stress. Notably, these pathologic alterations were present in the 8-month-old SR −/− mice but not 2- to 3-month-old SR −/− mice (Benneyworth, Roseman, Basu, & Coyle, 2011), consistent with the evidence that the pathology of schizophrenia evolves over the years from first episode to chronic state (Krystal & Anticevic, 2015).

NMDARs play a fundamental role in the functional neuroplastic response, long-term potentiation (LTP), which has been considered the molecular substrate of learning and memory (Malenka & Nicoll, 1993). The SR −/− male mouse exhibited substantial impairments of LTP (~70% or more) at CA3–CA1 synapse in the hippocampus (Basu et al., 2009), at the thalamic synapse in the lateral nucleus of the amygdala (Li et al., 2013), and at the perforant path-dentate gyrus synapse (Balu et al., 2013). Notably, the deficit could be overcome by high-frequency stimulation, consistent with recruitment of glycine from astrocytes (Li et al., 2013), by perfusion with exogenous D-serine (Basu et al., 2009), or by treatment with D-serine to restore brain levels prior to sacrifice (Balu et al., 2013). Frantseva et al. (2008) used transcranial magnetic stimulation over the contralateral motor cortex to demonstrate impaired motor evoked potentials, which may represent LTP, and this deficit correlated with impaired motor-skilled learning. Postmortem studies of the neurochemistry and gene expression in schizophrenia have revealed alterations consistent with NMDAR hypofunction, such as reduced BDNF/Akt/mammalian target of rapamycin (mTOR) signaling in the hippocampus, which is replicated in the male SR −/− mouse (Balu et al., 2013).

The decision to choose knocking-out SR as a strategy to impair NMDAR function proved to be propitious. The largest genome-wide association study (GWAS) of risk genes for schizophrenia including over 100,000 controls and nearly 40,000 subjects with schizophrenia yielded 108 sites on the genome that achieved GWAS significance of 5×10^{-8}, supporting the evidence that schizophrenia is a disorder of complex genetics with multiple risk alleles of modest effect interacting with the environment to cause the phenotype (Ripke, Neale, Corvin, et al., 2014). Notably, one of these sites contained the *SRR* gene; and the allelic variant in a noncoding region (as were the vast majority of the SNPs) reduced SR expression (Birnbaum, Zhang, Hyde, Kleinman, Weinberger, 2014). Furthermore, over a dozen other sites are associated with genes encoding proteins that are within 2 degrees of separation from the NMDAR, including *GRIN2A*, *GRIA1*, *Arc*, and *GRM3* (Balu & Coyle, 2015).

An important strategy for validating the hypothesized reduced NMDAR function in schizophrenia is to demonstrate that enhancing NMDAR function reduces core symptoms of the disorder. While there were no drugs developed to enhance NMDAR function, DCS, a drug developed to treat tuberculosis by inhibiting alanine racemase and D-alanine: D-alanine ligase, is also a partial agonist at the GMS on the NMDAR (Anon, 2008; Watson, Bolanowski, Baganoff, Deppeler, & Lanthorn, 1990). DCS was subsequently shown to have cognitive enhancing effects in animal models of dementia (Flood, Morley, & Lanthorn, 1992; Schuster & Schmidt, 1992). A double-blind dose finding study of DCS in patients with schizophrenia, who were on stable doses of antipsychotic drugs, was carried out to determine its effects on cognition and negative symptoms (Goff et al., 1995). The patients were maintained on antipsychotic drugs because the outcome was uncertain. Thus, there were ethical concerns about terminating an effective treatment and because negative and cognitive symptoms were unaffected by antipsychotic drugs. DCS exhibited a U-shaped dose response curve with decreased negative symptoms and improved cognition at a dose of 50 mg/day (Goff et al., 1995).

A subsequent 8-week, placebo-controlled clinical trial of 50 mg/day of DCS failed to demonstrate an effect on cognition, although negative symptoms were reduced by a significant 23% (Goff et al., 1999). In retrospect, such loss of DCS efficacy on cognition with chronic treatment was not surprising as it has been well documented in experimental animals (Parnas, Weber, & Richardson, 2005; Quartermain, Mower, Rafferty, Herting, & Lanthorn, 1994). The problem of NMDAR desensitization prompted Goff to carry-out a clinical trial with once a week treatment with DCS in patients with schizophrenia, who were stabilized on antipsychotic drugs (Goff et al., 2008). He replicated the effects of DCS on negative symptoms, but found that a cognitive task improved only after the first dose. Yurgelun-Todd et al. (2005) found that 8-week treatment of schizophrenic subjects stabilized on antipsychotic drugs with 50 mg/day of DCS also exhibited a significant reduction of negative symptoms that correlated significantly with increased activation of the left superior temporal gyrus when performing a memory task.

Javitt and his colleagues have carried out a series of clinical trials of glycine, a full agonist at the GMS on the NMDAR, which poorly crosses the blood–brain barrier and thus requires substantial doses (30–60 g/day) for efficacy (Javitt, 2006). Tsai has carried out clinical trials with D-serine, D-alanine, and sarcosine, which is an inhibitor of the glycine transporter, glycine transporter 1 (GlyT1), and a GMS agonist, and summarized the findings from his studies and those of others in a metaanalysis (Tsai & Lin, 2010). Their findings indicate that GMS agonists significantly reduce negative symptoms, positive symptoms, and improve cognition in patients with schizophrenia receiving antipsychotic drugs with effect sizes of 0.38–0.26. Finally, they have been studying the efficacy of sodium benzoate, an inhibitor of DAAO. The addition of 1 g per day of sodium benzoate to a stable regimen of antipsychotic drugs resulted in significant reduction in negative symptoms and improvement processing speed and visual learning (Lane et al., 2013). This finding strongly supports the primacy of D-serine as the GMS agonist critical to the core symptoms of schizophrenia.

3. ADDICTIONS

The cooccurrence of substance abuse and psychotic disorders, especially schizophrenia, presents serious challenges with treatment noncompliance, violence, confinement within the legal justice system, and poor clinical outcomes (Green, Canuso, Brenner, & Wojcik, 2003). The risk for substance abuse in individuals diagnosed with schizophrenia is three- to fourfold greater than in the general population, excluding nicotine dependence (Kavanagh, McGrath, Saunders, Dore, & Clark, 2002). In the case of nicotine dependence, up to 85% of individuals with schizophrenia have nicotine dependence, especially those with negative symptoms and chronicity (Cantor-Graae, Nordström, & McNeil, 2001). After nicotine, ethanol, cannabis, and stimulants appear to be the most commonly abused substances. In circumstances where cocaine is readily available, abuse can be high (Cantor-Graae et al., 2001). As recent research has revealed the central role of glutamatergic neurotransmission (for review, Carlezon & Thomas, 2009), especially mediated by NMDARs, in substance abuse and dependence, Coyle (2006) hypothesized that the high prevalence of comorbid substance abuse in schizophrenia result from share molecular mechanisms and not merely adverse social circumstances.

Substance abuse and dependence involve alterations in motivation, loss of behavioral inhibition, craving in the absence of withdrawal, and altered responsiveness to stressors and drug-associated stimuli (Carlezon & Thomas, 2009). Repeated administration of most drugs of abuse produces a state of behavioral sensitization that can be manifested in numerous behavioral tests (Carlezon & Nestler, 2002). Several studies now show that extinction of drug-mediated conditioned place preference (CPP) is NMDAR-dependent and is enhanced with treatment with DCS (Paolone, Botreau, & Stewart, 2009; Thanos, Bermeo, Wang, & Volkow, 2010). DCS also facilitates the extinction of morphine withdrawal-induced conditioned place aversion (Myers & Carlezon, 2010), suggesting that NMDAR function has a broad influence on how drug-related cues contribute to the development and maintenance of addictive behaviors. Interestingly, DCS can either weaken (by facilitating extinction) or strengthen (by facilitating reconsolidation) drug-related cues, depending on the timing of treatment (Myers & Carlezon, 2012).

In this context, Benneyworth and Coyle (2012) studied behavioral sensitization to D-amphetamine in mice with genetically altered GMS activation, the SR −/− mouse, and the GlyT1 hypomorph mouse that exhibits increased NMDAR GMS activation (Tsai et al., 2004). Repeated psychostimulant treatment results in behavioral sensitization as measured as increased efficacy of the drug to stimulate locomotor activity (Vezina & Leyton, 2009). The acquisition of sensitization is facilitated by associative learning that links a specific context to drug exposure (Badiani, Anagnostaras, & Robinson, 1995). SR −/− mice showed reduced expression of context-specific sensitization and conditioned hyperactivity. Nevertheless, this attenuated conditioned hyperactivity was completely resistant to extinction. Furthermore, while extinction in wild type (WT) mice with repeated context exposure reversed the increased spine density in the nucleus accumbens (NAc), the increased NAc spine density in SR −/− mice was unaffected by this extinction protocol. The GlyT1 +/− mice with enhanced GMS exhibited a more rapid acquisition of sensitization with amphetamine, but no apparent alteration in the extinction of conditioned hyperactivity. This finding is consistent with the report of Curcio et al. (2013), who found that administration of D-serine into the NAc enhanced behavioral sensitization to cocaine. Thus, based on the results with SR −/−

mice, it would appear that one possible explanation for the increased prevalence of substance abuse in schizophrenia may be impaired extinction that interferes with remaining abstinent.

CPP may be a homolog of drug craving in experimental animals. Recent studies indicate that enhancement of NMDAR GMS activity by treatment with DCS (Paolone et al., 2009; Thanos et al., 2010) or D-serine (Hammond, Seymour, Burger, & Wagner, 2013) accelerates extinction of cocaine-induced CPP and of cocaine self-administration. Accordingly, we studied CPP in the SR −/− and GlyT1 +/− mice. Compared with WT mice, GlyT1 +/− mice displayed more rapid extinction of CPP and more robust cocaine-induced reinstatement than in WT mice (Puhl et al., 2015). SR −/− appeared to immediately "forget" the learned cocaine-cued place preference because they did not exhibit cocaine-induced reinstatement and also exhibited attenuated locomotor sensitization, as also was observed with D-amphetamine (Benneyworth & Coyle, 2012). The lack of reinstatement in SR −/− mice is consistent with critical role played by NMDARs in this process (Ma, Cepeda, & Cui, 2009). Interestingly, treatment of SR −/− mice with 300 mg/kg/day of D-serine, a dose that normalizes cortical D-serine levels (Balu et al., 2013), caused SR −/− mice to avoid the cocaine-paired side of the chamber during extinction. This counterintuitive behavior may reflect increased drug seeking after the cocaine reward was not obtained on the side previously rewarded with cocaine.

In ongoing studies, intracranial self-stimulation (ICSS) has been used to assess the hedonic properties of cocaine. In this test, rodents self-administer rewarding electrical stimuli to the medial forebrain bundle, which contains the NAc dopaminergic afferents (Markou & Koob, 1991). Drugs of abuse reduce the threshold for ICSS responding, suggesting that the rewarding effects of the drugs have additive effects with the rewarding effects of the stimulation. On the other hand, treatments that produce dysphoria (e.g., withdrawal and stress) increase thresholds for ICSS responding, suggesting that aversion can detract from reward in this test (Carlezon & Chartoff, 2007). Consistent with prior results, after stable self-stimulation thresholds were established, the addition of cocaine decreased the threshold in a dose-dependent manor in WT mice. In contrast, at the doses found to be effective in WT mice, cocaine had no effect on self-stimulation thresholds in SR −/− mice (Puhl et al., in press). Thus, the SR −/− mice exhibit profound anhedonia and require much higher doses of cocaine to achieve a hedonic response.

In summary, the role of the NMDARs in substance abuse behaviors observed with the SR −/− and GlyT1 +/− mice are consistent with the results of prior studies in which NMDAR function was manipulated pharmacologically (Ma et al., 2009). Given how closely the SR −/− mouse mimics the neuropathology and cognitive deficits of schizophrenia (Balu et al., 2013), these findings suggest that the very high prevalence of substance abuse in schizophrenia results from their lower hedonic responses to abused substances including nicotine, stimulants, opiates, and alcohol so that they require much higher doses to achieve a pleasurable response comparable to controls. As a consequence, they become much more physically dependent on the addictive substance and thus suffer substantial withdrawal symptoms if they cease taking the drug. The results also suggest that pharmacologic interventions to normalize NMDAR function might not only diminish cognitive and negative symptoms, but also reduce the risk for substance abuse in schizophrenia.

4. ANXIETY DISORDERS

Anxiety disorders include several disparate conditions including generalized anxiety disorder, panic disorder, and posttraumatic stress disorder. Michael Davis and colleagues have played a major role in implicating NMDAR function in anxiety disorders by studying the acquisition and extinction of conditioned fear using a Pavlovian strategy (Pavlov, 1927; for review, Davis, 2011). Classical fear conditioning occurs when an affectively neutral stimulus (unconditioned stimulus; UC) is coupled with a noxious aversive stimulus (conditioned stimulus; CS) such as a foot-shock. The fear-eliciting effects of the CS, often measured in rodents as the duration of "freezing" can be extinguished by repeatedly presenting the CS without the accompanying UC. Extinction does not result from "unlearning," but rather the learning of a new association (Falls & Davis, 1995). The amygdala is the brain structure that sits at the epicenter of fear conditioning as demonstrated by lesions of the amygdala (Falls & Davis, 1995), direct injection of NMDAR antagonists (Falls, Miserendino, & Davis, 1992), and functional brain imaging (Fredrikson & Faria, 2013).

However, the relative contribution of glycine or D-serine to GMS occupancy at critical NMDARs in the amygdala mediating LTP coupled to the CS–UC association remained ill-defined. Experiments using SR −/− mice and in vitro enzymatic degradation of D-serine with DAAO demonstrated the importance of this amino acid for the NMDAR-mediated component of excitatory postsynaptic currents (EPSCs) at thalamo-LA (lateral nucleus of the amygdala) synapses and NMDAR-dependent thalamo-BLA LTP (Li et al., 2013). Specifically, tonic activation of NMDARs at synapses in the amygdala under low-activity conditions is supported by ambient D-serine as demonstrated by its elimination with perfusion of the slice with DAAO. In contrast, strong afferent stimulation was insensitive to DAAO, but was abolished by perfusion with glycine oxidase. Consistent with these in vitro slice findings, SR −/− mice displayed impairments in fear memory retrieval when reexposed to the conditioning context 24 h after trace-fear conditioning (Balu et al., 2013, 2016; Basu, Puhl, & Coyle, 2016). That this impairment was specifically related to loss of D-serine was demonstrated by the fact that treatment of SR −/− with 150 mg/kg D-serine for 3 weeks restored contextual-related freezing to WT levels.

Preclinical animal studies using Pavlovian fear conditioning have been used to test ability of drugs to facilitate extinction learning. For example, intraamygdalar infusion of DCS facilitated the extinction of fear conditioning in a dose-dependent way that was prevented by coinfusion of the GMS antagonist, HA-966 (Walker, Ressler, Lu, & Davis, 2002). Enhancement of NMDAR function with DCS appears to act specifically on the consolidation of the memory (Richardson, Ledgerwood, & Cranney, 2004).

Demonstrating the translational potential of these animal studies, Ressler and colleagues pioneered the use of DCS to augment exposure therapy to treat anxiety disorders building upon the animal studies with extinction in fear conditioning paradigms (Morrison & Ressler, 2014). His first demonstration of the efficacy of DCS with exposure therapy cleverly exploited virtual glass Hyatt elevators in patients with acrophobia (Ressler et al., 2004). Coupling exposure therapy with DCS resulted in those acrophobics being able to tolerate significantly higher virtual floors as compared to those receiving placebo and exposure. Importantly, this reduction in anxiety persisted for 3 months. In their metaanalysis, Norberg, Krystal, and Tolin (2008) found that DCS significantly facilitated fear extinction and exposure therapy for anxiety disorders, that the effects generally persisted, that desensitization to the effects of DCS appeared with chronic treatment, and that DCS administration was most effective when closely timed to the intervention. A more recent metaanalysis by Mataix-Cols et al. (2017) found that DCS treatment was associated with a small augmentation effect on exposure-based cognitive behavior therapy for anxiety, obsessive–compulsive, and posttraumatic stress disorders, an effect that was not moderated by the concurrent use of antidepressants.

5. BRAIN DAMAGE

Excessive activation of glutamate ionotropic receptors, especially NMDARs, has long been known to cause oxidative stress, thereby compromising neuronal function and ultimately causing neuronal death (Coyle & Puttfarcken, 1993). The GMS on the NMDAR is thus a target for neuroprotection, as GMS antagonists prevent NMDAR-mediated excitotoxic neuronal degeneration (Wu, Lee, & Schwarcz, 2000). However, the relative roles of D-serine or glycine as the endogenous coagonist-mediating excitotoxic neuronal degeneration were unexplored. Mustafa et al. (2010) used SR −/− mice to define the role of D-serine in excitotoxicity in vitro and in vivo. As reviewed by Jaffrey and Snyder (1995), nitric oxide appears to be the proximate mediator of excitotoxic neuronal degeneration in stroke and ischemia. Consistent with this, cerebral cortex cultures from SR −/− mice produce ~60% less NO than do those from litter mate WT mice, although there is no difference in the expression of neuronal nitric oxide synthase. When subject to glucose–oxygen deprivation, an in vitro model of ischemia, the SR −/− culture exhibited a ~50% reduction in neuronal degeneration. Similarly, after middle cerebral artery occlusion, the SR −/− adult mice had a ~50% reduction in infarct volume.

Traumatic brain injury results in neuronal dysfunction and even excitotoxic neuronal degeneration. The Liebl laboratory has been studying a model of closed head injury that results in compromised hippocampal neuronal function and cognitive impairment, without neuronal degeneration (Perez et al., 2016). After controlled cortical impact (CCI), hippocampal neurons downregulated their expression of SR and D-serine levels, whereas the reactive astrocytes that propagated in the damaged hippocampus after CCI expressed SR and synthesized D-serine (Perez et al., 2017). Notably, Western blots showed little change in the overall expression of SR in the hippocampus, demonstrating the importance of documenting cellular localization of SR immunohistochemically. Previous studies have demonstrated that cultured astrocytes, which assume the features of reactive astrocytes, express SR (Zhuang et al., 2010). The critical role that astrocytic D-serine release plays in impairing synaptic plasticity and cognition after CCI was established by showing that mice with SR selectively eliminated in glial fibrillary associated protein (GFAP)-containing astrocytes were protected from the deleterious effects of CCI. Thus, the tonic release of D-serine from postinjury proliferating reactive astrocytes, which would preferentially act at extrasynaptic NMDARs known to mediate excitotoxicity, may be largely responsible for the symptoms of concussive closed head injury (Perez et al., 2017). Notably, cultured astrocytes exhibit characteristics of A1 reactive astrocytes that have neurotoxic as opposed to A2 neurotrophic astrocytes

(Liddelow et al., 2017) effects and express SR (S. Li, T. Anderson, J.T. Coyle, et al., unpublished).

6. CONCLUSION

It appears that SR through its product, D-serine, plays a dominant role in modulating NMDAR function in forebrain. In fact, it would not be an overstatement that D-serine is the "gate-keeper" for NMDAR function in forebrain and can be linked to most pathologic processes known to involve forebrain NMDARs. That the GMS, where D-serine acts in forebrain, might be a target for pharmacologic intervention to modify NMDAR activity has been addressed by the Schwarcz laboratory (Schwarcz, Bruno, Muchowski, & Wu, 2012). Kynurenic acid (Kyna) blocks the GMS on the NMDAR, but also is a noncompetitive inhibitor at an allosteric site on the α-7-nicotinic receptor. Altering the levels of Kyna, an endogenous metabolite of tryptophan, shifts vulnerability to excitotoxic neuronal degeneration and seizures. The derivative of Kyna, 7-chlorokynurenic acid, is a potent and selective GMS antagonist (Croucher & Bradford, 1990).

Of course, strategies to manipulate the effects of D-serine in disease processes presume that the site of synthesis and release are well understood. Many publications have indicated that D-serine is a "glio-transmitter," the release of which is coordinated by synaptic glutamate to ensure NMDAR activation (Gundersen, Storm-Mathisen, & Bergersen, 2015). As reviewed by Wolosker, Balu, and Coyle (2016), this concept arose out of a series of unforeseen artifacts: lack of specificity of SR antibodies, expression of SR in cultured "reactive" astrocytes, and high concentrations of L-serine in astrocytes causing deceptive immune cross-reactivity with D-serine antiserum in immunocytochemical studies. These artifacts were uncovered by the use of SR−/− mice to verify specificity of SR antibodies (Balu, Takagi, Puhl, Benneyworth, & Coyle, 2014; Miya et al., 2008) and of L-serine blocking conditions to ensure D-serine immune-specificity (Balu et al., 2014), as well as conditional knock-out methods that showed negligible effects on SR expression and NMDAR-dependent neurotransmission when silencing SR in astrocytes (Benneyworth & Coyle, 2012; Ishiwata, Umino, Balu, Coyle, & Nishikawa, 2015; Perez et al., 2017).

The neuronal localization of SR and D-serine raised the possibility that D-serine was a "cotransmitter" with glutamate, much like neuropeptides are exocytotically released with simple neurotransmitters like GABA and dopamine. However, immunohistochemical studies indicated that SR and

D-serine are also localized to GABAergic neurons, in addition to glutamatergic neurons across the forebrain (Balu et al., 2014; Miya et al., 2008). Initially, this localization to GABAergic neurons seemed puzzling since postsynaptic GABA receptors do not possess a GMS. However, Lin, Jacobi, Anderson, and Lynch (2016) found that endogenous D-serine and SR colocalize with the PSD-95 in glutamatergic synapses on both excitatory and inhibitory neurons, but not with the presynaptic vesicular glutamate transporter-1, VGluT1. Thus, D-serine appears to function in an autocrine fashion, being released from the postsynaptic neuron, thereby ensuring that the postsynaptic NMDARs' GMS are occupied with D-serine to respond immediately to released glutamate (Fig. 1).

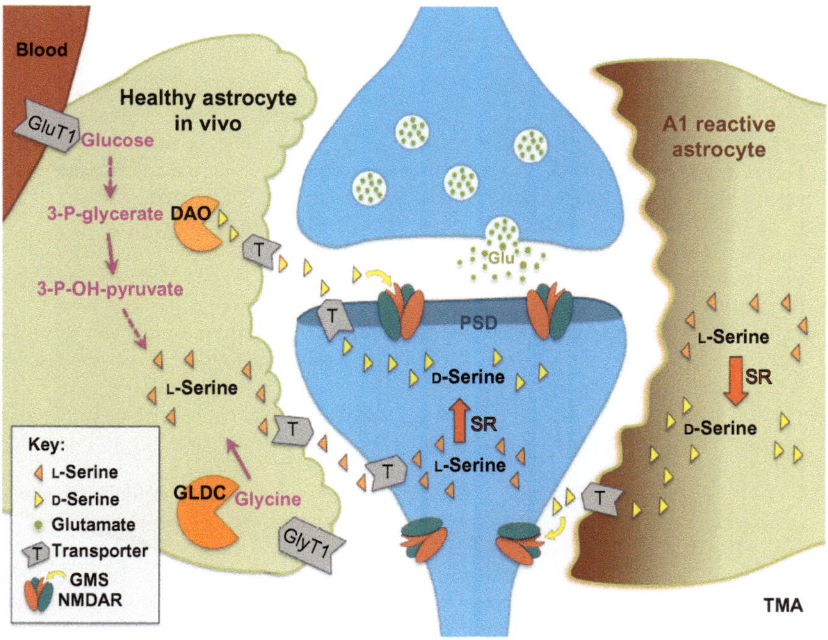

Fig. 1 Schematic representation of D-serine pathways in health and disease. Resting astrocytes synthesize L-serine from glucose, which is then transported into neurons to be converted to D-serine by serine racemase, a process known as the "serine shuttle" (Wolosker et al., 2016). Serine racemase and D-serine are concentrated at the postsynaptic densities in glutamatergic and serine racemase-expressing GABAergic neurons (Li et al., 2013), where D-serine binds to the glycine modulatory sites on synaptic NMDA receptors, rendering them "primed" to respond to synaptic glutamate. D-serine is transported into astrocytes where it is catabolized by D-amino acid oxidase (DAAO). Inflammatory insults such as traumatic brain injury cause the proliferation of reactive or A1 "toxic" astrocytes (Liddelow et al., 2017) that express serine racemase and release D-serine, which activates extrajunctional receptors causing neurotoxicity (Perez et al., 2017).

Our 20-year pursuit of the hypothesis that NMDAR hypofunction is a fundamental pathophysiologic mechanism in schizophrenia (Coyle, 1996) has led to many surprises and counter-intuitive discoveries. But the route was laid out by the lessons of my mentor, Sol Snyder: try to ask important questions, do good basic science, keep your eye on clinical relevance, and follow the evidence.

CONFLICT OF INTEREST

J.T.C. reports holding a patent on the clinical use of D-serine that is owned by Massachusetts General Hospital but could yield royalties to J.T.C. D.T.B. reports no conflicts.

ACKNOWLEDGMENTS

Some of the research described in this review was supported by NIH research grants including R01MH05190 and 1R21DA035427 and K99MH099252 and R00MH099252 to D.T.B.

REFERENCES

Anis, N. A., Berry, S. C., Burton, N. R., & Lodge, D. (1983). The dissociative anaesthetics, ketamine and phencyclidine, selectively reduce excitation of central mammalian neurones by N-methyl-aspartate. *British Journal of Pharmacology*, *79*(2), 565–575.

Anon. (2008). Cycloserine. *Tuberculosis (Edinburgh, Scotland)*, *88*(2), 100–101.

Badiani, A., Anagnostaras, S. G., & Robinson, T. E. (1995). The development of sensitization to the psychomotor stimulant effects of amphetamine is enhanced in a novel environment. *Psychopharmacology* (Berlin), *117*(4), 443–452.

Bakshi, V. P., & Geyer, M. A. (1995). Antagonism of phencyclidine-induced deficits in prepulse inhibition by the putative atypical antipsychotic olanzapine. *Psychopharmacology*, *122*(2), 198–201.

Balu, D. T., Basu, A. C., Corradi, J. P., Cacace, A. M., & Coyle, J. T. (2012). The NMDA receptor co-agonists, D-serine and glycine, regulate neuronal dendritic architecture in the somatosensory cortex. *Neurobiology of Disease*, *45*(2), 671–682.

Balu, D. T., & Coyle, J. T. (2015). The NMDA receptor 'glycine modulatory site' in schizophrenia: D-serine, glycine, and beyond. *Current Opinion in Pharmacology*, *20*, 109–115.

Balu, D. T., Li, Y., Puhl, M. D., Benneyworth, M. A., Basu, A. C., Takagi, S., et al. (2013). Multiple risk pathways for schizophrenia converge in serine racemase knockout mice, a mouse model of NMDA receptor hypofunction. *Proceedings of the National Academy of Sciences of the United States of America*, *110*(26), E2400–E2409. https://doi.org/10.1073/pnas.1304308110.

Balu, D. T., Li, Y., Takagi, S., Presti, K. T., Ramikie, T. S., Rook, J. M., et al. (2016). An mGlu5-positive allosteric modulator rescues the neuroplasticity deficits in a genetic model of NMDA receptor hypofunction in schizophrenia. *Neuropsychopharmacology*, *41*(8), 2052–2061.

Balu, D. T., Takagi, S., Puhl, M. D., Benneyworth, M. A., & Coyle, J. T. (2014). D-serine and serine racemase are localized to neurons in the adult mouse and human forebrain. *Cellular and Molecular Neurobiology*, *34*(3), 419–435.

Basu, A. C., Puhl, M. D., & Coyle, J. T. (2016). Endogenous co-agonists of the NMDA receptor modulate contextual fear in trace conditioning. *Neurobiology of Learning and Memory*, *136*, 244–250.

Basu, A. C., Tsai, G. E., Ma, C. L., Ehmsen, J. T., Mustafa, A. K., Han, L., et al. (2009). Targeted disruption of serine racemase affects glutamatergic neurotransmission and behavior. *Molecular Psychiatry*, *14*(7), 719–727.

Benneyworth, M. A., & Coyle, J. T. (2012). Altered acquisition and extinction of amphetamine-paired context conditioning in genetic mouse models of altered NMDA receptor function. *Neuropsychopharmacology*, *37*(11), 2496–2504.

Benneyworth, M. A., Roseman, A. S., Basu, A. C., & Coyle, J. T. (2011). Failure of NMDA receptor hypofunction to induce a pathological reduction in PV-positive GABAergic cell markers. *Neuroscience Letters*, *488*(3), 267–271.

Bergeron, R., & Coyle, J. T. (2012). NAAG, NMDA receptor and psychosis. *Current Medicinal Chemistry*, *19*(9), 1360–1364.

Bergeron, R., Coyle, J. T., Tsai, G., & Greene, R. W. (2005). NAAG reduces NMDA receptor current in CA1 hippocampal pyramidal neurons of acute slices and dissociated neurons. *Neuropsychopharmacology*, *30*(1), 7–16.

Birnbaum, R., Zhang, F., Hyde, T. M., Kleinman, J. E., & Weinberger, D. R. (2014). Serine racemase (SRR) and schizophrenia risk: Functional genomic characterization of SCZ GWAS risk SNP rs4523957 by RNA sequencing. *American College of Neuropsychopharmacology* (Abstracts).

Bredt, D. S., & Snyder, S. H. (1969). Nitric oxide mediates glutamate-linked enhancement of cGMP levels in the cerebellum. *Proceedings of the National Academy of Sciences of the United States of America*, *86*(22), 9030–9033.

Cantor-Graae, E., Nordström, L. G., & McNeil, T. F. (2001). Substance abuse in schizophrenia: A review of the literature and a study of correlates in Sweden. *Schizophrenia Research*, *48*(1), 69–82.

Carlezon, W. A., Jr., & Chartoff, E. H. (2007). Intracranial self-stimulation (ICSS) in rodents to study the neurobiology of motivation. *Nature Protocols*, *2*(11), 2987–2995.

Carlezon, W. A., Jr., & Nestler, E. J. (2002). Elevated levels of GluR1 in the midbrain: A trigger for sensitization to drugs of abuse? *Trends in Neurosciences*, *25*(12), 610–615.

Carlezon, W. A., Jr., & Thomas, M. J. (2009). Biological substrates of reward and aversion: A nucleus accumbens activity hypothesis. *Neuropharmacology*, *56*(Suppl. 1), 122–132.

Coyle, J. T. (1996). The glutamatergic dysfunction hypothesis for schizophrenia. *Harvard Review of Psychiatry*, *3*(5), 241–253.

Coyle, J. T. (2006). Substance use disorders and Schizophrenia: A question of shared glutamatergic mechanisms. *Neurotoxicity Research*, *10*(3–4), 221–233.

Coyle, J. T., Basu, A., Benneyworth, M., Balu, D., & Konopaske, G. (2012). Glutamatergic synaptic dysregulation in schizophrenia: Therapeutic implications. *Handbook of Experimental Pharmacology*, *213*, 267–295.

Coyle, J. T., & Puttfarcken, P. (1993). Oxidative stress, glutamate, and neurodegenerative disorders. *Science*, *262*(5134), 689–695.

Croucher, M. J., & Bradford, H. F. (1990). 7-Chlorokynurenic acid, a strychnine-insensitive glycine receptor antagonist, inhibits limbic seizure kindling. *Neuroscience Letters*, *118*(1), 29–32.

Curcio, L., Podda, M. V., Leone, L., Piacentini, R., Mastrodonato, A., Cappelletti, P., et al. (2013). Reduced D-serine levels in the nucleus accumbens of cocaine-treated rats hinder the induction of NMDA receptor-dependent synaptic plasticity. *Brain*, *136*, 1216–1230.

Davis, M. (2011). NMDA receptors and fear extinction: Implications for cognitive behavioral therapy. *Dialogues in Clinical Neuroscience*, *13*(4), 463–474.

Davis, K. L., Buchsbaum, M. S., Shihabuddin, L., Spiegel-Cohen, J., Metzger, M., Frecska, E., et al. (1998). Ventricular enlargement in poor-outcome schizophrenia. *Biological Psychiatry*, *43*(11), 783–793.

DeVito, L. M., Balu, D. T., Kanter, B. R., Lykken, C., Basu, A. C., Coyle, J. T., et al. (2011). Serine racemase deletion disrupts memory for order and alters cortical dendritic morphology. *Genes, Brain, and Behavior, 10*(2), 210–222.

Erlenmeyer-Kimling, L., Rock, D., Roberts, S. A., Janal, M., Kestenbaum, C., Cornblatt, B., et al. (2000). Attention, memory, and motor skills as childhood predictors of schizophrenia-related psychoses: The New York High-Risk Project. *The American Journal of Psychiatry, 157*(9), 1416–1422.

Falls, W. A., & Davis, M. (1995). Lesions of the central nucleus of the amygdala block conditioned excitation, but not conditioned inhibition of fear as measured with the fear-potentiated startle effect. *Behavioral Neuroscience, 109*(3), 379–387.

Falls, W. A., Miserendino, M. J., & Davis, M. (1992). Extinction of fear-potentiated startle: Blockade by infusion of an NMDA antagonist into the amygdala. *Journal of Neuroscience, 12*(3), 854–863.

Farber, N. B., Wozniak, D. F., Price, M. T., Labruyere, J., Huss, J., St Peter, H., et al. (1995). Age-specific neurotoxicity in the rat associated with NMDA receptor blockade: Potential relevance to schizophrenia? *Biological Psychiatry, 38*(12), 788–796.

Flood, J. F., Morley, J. E., & Lanthorn, T. H. (1992). Effect on memory processing by D-cycloserine, an agonist of the NMDA/glycine receptor. *European Journal of Pharmacology, 221*(2–3), 249–254.

Frantseva, M. V., Fitzgerald, P. B., Chen, R., Möller, B., Daigle, M., & Daskalakis, Z. J. (2008). Evidence for impaired long-term potentiation in schizophrenia and its relationship to motor skill learning. *Cerebral Cortex, 18*(5), 990–996.

Fredrikson, M., & Faria, V. (2013). Neuroimaging in anxiety disorders. *Modern Trends in Pharmacopsychiatry, 29*, 47–66.

Ginovart, N., & Kapur, S. (2012). Role of dopamine D(2) receptors for antipsychotic activity. *Handbook of Experimental Pharmacology, 212*, 27–52.

Goff, D. C., Cather, C., Gottlieb, J. D., Evins, A. E., Walsh, J., Raeke, L., et al. (2008). Once-weekly D-cycloserine effects on negative symptoms and cognition in schizophrenia: An exploratory study. *Schizophrenia Research, 106*(2–3), 320–327.

Goff, D. C., Tsai, G., Levitt, J., Amico, E., Manoach, D., Schoenfeld, D. A., et al. (1999). A placebo-controlled trial of D-cycloserine added to conventional neuroleptics in patients with schizophrenia. *Archives of General Psychiatry, 56*(1), 21–27.

Goff, D. C., Tsai, G., Manoach, D. S., & Coyle, J. T. (1995). Dose-finding trial of D-cycloserine added to neuroleptics for negative symptoms in schizophrenia. *The American Journal of Psychiatry, 152*(8), 1213–1215.

Green, A. I., Canuso, C. M., Brenner, M. J., & Wojcik, J. D. (2003). Detection and management of comorbidity in patients with schizophrenia. *The Psychiatric Clinics of North America, 26*(1), 115–139.

Gundersen, V., Storm-Mathisen, J., & Bergersen, L. H. (2015). Neuroglial transmission. *Physiological Reviews, 95*(3), 695–726.

Hammond, S., Seymour, C. M., Burger, A., & Wagner, J. J. (2013). D-Serine facilitates the effectiveness of extinction to reduce drug-primed reinstatement of cocaine-induced conditioned place preference. *Neuropharmacology, 64*, 464–471.

Hashimoto, K., Engberg, G., Shimizu, E., Nordin, C., Lindström, L. H., & Iyo, M. (2005). Reduced D-serine to total serine ratio in the cerebrospinal fluid of drug naive schizophrenic patients. *Progress in Neuro-Psychopharmacology & Biological Psychiatry, 29*(5), 767–769.

Hashimoto, A., Nishikawa, T., Hayashi, T., Fujii, N., Harada, K., Oka, T., et al. (1992). The presence of free D-serine in rat brain. *FEBS Letters, 296*(1), 33–36.

Ishiwata, S., Umino, A., Balu, D. T., Coyle, J. T., & Nishikawa, T. (2015). Neuronal serine racemase regulates extracellular D-serine levels in the adult mouse hippocampus. *Journal of Neural Transmission (Vienna), 122*(8), 1099–1103.

Jackson, P. F., & Slusher, B. S. (2001). Design of NAALADase inhibitors: A novel neuroprotective strategy. *Current Medicinal Chemistry*, *8*(8), 949–957.
Jaffrey, S. R., & Snyder, S. H. (1995). Nitric oxide: A neural messenger. *Annual Review of Cell and Developmental Biology*, *11*, 417–440.
Javitt, D. C. (2006). Is the glycine site half saturated or half unsaturated? Effects of glutamatergic drugs in schizophrenia patients. *Current Opinion in Psychiatry*, *19*(2), 151–157.
Javitt, D. C., & Zukin, S. R. (1991). Recent advances in the phencyclidine model of schizophrenia. *The American Journal of Psychiatry*, *148*(10), 1301–1308.
Johnson, J. W., & Ascher, P. (1987). Glycine potentiates the NMDA response in cultured mouse brain neurons. *Nature*, *325*(6104), 529–531.
Johnstone, E. C., Owens, D. G., Bydder, G. M., Colter, N., Crow, T. J., & Frith, C. D. (1989). The spectrum of structural brain changes in schizophrenia: Age of onset as a predictor of cognitive and clinical impairments and their cerebral correlates. *Psychological Medicine*, *19*(1), 91–103.
Kavanagh, D. J., McGrath, J., Saunders, J. B., Dore, G., & Clark, D. (2002). Substance misuse in patients with schizophrenia: Epidemiology and management. *Drugs*, *62*(5), 743–755.
Kleckner, N. W., & Dingledine, R. (1988). Requirement for glycine in activation of NMDA-receptors expressed in Xenopus oocytes. *Science*, *241*(4867), 835–837.
Krystal, J. H., & Anticevic, A. (2015). Toward illness phase-specific pharmacotherapy for schizophrenia. *Biological Psychiatry*, *78*(11), 738–740.
Lane, H. Y., Lin, C. H., Green, M. F., Hellemann, G., Huang, C. C., Chen, P. W., et al. (2013). Add-on treatment of benzoate for schizophrenia: a randomized, double-blind, placebo-controlled trial of D-amino acid oxidase inhibitor. *JAMA Psychiatry*, *70*(12), 1267–1275.
Lewis, D. A. (2014). Inhibitory neurons in human cortical circuits: Substrate for cognitive dysfunction in schizophrenia. *Current Opinion in Neurobiology*, *26*, 22–26.
Li, Y., Sacchi, S., Pollegioni, L., Basu, A. C., Coyle, J. T., & Bolshakov, V. Y. (2013). Identity of endogenous NMDAR glycine site agonist in amygdala is determined by synaptic activity level. *Nature Communications*, *4*, 1760. https://doi.org/10.1038/ncomms2779.
Liddelow, S. A., Guttenplan, K. A., Clarke, L. E., Bennett, F. C., Bohlen, C. J., Schirmer, L., et al. (2017). Neurotoxic reactive astrocytes are induced by activated microglia. *Nature*, *541*(7638), 481–487.
Lim, J., Lee, S. A., Lam, M., Rapisarda, A., Kraus, M., Keefe, R. S., et al. (2016). The relationship between negative symptom subdomains and cognition. *Psychological Medicine*, *46*(10), 2169–2177.
Lin, H., Jacobi, A. A., Anderson, S. A., & Lynch, D. R. (2016). D-Serine and serine racemase are associated with PSD-95 and glutamatergic synapse stability. *Frontiers in Cellular Neuroscience*, *10*, 34.
Ma, Y. Y., Cepeda, C., & Cui, C. L. (2009). The role of striatal NMDA receptors in drug addiction. *International Review of Neurobiology*, *89*, 131–146.
Malenka, R. C., & Nicoll, R. A. (1993). NMDA-receptor-dependent synaptic plasticity: Multiple forms and mechanisms. *Trends in Neurosciences*, *16*(12), 521–527.
Markou, A., & Koob, G. F. (1991). Postcocaine anhedonia. An animal model of cocaine withdrawal. *Neuropsychopharmacology*, *4*(1), 17–26.
Mataix-Cols, D., et al. (2017). D-Cycloserine augmentation of exposure-based cognitive behavior therapy for anxiety, obsessive-compulsive, and posttraumatic stress disorders: A systematic review and meta-analysis of individual participant data. *JAMA Psychiatry*, *74*(5), 501–510.
Meunier, C. N., Dallérac, G., Le Roux, N., Sacchi, S., Levasseur, G., Amar, M., et al. (2016). D-Serine and glycine differentially control neurotransmission during visual cortex critical period. *PLoS One*, *11*(3), e0151233.

Miya, K., Inoue, R., Takata, Y., Abe, M., Natsume, R., Sakimura, K., et al. (2008). Serine racemase is predominantly localized in neurons in mouse brain. *The Journal of Comparative Neurology*, *510*(6), 641–654.
Moghaddam, B., & Krystal, J. H. (2012). Capturing the angel in "angel dust": Twenty years of translational neuroscience studies of NMDA receptor antagonists in animals and humans. *Schizophrenia Bulletin*, *38*(5), 942–949.
Morrison, F. G., & Ressler, K. J. (2014). From the neurobiology of extinction to improved clinical treatments. *Depression and Anxiety*, *31*(4), 279–290.
Mothet, J. P., Parent, A. T., Wolosker, H., Brady, R. O., Jr., Linden, D. J., Ferris, C. D., et al. (2000). D-serine is an endogenous ligand for the glycine site of the *N*-methyl-D-aspartate receptor. *Proceedings of the National Academy of Sciences of the United States of America*, *97*(9), 4926–4931.
Moyer, C. E., Shelton, M. A., & Sweet, R. A. (2015). Dendritic spine alterations in schizophrenia. *Neuroscience Letters*, *601*, 46–53.
Mustafa, A. K., Ahmad, A. S., Zeynalov, E., Gazi, S. K., Sikka, G., Ehmsen, J. T., et al. (2010). Serine racemase deletion protects against cerebral ischemia and excitotoxicity. *The Journal of Neuroscience*, *30*(4), 1413–1416.
Myers, K. M., & Carlezon, W. A., Jr. (2010). Extinction of drug- and withdrawal-paired cues in animal models: Relevance to the treatment of addiction. *Neuroscience & Biobehavioral Reviews*, *35*(2), 285–302.
Myers, K. M., & Carlezon, W. A., Jr. (2012). D-Cycloserine effects on extinction of conditioned responses to drug-related cues. *Biological Psychiatry*, *71*(11), 947–955.
Neims, A. H., Zieverink, W. D., & Smilack, J. D. (1966). Distribution of D-amino acid oxidase in bovine and human nervous tissues. *Journal of Neurochemistry*, *13*(3), 163–168.
Norberg, M. M., Krystal, J. H., & Tolin, D. F. (2008). A meta-analysis of D-cycloserine and the facilitation of fear extinction and exposure therapy. *Biological Psychiatry*, *63*(12), 1118–1126.
Paolone, G., Botreau, F., & Stewart, J. (2009). The facilitative effects of D-cycloserine on extinction of a cocaine-induced conditioned place preference can be long lasting and resistant to reinstatement. *Psychopharmacology*, *202*(1–3), 403–409.
Parnas, A. S., Weber, M., & Richardson, R. (2005). Effects of multiple exposures to D-cycloserine on extinction of conditioned fear in rats. *Neurobiology of Learning and Memory*, *83*(3), 224–231.
Pavlov, I. P. (1927). *Conditioned reflexes: An investigation of the physiological activity of the cerebral cortex*. Oxford, United Kingdom: Oxford University Press.
Perez, E. J., Cepero, M. L., Perez, S. U., Coyle, J. T., Sick, T. J., & Liebl, D. J. (2016). EphB3 signaling propagates synaptic dysfunction in the traumatic injured brain. *Neurobiology of Disease*, *94*, 73–84.
Perez, E. J., Tapanes, S. A., Loris, Z. B., Sick, T. J., Coyle, J. T., & Liebl, D. J. (2017). Enhanced astrocytic D-serine underlies synaptic damage after traumatic brain injury. *The Journal of Clinical Investigation*, *127*, 3114–3125.
Puhl, M. D., Desai, R. I., Takagi, S., Presti, K. T., Doyle, M. R., Donahue, R. J., et al. N-methyl-D-aspartate receptor co-agonist availability affects behavioral and neurochemical responses to cocaine: Insights into co-morbid schizophrenia and substance abuse. *Addiction Biology*, in press.
Puhl, M. D., Mintzopoulos, D., Jensen, J. E., Gillis, T. E., Konopaske, G. T., Kaufman, M. J., et al. (2015). In vivo magnetic resonance studies reveal neuroanatomical and neurochemical abnormalities in the serine racemase knockout mouse model of schizophrenia. *Neurobiology of Disease*, *73*, 269–274.
Quartermain, D., Mower, J., Rafferty, M. F., Herting, R. L., & Lanthorn, T. H. (1994). Acute but not chronic activation of the NMDA-coupled glycine receptor with D-cycloserine facilitates learning and retention. *European Journal of Pharmacology*, *257*(1–2), 7–12.

Ressler, K. J., Rothbaum, B. O., Tannenbaum, L., Anderson, P., Graap, K., Zimand, E., et al. (2004). Cognitive enhancers as adjuncts to psychotherapy: Use of D-cycloserine in phobic individuals to facilitate extinction of fear. *Archives of General Psychiatry, 61*(11), 1136–1144.

Richardson, R., Ledgerwood, L., & Cranney, J. (2004). Facilitation of fear extinction by D-cycloserine: Theoretical and clinical implications. *Learning & Memory, 11*(5), 510–516.

Ripke, S., Neale, B. M., Corvin, A., et al. (2014). Biological insights from 108 schizophrenia-associated genetic loci. *Nature, 511*(7510), 421–427.

Schell, M. J., Molliver, M. E., & Snyder, S. H. (1995). D-Serine, an endogenous synaptic modulator: Localization to astrocytes and glutamate-stimulated release. *Proceedings of the National Academy of Sciences of the United States of America, 92*(9), 3948–3952.

Schuster, G. M., & Schmidt, W. J. (1992). D-Cycloserine reverses the working memory impairment of hippocampal-lesioned rats in a spatial learning task. *European Journal of Pharmacology, 224*(1), 97–98.

Schwarcz, R., Bruno, J. P., Muchowski, P. J., & Wu, H. Q. (2012). Kynurenines in the mammalian brain: When physiology meets pathology. *Nature Reviews. Neuroscience, 13*(7), 465–477.

Selemon, L. D., & Goldman-Rakic, P. S. (1999). The reduced neuropil hypothesis: A circuit based model of schizophrenia. *Biological Psychiatry, 45*(1), 17–25.

Snyder, S. H. (1976). The dopamine hypothesis of schizophrenia: Focus on the dopamine receptor. *The American Journal of Psychiatry, 133*(2), 197–202.

Steullet, P., Cabungcal, J. H., Coyle, J., Didriksen, M., Gill, K., Grace, A. A., et al. (2017). Oxidative stress-driven parvalbumin interneuron impairment as a common mechanism in models of schizophrenia. *Molecular Psychiatry, 22*(7), 936–943.

Thanos, P. K., Bermeo, C., Wang, G. J., & Volkow, N. D. (2010). D-Cycloserine facilitates extinction of cocaine self-administration in rats. *Synapse, 65*(9), 938–944.

Tsai, G. E., & Lin, P. Y. (2010). Strategies to enhance *N*-methyl-D-aspartate receptor-mediated neurotransmission in schizophrenia, a critical review and meta-analysis. *Current Pharmaceutical Design, 16*(5), 522–537.

Tsai, G., Passani, L. A., Slusher, B. S., Carter, R., Baer, L., Kleinman, J. E., et al. (1995). Abnormal excitatory neurotransmitter metabolism in schizophrenic brains. *Archives of General Psychiatry, 52*(10), 829–836.

Tsai, G., Ralph-Williams, R. J., Martina, M., Bergeron, R., Berger-Sweeney, J., Dunham, K. S., et al. (2004). Gene knockout of glycine transporter 1: Characterization of the behavioral phenotype. *Proceedings of the National Academy of Sciences of the United States of America, 101*(22), 8485–8490.

Tsai, G., Yang, P., Chung, L. C., Lange, N., & Coyle, J. T. (1998). D-serine added to antipsychotics for the treatment of schizophrenia. *Biological Psychiatry, 44*(11), 1081–1089.

Verma, A., Hirsch, D. J., Glatt, C. E., Ronnett, G. V., & Snyder, S. H. (1993). Carbon monoxide: A putative neural messenger. *Science, 259*(5093), 381–384.

Vezina, P., & Leyton, M. (2009). Conditioned cues and the expression of stimulant sensitization in animals and humans. *Neuropharmacology, 56*(Suppl. 1), 160–168.

Walker, D. L., Ressler, K. J., Lu, K. T., & Davis, M. (2002). Facilitation of conditioned fear extinction by systemic administration or intra-amygdala infusions of D-cycloserine as assessed with fear-potentiated startle in rats. *The Journal of Neuroscience, 22*(6), 2343–2351.

Watson, G. B., Bolanowski, M. A., Baganoff, M. P., Deppeler, C. L., & Lanthorn, T. H. (1990). D-Cycloserine acts as a partial agonist at the glycine modulatory site of the NMDA receptor expressed in Xenopus oocytes. *Brain Research, 510*(1), 158–160.

Wolosker, H., Balu, D. T., & Coyle, J. T. (2016). The rise and fall of the D-Serine-mediated gliotransmission hypothesis. *Trends in Neurosciences, 39*(11), 712–721.

Wolosker, H., Blackshaw, S., & Snyder, S. H. (1999). Serine racemase: A glial enzyme synthesizing D-serine to regulate glutamate-*N*-methyl-D-aspartate neurotransmission. *Proceedings of the National Academy of Sciences of the United States of America, 96*(23), 13409–13414.

Wolosker, H., Sheth, K. N., Takahashi, M., Mothet, J. P., Brady, R. O., Jr., Ferris, C. D., et al. (1999). Purification of serine racemase: Biosynthesis of the neuromodulator D-serine. *Proceedings of the National Academy of Sciences of the United States of America, 96*(2), 721–725.

Wu, H. Q., Lee, S. C., & Schwarcz, R. (2000). Systemic administration of 4-chlorokynurenine prevents quinolinate neurotoxicity in the rat hippocampus. *European Journal of Pharmacology, 390*(3), 267–274.

Yurgelun-Todd, D. A., Coyle, J. T., Gruber, S. A., Renshaw, P. F., Silveri, M. M., Amico, E., et al. (2005). Functional magnetic resonance imaging studies of schizophrenic patients during word production: Effects of D-cycloserine. *Psychiatry Research, 138*(1), 23–31.

Zhuang, Z., Yang, B., Theus, M. H., Sick, J. T., Bethea, J. R., Sick, T. J., et al. (2010). EphrinBs regulate D-serine synthesis and release in astrocytes. *The Journal of Neuroscience, 30*(47), 16015–16024.

CHAPTER FOUR

Nitric Oxide Signaling in Neurodegeneration and Cell Death

Ted M. Dawson[*,†,‡,§,1], **Valina L. Dawson**[*,†,‡,§,1]
[*]Neuroregeneration and Stem Cell Programs, Institute for Cell Engineering, Johns Hopkins University School of Medicine, Baltimore, MD, United States
[†]Johns Hopkins University School of Medicine, Baltimore, MD, United States
[‡]Adrienne Helis Malvin Medical Research Foundation, New Orleans, LA, United States
[§]Diana Helis Henry Medical Research Foundation, New Orleans, LA, United States
[1]Corresponding authors: e-mail address: tdawson@jhmi.edu; vdawson1@jhmi.edu

Contents

Abstract

In this tribute to Solomon H. Snyder (Sol) we discuss the mechanisms by which nitric oxide (NO) kills neurons. We provide a historical perspective regarding the discovery that glutamate excitotoxicity is mediated by NO. It also contains a discussion of the discovery that neuronal nitric oxide synthase (nNOS) catalytic activity accounts for NADPH diaphorase activity and its localization in the central nervous system. NADPH diaphorase/nNOS neurons are unique in that they are resistant to toxic effects of excess glutamate and that they are resistant to neurodegeneration in a variety of neurodegenerative diseases. NADPH diaphorase/nNOS neurons are resistant to neurotoxicity and neurodegeneration through the overexpression of manganese superoxide dismutase. The review also delves into the mechanisms by which NO kills neurons including NO's activation of the glyceraldehyde-3-phosphate dehydrogenase-dependent cell pathway. In addition, there is a review of parthanatos in which NO combines with the superoxide anion ($O_2^{\cdot -}$) to form peroxynitrite ($ONOO^-$) that damages DNA and activates poly

Advances in Pharmacology, Volume 82
ISSN 1054-3589
https://doi.org/10.1016/bs.apha.2017.09.003

(ADP-ribose) (PAR) polymerase (PARP). This ultimately leads to activation of the PARP-dependent apoptosis-inducing factor-associated nuclease, the final executioner in NO-dependent cell death. Finally, there is a discussion of potential targets that are under development that target the mechanisms by which NO kills neurons.

ABBREVIATIONS

Ψ	mitochondrial membrane potential
AD	Alzheimer's disease
ADP	adenosine diphosphate
AIDS	acquired immune deficiency syndrome
AIF	apoptosis-inducing factor
AIMP2	aminoacyl tRNA synthetase complex interacting multifunctional protein
ALS	amyotrophic lateral sclerosis
AMPA	α-amino-3-hydroxy-5-methyl-4-isoxazoleproprionate
ANT	adenine nucleotide translocase
AOB	accessory olfactory bulb
ARH3	ADP-ribosyl-acceptor hydrolase 3
C	colliculi
CB	cerebellum
CBP	CREB-binding protein
cGMP	cyclic guanosine monophosphate
CP	caudate putamen
CREB	cAMP response element-binding protein
CX	cortex
CyPD	cyclophilin D
DA	dopamine
DG	dentate gyrus
Drp1	dynamin-related protein
EAE	experimental allergic encephalomyelitis
eNOS	endothelial nitric oxide synthase
F_1F_0-ATPase	ATP synthase
GABAergic	gamma-aminobutyric acid-ergic
GAPDH	glyceraldehyde-3-phosphate dehydrogenase
GAPDH-SNO	*S*-nitrosylated GAPDH
GOSPEL	GAPDH's competitor of Siah protein enhances life
GOSPEL-SNO	*S*-nitrosylate GOSPEL
HB	hemoglobin
HD	Huntington's disease
HIV	human immunodeficiency virus
HK	hexokinase
HYB	hybridization
IC	islands of Callejae
iNOS	inducible nitric oxide synthase
JW	James K. Wamsley

L-Arg	L-arginine
LPS	lipopolysaccharide
MCAO	middle cerebral artery occlusion
MD	Marc Dichter
MIF	macrophage migration inhibitor factor
MK	Michael Kuhar
MnSOD	manganese superoxide dismutase
MPT	mitochondrial membrane permeability transition
MPTP	1-methyl-4-phenyl-1,2,3,6-tetrahydropyridine
NAD^+	nicotinamide adenine dinucleotide
NADH	nicotinamide adenine dinucleotide + hydrogen
NADPH	nicotinamide adenine dinucleotide phosphate
N-Arg	N^G-nitro-L-arginine
NMDA	*N*-methyl-D-aspartate
NO	nitric oxide
NOS	nitric oxide synthase
nNOS	neuronal nitric oxide synthase
$O_2^{\bullet -}$	superoxide anion
OB	olfactory bulb
$ONOO^-$	peroxynitrite
PAAN	PARP-1-dependent AIF-associated nuclease
PAR	poly (ADP-ribose)
PARG	poly (ADP-ribose) glycohydrolase
PARP	poly (ADP-ribose) polymerase
PD	Parkinson's disease
PPN	pedunculopontine nucleus
PRAT	Postdoctoral Research Associate
PSD-95	postsynaptic density-95
SIAH	Seven in Absentia Homolog
SO	supraoptic nucleus
Sol	Solomon H. Snyder
TBI	traumatic brain injury
TLR4	toll-like receptor 4
TNFα	tumor necrosis factor α
VDAC	voltage-dependent anion channel
XIAP	X-linked inhibitor of apoptosis

1. INTRODUCTION

In this tribute to Solomon H. Snyder (Sol) we focus on our discovery that we made as postdoctoral fellows that nitric oxide (NO) mediates glutamate excitotoxicity and that NO synthase activity accounted for nicotinamide adenine dinucleotide (NAD^+) phosphate (NADPH) diaphorase activity. We also discuss our own laboratories' work and those of others that followed on the role of NO in neuronal cell death.

2. HISTORICAL PERSPECTIVE

While we were graduate students at the University of Utah, both of us worked on neurotransmitter receptor and enzyme localization using receptor autoradiography in James K. Wamsley's (JW) laboratory (Dawson, Dawson, Filloux, & Wamsley, 1988; Dawson, Dawson, & Wamsley, 1990; Dawson, Gehlert, McCabe, Barnett, & Wamsley, 1986). JW had just finished a postdoctoral fellowship with Michael Kuhar (MK) at Johns Hopkins where receptor autoradiography was just developed (Kuhar & Aghajanian, 1973; Kuhar & Yamamura, 1975; Wamsley, Zarbin, Birdsall, & Kuhar, 1980; Young, Wamsley, Zarbin, & Kuhar, 1980). It was our work with receptor neurotransmitters that cemented our interest, particularly for Ted in working with Sol. Ted's first introduction to Sol was through a reading assignment at Montana State University in Bozeman, Montana, where Ted reviewed and wrote a short treatise on Pert and Snyder's *Science* paper on the discovery of the opiate receptor (Pert & Snyder, 1973). Little did Ted know that would ultimately lead to his interest in working with Sol.

As Valina was finishing her Ph.D. at the University of Utah, Ted was a neurology resident at the Hospital of the University of Pennsylvania in Philadelphia. Valina joined Ted in Philadelphia during his last year (1989–90) as a neurology resident where she worked as a postdoctoral fellow with Marc Dichter (MD) on the characterization of the polyamine recognition site of the *N*-methyl-D-aspartate (NMDA) receptor (Williams, Dawson, Romano, Dichter, & Molinoff, 1990). MD's laboratory pioneered the use of rodent cultures to study electrophysiology (Dichter, 1978) and this is where Valina became proficient in primary rodent neuronal cultures. This would turn out to be quite fortuitous. During this year together in Philadelphia, we began to explore opportunities for further scientific training. Since we had been apart while Valina was in Utah and Ted in Philadelphia, in addition to our criteria of our learning different skills from our future postdoctoral mentors, we wanted to be in the same geographical location. Fortune would have it that was Ted was accepted into Sol's lab and Valina was awarded a NIH

Postdoctoral Research Associate (PRAT) fellowship, which provided her the opportunity to work at the National Institute of Drug Abuse in Baltimore.

While Ted was considering his postresidency training options, Sol flooded Ted with many of his laboratory's recent papers. Among them was a paper entitled "Nitric oxide mediates glutamate-linked enhancement of cyclic guanosine monophosphate (cGMP) levels in the cerebellum" (Bredt & Snyder, 1989) and "Isolation of nitric oxide synthetase, a calmodulin-requiring enzyme" (Bredt & Snyder, 1990). We read these and other papers, but the work on NO was particularly exciting. In addition to the publications that suggested that glutamate could stimulate NO production (Bredt & Snyder, 1989; Garthwaite, Charles, & Chess-Williams, 1988; Knowles, Palacios, Palmer, & Moncada, 1989), there were publications that indicated that NO was, in part, responsible for the cytotoxicity of macrophages (Hibbs, Taintor, & Vavrin, 1987; Hibbs, Taintor, Vavrin, & Rachlin, 1988). These reports coupled with the emerging evidence that excessive glutamate receptor stimulation killed neurons (B. Meldrum & Garthwaite, 1990) prompted us to wonder whether glutamate-stimulated NO production was responsible for glutamate induced cell death. Since some of the papers that Sol shared with us were unpublished, we waited until we were settled in Baltimore to test our idea that NO mediates glutamate toxicity in neurons.

3. NITRIC OXIDE MEDIATES GLUTAMATE EXCITOTOXICITY

Both of us were initially given different projects in our respective laboratories (Arriza et al., 1992; Attramadal et al., 1992; Fotuhi et al., 1993; Kusama et al., 1993; Mourey, Dawson, Barrow, Enna, & Snyder, 1992; Sharp et al., 1993; Steiner et al., 1992), but we knew that our idea that NO may play a role in glutamate toxicity was an idea that needed to be tested. In addition, we had a strong desire to work together like we had done in our graduate work. Since there were a few competitive NO synthase (NOS) inhibitors that could be readily obtained from biological supply companies, we obtained N^{ω}-monomethyl-L-arginine and N^{ω}-nitro-L-arginine, two water soluble NOS inhibitors that we used to test the role of NO in glutamate toxicity (Dawson, Dawson, London, Bredt, & Snyder, 1991). Valina led these efforts due to her expertise in primary neuronal culture that she learned while in MD's laboratory. Unbeknownst to us at the time was that MD's culture protocol was critical to the success of our future experiments since they expressed both relatively mature inhibitory and excitatory neurons similar to the adult cortex, which we now know is essential for glutamate to mediate its full neurotoxic potential (Dawson, Dawson, Bartley, Uhl, & Snyder, 1993; Dawson, Kizushi, Huang, Snyder, & Dawson, 1996; Samdani, Newcamp, et al., 1997; Xu et al., 2016). Among the inhibitory neurons were a rare population of neurons that expressed neuronal nitric oxide synthase (nNOS) (Dawson, Bredt, Fotuhi, Hwang, & Snyder, 1991). The use of N^{ω}-monomethyl-L-arginine and N^{ω}-nitro-L-arginine allowed us to show that NO mediates glutamate neurotoxicity in primary neuronal cultures (Fig. 1) (Dawson, Dawson, et al., 1991). The potency of these two inhibitors was directly proportional to their potency in inhibiting NOS and cell death could be prevented by excess L-arginine, the substrate of NOS, consistent with the competitive nature

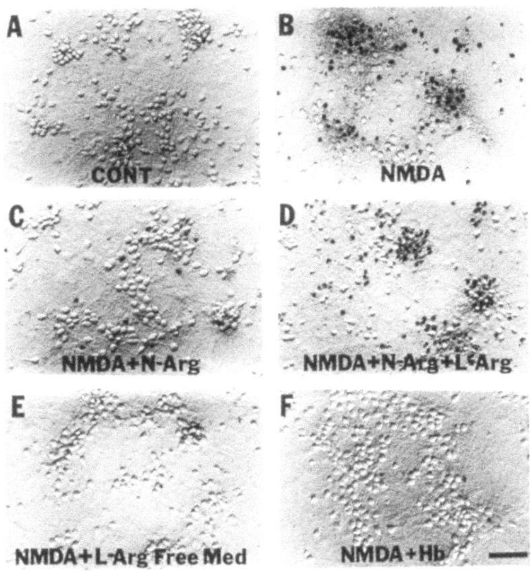

Fig. 1 Nitric oxide (NO) mediates glutamate excitotoxicity. (A) Control (CONT) with normal appearing neurons. (B) A sister culture treated with 300 μM NMDA plus 10 μM glycine for 5 min. Cell death was assessed 24 h later by trypan blue exclusion. Dead cells appear as *black dots.* (C) 100 μM N^{G}-nitro-L-arginine (N-Arg) protects against NMDA neurotoxicity. (D) Reversal of N^{G}-nitro-L-arginine protection against NMDA neurotoxicity by 1 mM L-arginine (L-Arg), the substrate of nNOS. (E) NMDA neurotoxicity is prevented by growing neurons in an L-arginine-free media. (F) Reduced hemoglobin (Hb), which scavenges NO, prevents NMDA excitotoxicity. *Reproduced from Dawson, V. L., Dawson, T. M., London, E. D., Bredt, D. S., & Snyder, S. H. (1991). Nitric oxide mediates glutamate neurotoxicity in primary cortical cultures.* Proceedings of the National Academy of Sciences of the United States of America, 88*(14), 6368–6371.*

of the inhibitors. In addition, removal of arginine from the culture media by either treating the cultures with arginase or growing the neurons in arginine-free media attenuated the glutamate toxicity. Exogenous NO was also toxic to neurons and reduced hemoglobin, which binds NO, markedly prevented both glutamate neurotoxicity and exogenous NO toxicity. This was the first report that NO mediates glutamate excitotoxicity, and according to Google Scholar it has been cited 2463 times as of June 2017.

This work was not without controversy, in that some laboratories were unable to replicate our findings, some of them from prominent glutamate toxicity laboratories (Dawson & Snyder, 1994; Samdani, Dawson, & Dawson, 1997). Sol fueled this controversy during his lecture entitled "Nitric Oxide: A Novel Neuronal Messenger" at the 1992 22nd Annual Society for Neuroscience Meeting in Anaheim, California, by stating that "if you do the experiment right you will observe the NO mediates glutamate excitotoxicity." This created camps of investigators that were protagonists and antagonists of the role of NO in mediating glutamate neurotoxicity. Subsequent work validated his statement and cemented the importance of NO in mediating glutamate excitotoxicity and launched our future scientific careers. It was shown, by a variety of laboratories that agents that decreased NOS catalytic activity including calcineurin inhibitors, agents that bind or antagonize calmodulin, flavoprotein inhibitors, and arginine analogue NOS inhibitors were neuroprotective in glutamate excitotoxicity paradigms (Brown & Vilalta, 2015; Dawson & Dawson, 1996, 2017; Dawson & Snyder, 1994; Mukherjee, Cinelli, Kang, & Silverman, 2014; Samdani, Dawson, et al., 1997; Yun, Dawson, & Dawson, 1996). Gene-targeting approaches confirmed that elimination of nNOS protected against glutamate excitotoxicity and the source of neurotoxic NO was from nNOS (Dawson et al., 1996).

While there is now no doubt now that NO mediates glutamate neurotoxicity; as noted earlier there were antagonists to this idea. In particular, there were reports that failed to observe a role for NO in glutamate excitotoxicity (Dawson & Dawson, 1996; Dawson & Snyder, 1994; Samdani, Dawson, et al., 1997; Yun et al., 1996). It was subsequently shown that most of the failures to see an NO component to glutamate neurotoxicity was due to lack of expression of nNOS. Glutamate neurotoxicity is dependent on the number of nNOS neurons and the level of nNOS (Dawson, Dawson, Bartley, et al., 1993; Samdani, Newcamp, et al., 1997). The culture paradigm also determines the level of nNOS expression and the susceptibility to glutamate and NO-mediated neurotoxicity. Neurons grown on glial feeder layers express low levels of nNOS, whereas neurons using MD's culture methods express high levels of nNOS, hence the fortuitous postdoctoral experience for Valina in MD's laboratory (Samdani, Dawson, et al., 1997; Samdani, Newcamp, et al., 1997). As primary neuronal culture systems have transitioned from rodent neuronal cultures to human neuronal cultures, the importance of nNOS expression in glutamate toxicity was confirmed (Xu et al., 2016). Additionally, depending on the oxidation or reduction status of NO, it has either neurodestructive or neuroprotective properties (Lipton et al., 1993).

4. nNOS CONTRIBUTES TO NEURONAL TOXICITY

Immunohistochemistry for nNOS revealed that it is expressed exclusively in neurons (Dawson, Bredt, et al., 1991; Dawson & Snyder, 1994). Only 1%–2% of all neurons in the cortex and corpus striatum express nNOS. In the hypothalamus, nNOS is localized to paraventricular magnocellular neurons and the supraoptic neurons that project to the posterior pituitary. In the hippocampus, it is expressed in the granule cells of the dentate gyrus, while the remainder of the hippocampus it is expressed in 1%–2% of neurons. In the cerebellum, nNOS is enriched in basket and granule neurons. The superior and inferior colliculi express a dense plexus of nNOS neurons within their superficial layers. nNOS is not enriched in any specific neurotransmitter system. Cerebellar glutaminergic granule and gamma-aminobutyric acid-ergic (GABAergic) basket neurons express nNOS, while in the cortex and corpus striatum, somatostatin and neuropeptide Y express nNOS. In the brainstem nNOS is expressed in choline acetyl transferase neurons that lack somatostatin and neuropeptide Y (Dawson, Bredt, et al., 1991; Dawson & Snyder, 1994). Despite lacking a specific neurotransmitter phenotype, all nNOS neurons express NADPH diaphorase (Bredt et al., 1991; Dawson, Bredt, et al., 1991; Hope, Michael, Knigge, & Vincent, 1991).

A blue formazan precipitant results from tetrazolium dyes being reduced by NAPDH diaphorase in the presence of NADPH, but not NAD^{+} + hydrogen (NADH) (Thomas & Pearse, 1961, 1964). Transient expression of nNOS in human kidney 293 cells, which do not endogenously express nNOS, led to cells that exhibited both nNOS and NADPH diaphorase staining establishing that NADPH diaphorase staining was due to nNOS (Fig. 2) (Dawson, Bredt, et al., 1991). The majority of NADPH diaphorase activity in brain homogenates is not due to nNOS (Hope et al., 1991), while in paraformaldehyde-fixed tissue nNOS immunoreactivity is identical to NADPH diaphorase staining. nNOS is resistant to inactivation by

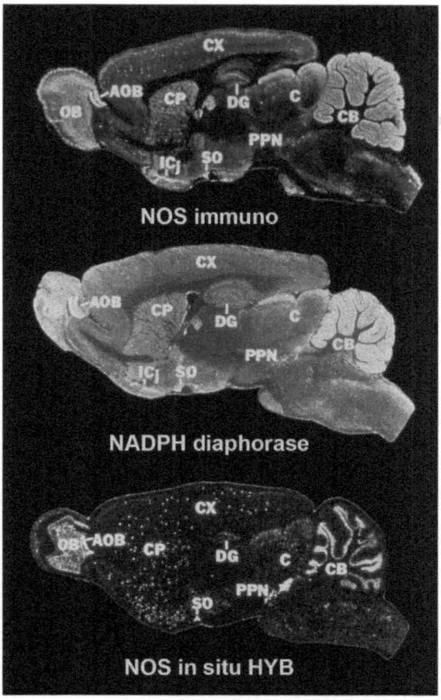

Fig. 2 Neuronal nitric oxide synthase catalytic activity accounts for NAPPH diaphorase staining. Darkfield photomicrographs of neuronal nitric oxide synthase (NOS) immunoreactivity (*top*), NADPH diaphorase staining (*middle*), and neuronal NOS messenger RNA via in situ hybridization (HYB) (*bottom*). Note the identical distribution of NADPH diaphorase and neuronal NOS. *AOB*, accessory olfactory bulb; *C*, colliculi; *CB*, cerebellum; *CP*, caudate putamen; *CX*, cortex; *DG*, dentate gyrus; *HYB*, hybridization; *IC*, islands of Callejae; *OB*, olfactory bulb; *PPN*, pedunculopontine nucleus; *SO*, supraoptic nucleus. *Reproduced from Bredt, D. S., Glatt, C. E., Hwang, P. M., Fotuhi, M., Dawson, T. M., & Snyder, S. H. (1991). Nitric oxide synthase protein and mRNA are discretely localized in neuronal populations of the mammalian CNS together with NADPH diaphorase.* Neuron, *7(4), 615–624, also see Dawson, V. L., Dawson, T. M., London, E. D., Bredt, D. S., & Snyder, S. H. (1991). Nitric oxide mediates glutamate neurotoxicity in primary cortical cultures.* Proceedings of the National Academy of Sciences of the United States of America, 88*(14), 6368–6371.*

paraformaldehyde, while all other NADPH enzymes are inactivated, which accounts for the NADPH diaphorase stain exclusively recognizing nNOS neurons (Dawson, Bredt, et al., 1991; Dawson & Snyder, 1994). NAPPH diaphorase/nNOS neurons are relatively unique. They survive toxic insults that kill most neurons including cerebral ischemia and glutamate neurotoxicity. They also survive the neurodegeneration engendered by Alzheimer's disease (AD) and Huntington's disease (HD) (Dawson, Dawson, Bartley, et al., 1993; Ferrante et al., 1985; Hyman et al., 1992; Koh & Choi,

1988; Koh, Peters, & Choi, 1986; Uemura, Kowall, & Beal, 1990). Ted's report that nNOS accounts for NAPDH diaphorase has been cited 2127 times as of June 2017 according to Google Scholar. The resistance of nNOS/NADPH diaphorase neurons to toxic insults is due to their enrichment in mitochondrial manganese superoxide dismutase (MnSOD) since knockdown of MnSOD renders nNOS/NADPH diaphorase neurons susceptible to toxic insults, while overexpression of MnSOD renders non-nNOS/NADPH diaphorase resistant to the same toxic insults (Gonzalez-Zulueta et al., 1998). Since nNOS is expressed in only 1%–2% of neurons throughout the majority of the brain, how can it be responsible for neuronal toxicity? nNOS neurons have extensive neuronal processes and probably come in contact with most if not all neurons (Fig. 3).

The studies outlined earlier that solidified the role of nNOS-derived NO mediating glutamate neurotoxicity laid the foundation for the exploration of nNOS-derived NO contributions to neurodegenerative and neurologic

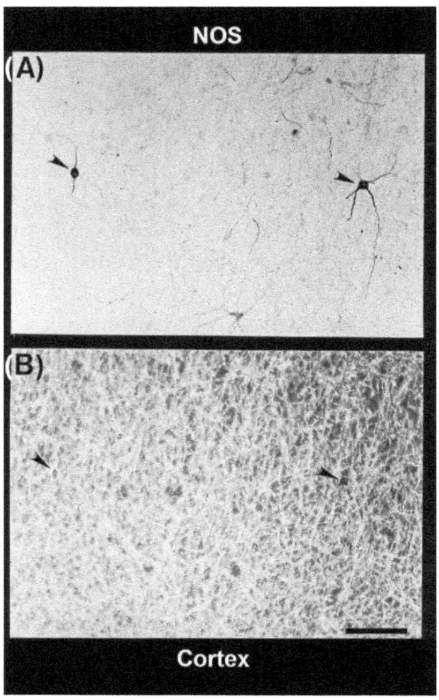

Fig. 3 Neuronal nitric oxide synthase neurons have extensive neuronal ramifications. (A) Brightfield photomicrograph illustrating the distribution of neuronal nitric oxide synthase (NOS) in the cortex. Note the sparse distribution of the neuronal NOS-positive neurons. (B) Darkfield photomicrograph showing the extensive ramifications of neuronal NOS neurons in the cortex. Although the neuronal NOS neurons only comprise 1%–2% of the neuronal population, their processes are able exert a wide influence due to their extensive ramifications. Bar = 100 μm.

disorders. In AD there are elevated levels of NO and tyrosine nitration, a marker of NO-mediated injury (Dorheim, Tracey, Pollock, & Grammas, 1994; Sultana et al., 2006). NO may be associated with hyperphosphorylation of tau (Saez, Pehar, Vargas, Barbeito, & Maccioni, 2004; Sultana et al., 2006). In PD there is marked elevation of indices of nitrosative stress including tyrosine nitration of α-synuclein (Giasson et al., 2000) and *S*-nitrosylation of parkin, an ubiquitin E3 ligase linked to PD (Chung et al., 2004). Nitration of α-synuclein causes it to aggregate and likely contributes to the toxicity of pathologic α-synuclein (Hodara et al., 2004). *S*-nitrosylation of parkin ultimately leads to its inactivation and loss of parkin's protective function, which contributes to PD (Chung et al., 2004; Yao et al., 2004). In the MPTP (1-methyl-4-phenyl-1,2,3,6-tetrahydropyridine) intoxication model of PD, selective nNOS inhibitors and knockout of nNOS reduce the loss of dopamine (DA) neurons (Kurosaki et al., 2002; Przedborski et al., 1996). Inhibitors of nNOS protect against motor neuron degeneration in the Wobbler mouse model of amyotrophic lateral sclerosis (ALS) (Ikeda, Iwasaki, & Kinoshita, 1998). The human immunodeficiency virus (HIV) coat protein, gp120 which plays a role in acquired immune deficiency syndrome (AIDS) dementia, kills neurons via NO (Dawson, Dawson, Uhl, & Snyder, 1993). NO derived from nNOS also plays a role in stroke since selective nNOS inhibitors and knockout of nNOS reduce infarct volume following middle cerebral artery occlusion (MCAO) (Dawson, 1994; Samdani, Dawson, et al., 1997; Yun et al., 1996). On the other hand, nonselective NOS inhibitors increase the severity of stroke through inhibition of endothelial NOS (eNOS) by reducing cerebral blood flow similar to what occurs in eNOS knockout mice (Huang et al., 1996; Samdani, Dawson, et al., 1997; Yun et al., 1996). Selective inhibition of nNOS reduces injury after traumatic brain injury (TBI) (Hall, Wang, & Miller, 2012; Khan et al., 2016). CNS oxygen toxicity may involve nNOS-derived NO (Oury, Ho, Piantadosi, & Crapo, 1992). The neuropathology of Huntington's disease may involve nNOS (Deckel, 2001). Since almost all neurodegenerative diseases involve glutamate excitotoxicity at one level (see below), inhibition of nNOS would be expected to have neuroprotective effects in these disorders (Dawson & Dawson, 1998).

5. INDUCIBLE NITRIC OXIDE SYNTHASE CONTRIBUTES TO NEURONAL TOXICITY

Healthy uninjured tissue does not express inducible NOS (iNOS). Under pathologic conditions iNOS is expressed in macrophages and microglia, as well as, neurons, astrocytes, and endothelial cells (Nathan & Xie, 1994; Samdani, Dawson, et al., 1997). Cytokines, LPS, and other inflammatory mediators induce iNOS in astrocytes and microglia (Murphy, 2000). Expression of iNOS causes delayed neuronal cell death (Chao, Hu, Molitor, Shaskan, & Peterson, 1992; Dawson, Brahmbhatt, Mong, & Dawson, 1994), and it can exacerbate glutamate neurotoxicity (Hewett, Csernansky, & Choi, 1994). NO from iNOS kills neurons through a variety of mechanism including mitochondrial respiration inhibition, glycolysis inhibition, and activation of both apoptosis and parthanatos (Brown & Vilalta, 2015). Following cerebral ischemia in the late stages, iNOS is expressed during inflammation leading to delayed neuronal cell death. Inhibitors of iNOS or iNOS knockouts have reduced infarct volumes after MCAO (Iadecola & Alexander, 2001; Libikova, Pogady, Wiedermann, & Breier, 1975; Sugimoto & Iadecola, 2002; Zhao, Haensel, Araki, Ross, & Iadecola, 2000). NO derived from iNOS also plays a role in PD (Dehmer, Lindenau, Haid, Dichgans, & Schulz, 2000; Liberatore et al., 1999) and multiple sclerosis (Bagasra et al., 1995; Bo et al., 1994; Santiago, Perez-Mediavilla, & Lopez-Moratalla, 1998). There is also a role for iNOS in the AIDS dementia (Adamson, Kopnisky, Dawson, & Dawson, 1999; Adamson et al., 1996; Rostasy et al., 1999), and it may participate in the pathogenesis of ALS (Almer, Vukosavic, Romero, & Przedborski, 1999; Chen, Northington, & Martin, 2010; Martin, 2007). Microglial and astrocyte activation contributes to most if not all neurodegenerative diseases as well as stroke, TBI, and infections of the nervous system (Ghasemi & Fatemi, 2014). There is also a potential role for iNOS in neurodevelopmental disorders (Ghasemi & Fatemi, 2014).

6. INHIBITORS OF NITRIC OXIDE SYNTHASE

Given the role of nNOS and iNOS in neurologic and neurodegenerative disorders, there is a strong rationale for developing selective nNOS and iNOS inhibitors that would avoid the deleterious effects on cerebral perfusion through inhibiting eNOS. As with all drug development this is an iterative process in which selective and safe inhibitors of nNOS and iNOS are still under development (Mukherjee et al., 2014; Tinker & Wallace, 2006). Since the crystal structures of all three isoforms of NOS have been solved, it is hoped that rationale drug design will progress and lead to the identification of excellent and safe nNOS and iNOS inhibitors (Mukherjee et al., 2014).

7. MECHANISM OF NITRIC OXIDE NEURONAL TOXICITY

Part of our scientific direction as we transitioned from Sol's laboratory and we developed our independent scientific careers was, in part, understanding the mechanisms by which NO kills neurons. Since glutamate excitotoxicity was thought to play an important role in variety of disorders including ischemia/stroke, seizures, PD, AD, ALS, HD, hepatic encephalopathy, multiple sclerosis, TBI, and metabolic disorders of the brain (Arundine & Tymianski, 2004; Kostic, Zivkovic, & Stojanovic, 2013; Lai, Zhang, & Wang, 2013; Mattson, 2003; Mehta, Prabhakar, Kumar, Deshmukh, & Sharma, 2013; Meldrum, 1990, 1992; Sepers & Raymond, 2014), understanding the molecular mechanisms by which glutamate excitotoxicity kills neurons seemed like a fruitful venture that was worth pursuing, particularly in light of our discovery that a major component of glutamate excitotoxicity was mediated by NO.

Glutamate acts by binding to four postsynaptic receptors including NMDA, α-amino-3-hydroxy-5-methyl-4-isoxazoleproprionate (AMPA), kainate, and metabotropic receptors (Nakanishi, 1992). Neuronal damage in glutamate excitotoxicity and following focal ischemia is mediated in large part through NMDA receptor activation (Arundine & Tymianski, 2004; Lai et al., 2013; Meldrum & Garthwaite, 1990). In stroke, postsynaptic density-95 (PSD-95) inhibitors, which uncouple the NMDA receptor from its signaling cascade, support a role for glutamate excitotoxicity. PSD-95 inhibitors unequivocally show protection in rodent brain (Aarts & Tymianski, 2003; Sattler et al., 1999; Soriano et al., 2008; Sun et al., 2008), high-order brains of old-world primates (Cook, Teves, & Tymianski, 2012a, 2012b) and in humans (Hill et al., 2012).

Our group has focused our research program on excitotoxicity that is mediated and initiated by glutamate activation of NMDA receptors, intracellular calcium flux, NO, and free radicals (Fig. 4) (Dawson, Bredt, et al., 1991; Dawson, Dawson, Bartley, et al., 1993; Dawson & Dawson, 2017). Over 20 years ago Choi and colleagues showed that a 5-min bath application NMDA (500 μM) elicits cell death in cortical cultures 24 h later. Irreversible processes are set in motion by the 5-min exposure to NMDA, which sets in motion irreversible processes. This type of toxicity has been called "delayed or rapidly triggered neurotoxicity" (Choi & Rothman, 1990). Calcium entry via NMDA receptors is critical to this form of toxicity and is linked to the coupling of NMDA receptor activation of nNOS and NO formation.

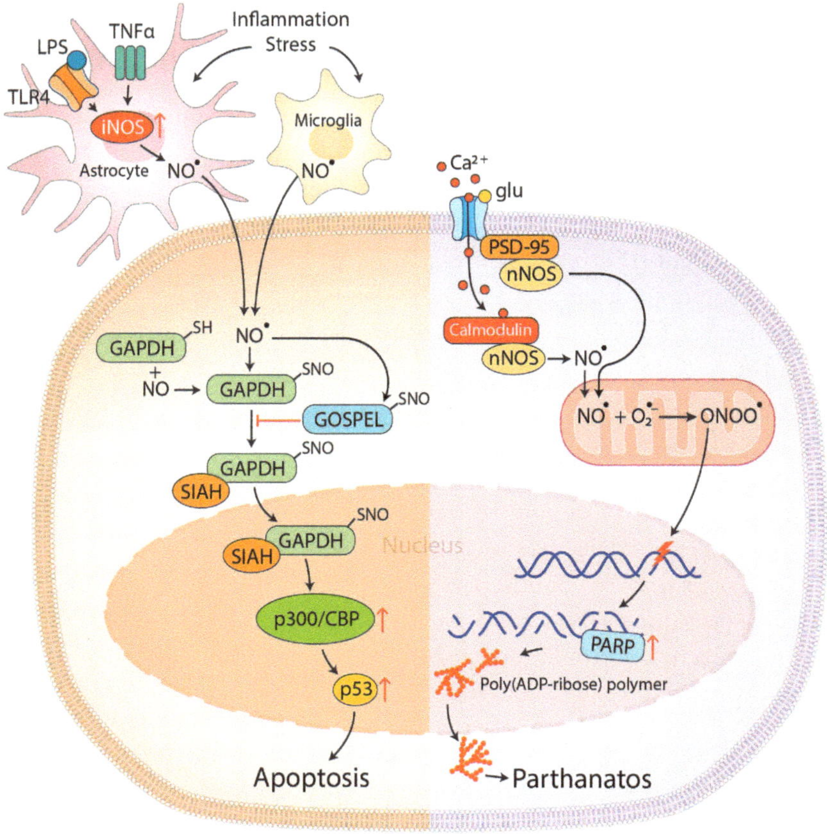

Fig. 4 Nitric oxide (NO) can kill neurons via both apoptosis and parthanatos. High levels of NO is generated from astrocytes and/or microglia that are activated by inflammation, stress, tumor necrosis factor α (TNFα), or lipopolysaccharide (LPS) binding to toll-like receptor 4 (TLR4) through turning on the expression of inducible nitric oxide synthase (iNOS). NO diffuses into neurons to *S*-nitrosylate GAPDH (GAPDH-SNO) which then binds SIAH. The GAPDH-SNO-SIAH protein complex translocate to the nucleus where it activates p300/CPB which increases the levels of p53 setting in motion p53-dependent apoptotic cell death. NO can also *S*-nitrosylate GOSPEL (GOSPEL-SNO) which inhibits the *S*-nitrosylation of GAPDH. Glutamate (glu) (*yellow circle*) activates NMDA receptors resulting in the influx of Ca^{2+} (*red circles*), which binds calmodulin and activates neuronal NO synthase (nNOS), to convert L-arginine to NO. PSD-95 protein tethers nNOS to the NMDA receptor. Excess NO can be neurotoxic, even though NO is an essential molecule in neuronal signal transduction. NO neurotoxicity is mediated by peroxynitrite $ONOO^-$, a reaction product from NO and superoxide anion ($O_2^{\cdot -}$). Peroxynitrite damages DNA, which results in over activation of PARP (PARP ↑) leading to generation of poly (ADP-ribose) polymer leading to parthanatos.

Treatment with NOS inhibitors, or disruption of the interaction between the NMDA receptor and nNOS or gene deletion of nNOS prevents cell death in cell culture, slice models, and in vivo models of stroke (Aarts & Tymianski, 2003; Cazevieille, Muller, Meynier, & Bonne, 1993; Dawson, Bredt, et al., 1991; Dawson, Dawson, Bartley, et al., 1993; Dawson & Dawson, 2017; Huang et al., 1994; Kollegger, McBean, & Tipton, 1993; Lustig, von Brauchitsch, Chan, & Greenberg, 1992; Moncada, Lekieffre, Arvin, & Meldrum, 1992).

NO itself is not directly toxic. NO is protective, in part, through inhibition of caspases or the NMDA receptor via *S*-nitrosylation (Brown, 2010). Instead it combines with the superoxide anion to form peroxynitrite ($ONOO^-$), which mediates most of the toxic actions of NO (Xia, Dawson, Dawson, Snyder, & Zweier, 1996). We and others have put forth the hypothesis that peroxynitrite modification of DNA and the subsequent DNA nicks trigger the next step in the excitotoxic death program by activating poly (ADP-ribose) polymerase-1 (PARP-1), a DNA damage-sensing enzyme, (de Murcia & Menissier de Murcia, 1994; de Murcia et al., 1994; Szabo & Dawson, 1998). In collaboration with Sol's lab we showed that inhibition of PARP-1 and knockout of PARP-1 profoundly protected against glutamate excitotoxicity and stroke (Eliasson et al., 1997; Zhang, Dawson, Dawson, & Snyder, 1994). Additional experimental and clinical studies supported the idea that overactivity of PARP-1 plays a prominent role in neuronal injury in stroke (Moroni, 2008; Pacher & Szabo, 2008). PARP-1 activation is also important in cell death following TBI, ischemia–reperfusion injury of the spleen, heart, skeletal muscle, and retina. It also plays a major role in arthritis, PD, β-islet cytotoxicity/diabetes mellitus, endotoxic shock, experimental allergic encephalomyelitis (EAE)/model of multiple sclerosis, liver damage, and multiple system organ failure (Virag & Szabo, 2002; Yu, Wang, Dawson, & Dawson, 2003). We recently showed that there is an alternative mechanism of PARP activation that does not require DNA damage, and it involves the direct activation of PARP by aminoacyl tRNA synthetase complex interacting multifunctional protein (AIMP2) (Dawson & Dawson, 2017; Lee et al., 2013). AIMP2 seems to play a particularly important role in PD (Lee et al., 2013).

Originally it was thought that the reduction of NAD^+ from PARP-1 activation and the ensuing energy collapse was cause of cell death to PARP-1 overactivation (Alano et al., 2010; Ha & Snyder, 1999). The bioenergetics collapse is actually due to free poly (ADP-ribose) (PAR) polymer, a cell death signal, which binds and inhibits hexokinase (HK) leading to inhibition of glycolysis followed by depletion of NAD^+ and ATP (Andrabi et al., 2014; Dawson & Dawson, 2017; Fouquerel et al., 2014). In addition to PAR polymer-binding HK, it also binds to apoptosis-inducing factor (AIF) causing its release from the mitochondria and translocation to the nucleus (Andrabi et al., 2006; Wang et al., 2011; Yu et al., 2006). AIF is required for PARP-1-dependent cell death (Dawson & Dawson, 2017; Fatokun, Liu, Dawson, & Dawson, 2013; Wang et al., 2011; Yu et al., 2002). PARP-1-dependent cell death is unique, in that morphologically the nuclei condense and shrink and cells take up propidium iodide. Broad spectrum caspase inhibitors are ineffective in PARP-1-dependent cell death. To classify this unique form of cell death, we coined the term parthanatos from *Thanatos*, the personification of death in Greek mythology (Dawson & Dawson, 2017; Fatokun et al., 2013) (Fig. 5). Parthanatos is characterized by rapid PARP-1 activation, PAR translocation from the nucleus to the mitochondria where it binds HK leading to the loss of cellular NAD^+ and ATP and mitochondrial depolarization as well as binding to AIF, which translocate to the nuclease initiating large-scale DNA fragmentation, the final step in the execution of parthanatos (Dawson & Dawson, 2017; Fatokun et al., 2013). Macrophage migration inhibitor factor (MIF) is the long-sought PARP-1-dependent AIF-associated nuclease (PAAN), which is required for cell death due to PARP-1 activation (Wang et al., 2016).

PAR glycohydrolase (PARG) and ADP-ribosyl-acceptor hydrolase 3 (ARH3) protect cells from parthanatos by degrading PAR and preventing the initiation of parthanatos (Dawson & Dawson, 2017; Feng et al., 2012; Koh et al., 2004; Mashimo, Kato, & Moss, 2013). In the course of investigating parthanatos, we discovered Iduna, a neuroprotective gene that is induced by preconditioning (Andrabi et al., 2011). Iduna is a first in class, PAR-dependent ubiquitin E3 ligase that is activated by binding PAR (DaRosa et al., 2015; Kang et al., 2011; Zhang et al., 2011). Iduna protects against parthanatos and DNA damage through its PAR-dependent E3 ligase activity (Kang et al., 2011).

Although potent and selective PARP inhibitors have been approved as synergizing agents in the treatment of refractory cancers and others are being evaluated (Berger et al., 2017; Hilton, Hadfield, Tran, & Shapiro, 2013), PARP inhibitors have not been advanced to clinical trials for neurologic disorders for a variety of reasons including poor brain penetrance. Due to the profound protection afforded by PARP inhibition in animal models of neuronal injury, there is a strong rational to consider

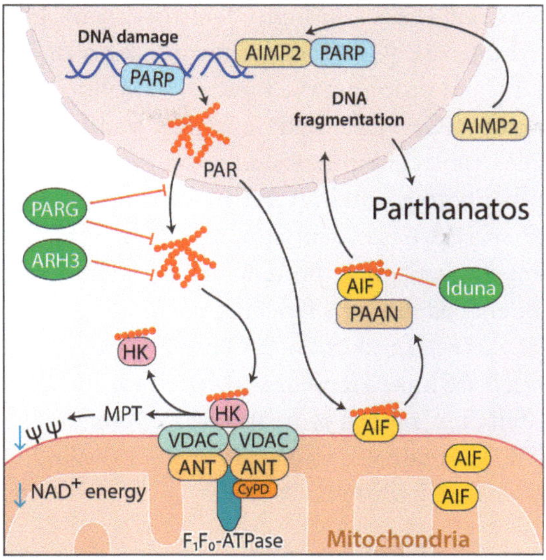

Fig. 5 Parthanatos. In parthanatos, a caspase-independent cell death program, apoptosis inducing factor (AIF) acts as the mitochondrial factor to mediate cell death. DNA damage or aminoacyl tRNA synthetase complex interacting multifunctional protein (AIMP2) activates poly (ADP-ribose) (PAR) polymerase 1 (PARP-1). PAR generated by activation of PARP-1 translocates from the nucleus to the mitochondria, where it binds AIF, inducing AIF release from the mitochondria. AIF then binds the parthanatos AIF-associated nuclease (PAAN) where they translocate to the nucleus and PAAN shreds genomic DNA acting as the final executioner in parthanatos. PAR polymer also binds and inactivates hexokinase (HK), which accounts for the energy depletion due to activation of PARP-1. PAR glycohydrolase (PARG) or ADP-ribosyl-acceptor hydrolase 3 (ARH3) degrades PAR polymer preventing parthanatos. Iduna, a PAR-dependent ubiquitin E3 ligase, is an inhibitor of parthanatos. Ψ, mitochondrial membrane potential; *ANT*, adenine nucleotide translocase; *CyPD*, cyclophilin D; *F_1F_0-ATPase*, ATP synthase; *MPT*, mitochondrial membrane permeability transition; *VDAC*, voltage-dependent anion channel. *Figure adapted from Dawson, T. M., & Dawson, V. L. (2017). Mitochondrial mechanisms of neuronal cell death: Potential therapeutics.* Annual Review of Pharmacology and Toxicology, 57, *437–454. doi:10.1146/annurev-pharmtox-010716-105001.*

repurposing these PARP inhibitors for neurologic disorders (Berger et al., 2017). In addition, development of PAAN inhibitors (Dawson & Dawson, 2017; Wang et al., 2016) is an attractive target since PAAN inhibitors would not be expected to interfere with DNA repair like PARP inhibitors. In addition, directly interfering with PAR polymer signaling offers an additional therapeutic avenue that does not involve PARP inhibition (Dawson & Dawson, 2017).

NO can also kill cells through *S*-nitrosylating glyceraldehyde-3-phosphate dehydrogenase (GAPDH). *S*-nitrosylation of GAPDH inhibits its catalytic activity and promotes the binding to Seven in Absentia Homolog 1 (Siah1), and the GAPDH-Siah1 complex transfers to nucleus where through a complex molecular process increases the activity of P300/cAMP response element-binding protein (CREB)-binding protein (CBP) leading to the activation of P53-dependent apoptosis (Sen et al., 2008). GOSPEL (GAPDH's competitor of Siah protein enhances life) is an inhibitor of GAPDH-dependent cell death by blocking the binding of GAPDH to Siah1 (Fig. 4) (Sen et al., 2009). In addition, NO can *S*-nitrosylate a variety of proteins some of which are linked to neuronal cell death and neurodegeneration such as parkin, dynamin-related protein (Drp1), X-linked inhibitor of apoptosis (XIAP), mitochondrial complex I, protein-disulfide isomerase, and mitochondrial complex I (Brown, 2010).

8. CONCLUSION

From our initial discovery that NO mediates glutamate neurotoxicity (Dawson, Dawson, et al., 1991) to elucidating the mechanism by which NO kills neurons through parthanatos (Dawson & Dawson, 2017), has been an exciting and fruitful scientific venture. All of it started with Sol. Although Valina was not directly in Sol lab, he adopted her as scientific mentee, where both of us learned how to ask and investigate important scientific questions. This work has led to many potential molecular targets to inhibit neurodegeneration. Prominent among them are PARP inhibitors (Berger et al., 2017), which hopefully will be repurposed for neurologic indications. Development of inhibitors of PAAN is also very promising and exploring the role of PAAN in neurologic diseases is the next exciting frontier.

CONFLICT OF INTEREST

T.M.D. and V.L.D. are founders of Valted, LLC and hold an ownership equity interest in the company. This arrangement has been reviewed and approved by the Johns Hopkins University in accordance with its conflict of interest policies.

ACKNOWLEDGMENTS

This work was supported by US National Institutes of Health Grants NS38377, NS67525, and DA00266 and by the JPB Foundation. The authors acknowledge the joint participation by the Adrienne Helis Malvin Medical Research Foundation and the Diana Helis Henry Medical Research Foundation through its direct engagement in the continuous active conduct of medical research in conjunction with the Johns Hopkins Hospital and the

Johns Hopkins University School of Medicine and the Foundation's Parkinson's Disease Programs M-1, M-2, M-2013, M-2014, M-2015, M-2016, and H-2014. The authors thank I-Hsun Wu for assistance with the illustrations. T.M.D. is the Leonard and Madlyn Abramson Professor in Neurodegenerative Diseases.

REFERENCES

Aarts, M. M., & Tymianski, M. (2003). Novel treatment of excitotoxicity: Targeted disruption of intracellular signalling from glutamate receptors. *Biochemical Pharmacology*, *66*(6), 877–886.

Adamson, D. C., Kopnisky, K. L., Dawson, T. M., & Dawson, V. L. (1999). Mechanisms and structural determinants of HIV-1 coat protein, gp41-induced neurotoxicity. *The Journal of Neuroscience*, *19*(1), 64–71.

Adamson, D. C., Wildemann, B., Sasaki, M., Glass, J. D., McArthur, J. C., Christov, V. I., et al. (1996). Immunologic NO synthase: Elevation in severe AIDS dementia and induction by HIV-1 gp41. *Science*, *274*(5294), 1917–1921.

Alano, C. C., Garnier, P., Ying, W., Higashi, Y., Kauppinen, T. M., & Swanson, R. A. (2010). NAD+ depletion is necessary and sufficient for poly(ADP-ribose) polymerase-1-mediated neuronal death. *The Journal of Neuroscience*, *30*(8), 2967–2978. https://doi.org/10.1523/JNEUROSCI.5552-09.2010.

Almer, G., Vukosavic, S., Romero, N., & Przedborski, S. (1999). Inducible nitric oxide synthase up-regulation in a transgenic mouse model of familial amyotrophic lateral sclerosis. *Journal of Neurochemistry*, *72*(6), 2415–2425.

Andrabi, S. A., Kang, H. C., Haince, J. F., Lee, Y. I., Zhang, J., Chi, Z., et al. (2011). Iduna protects the brain from glutamate excitotoxicity and stroke by interfering with poly (ADP-ribose) polymer-induced cell death. *Nature Medicine*, *17*(6), 692–699. https://doi.org/10.1038/nm.2387.

Andrabi, S. A., Kim, N. S., Yu, S. W., Wang, H., Koh, D. W., Sasaki, M., et al. (2006). Poly (ADP-ribose) (PAR) polymer is a death signal. *Proceedings of the National Academy of Sciences of the United States of America*, *103*(48), 18308–18313. https://doi.org/10.1073/pnas.0606526103.

Andrabi, S. A., Umanah, G. K., Chang, C., Stevens, D. A., Karuppagounder, S. S., Gagne, J. P., et al. (2014). Poly(ADP-ribose) polymerase-dependent energy depletion occurs through inhibition of glycolysis. *Proceedings of the National Academy of Sciences of the United States of America*, *111*(28), 10209–10214. https://doi.org/10.1073/pnas.1405158111.

Arriza, J. L., Dawson, T. M., Simerly, R. B., Martin, L. J., Caron, M. G., Snyder, S. H., et al. (1992). The G-protein-coupled receptor kinases beta ARK1 and beta ARK2 are widely distributed at synapses in rat brain. *The Journal of Neuroscience*, *12*(10), 4045–4055.

Arundine, M., & Tymianski, M. (2004). Molecular mechanisms of glutamate-dependent neurodegeneration in ischemia and traumatic brain injury. *Cellular and Molecular Life Sciences*, *61*(6), 657–668. https://doi.org/10.1007/s00018-003-3319-x.

Attramadal, H., Arriza, J. L., Aoki, C., Dawson, T. M., Codina, J., Kwatra, M. M., et al. (1992). Beta-arrestin2, a novel member of the arrestin/beta-arrestin gene family. *The Journal of Biological Chemistry*, *267*(25), 17882–17890.

Bagasra, O., Michaels, F. H., Zheng, Y. M., Bobroski, L. E., Spitsin, S. V., Fu, Z. F., et al. (1995). Activation of the inducible form of nitric oxide synthase in the brains of patients with multiple sclerosis. *Proceedings of the National Academy of Sciences of the United States of America*, *92*(26), 12041–12045.

Berger, N. A., Besson, V. C., Boulares, A. H., Burkle, A., Chiarugi, A., Clark, R. S., et al. (2017). Opportunities for the repurposing of PARP inhibitors for the therapy of non-oncological diseases. *British Journal of Pharmacology*. https://doi.org/10.1111/bph.13748 (Epub ahead of print).

Bo, L., Dawson, T. M., Wesselingh, S., Mork, S., Choi, S., Kong, P. A., et al. (1994). Induction of nitric oxide synthase in demyelinating regions of multiple sclerosis brains. *Annals of Neurology, 36*(5), 778–786. https://doi.org/10.1002/ana.410360515.

Bredt, D. S., Glatt, C. E., Hwang, P. M., Fotuhi, M., Dawson, T. M., & Snyder, S. H. (1991). Nitric oxide synthase protein and mRNA are discretely localized in neuronal populations of the mammalian CNS together with NADPH diaphorase. *Neuron, 7*(4), 615–624.

Bredt, D. S., & Snyder, S. H. (1989). Nitric oxide mediates glutamate-linked enhancement of cGMP levels in the cerebellum. *Proceedings of the National Academy of Sciences of the United States of America, 86*(22), 9030–9033.

Bredt, D. S., & Snyder, S. H. (1990). Isolation of nitric oxide synthetase, a calmodulin-requiring enzyme. *Proceedings of the National Academy of Sciences of the United States of America, 87*(2), 682–685.

Brown, G. C. (2010). Nitric oxide and neuronal death. *Nitric Oxide, 23*(3), 153–165. https://doi.org/10.1016/j.niox.2010.06.001.

Brown, G. C., & Vilalta, A. (2015). How microglia kill neurons. *Brain Research, 1628*(Pt. B), 288–297. https://doi.org/10.1016/j.brainres.2015.08.031.

Cazevieille, C., Muller, A., Meynier, F., & Bonne, C. (1993). Superoxide and nitric oxide cooperation in hypoxia/reoxygenation-induced neuron injury. *Free Radical Biology & Medicine, 14*(4), 389–395.

Chao, C. C., Hu, S., Molitor, T. W., Shaskan, E. G., & Peterson, P. K. (1992). Activated microglia mediate neuronal cell injury via a nitric oxide mechanism. *Journal of Immunology, 149*(8), 2736–2741.

Chen, K., Northington, F. J., & Martin, L. J. (2010). Inducible nitric oxide synthase is present in motor neuron mitochondria and Schwann cells and contributes to disease mechanisms in ALS mice. *Brain Structure & Function, 214*(2–3), 219–234. https://doi.org/10.1007/s00429-009-0226-4.

Choi, D. W., & Rothman, S. M. (1990). The role of glutamate neurotoxicity in hypoxic-ischemic neuronal death. *Annual Review of Neuroscience, 13*, 171–182. https://doi.org/10.1146/annurev.ne.13.030190.001131.

Chung, K. K., Thomas, B., Li, X., Pletnikova, O., Troncoso, J. C., Marsh, L., et al. (2004). S-nitrosylation of parkin regulates ubiquitination and compromises parkin's protective function. *Science, 304*(5675), 1328–1331. https://doi.org/10.1126/science.1093891.

Cook, D. J., Teves, L., & Tymianski, M. (2012a). A translational paradigm for the preclinical evaluation of the stroke neuroprotectant Tat-NR2B9c in gyrencephalic nonhuman primates. *Science Translational Medicine, 4*(154), 154ra133. https://doi.org/10.1126/scitranslmed.3003824.

Cook, D. J., Teves, L., & Tymianski, M. (2012b). Treatment of stroke with a PSD-95 inhibitor in the gyrencephalic primate brain. *Nature, 483*(7388), 213–217. https://doi.org/10.1038/nature10841.

DaRosa, P. A., Wang, Z., Jiang, X., Pruneda, J. N., Cong, F., Klevit, R. E., et al. (2015). Allosteric activation of the RNF146 ubiquitin ligase by a poly(ADP-ribosyl)ation signal. *Nature, 517*(7533), 223–226. https://doi.org/10.1038/nature13826.

Dawson, D. A. (1994). Nitric oxide and focal cerebral ischemia: Multiplicity of actions and diverse outcome. *Cerebrovascular and Brain Metabolism Reviews, 6*(4), 299–324.

Dawson, V. L., Brahmbhatt, H. P., Mong, J. A., & Dawson, T. M. (1994). Expression of inducible nitric oxide synthase causes delayed neurotoxicity in primary mixed neuronal-glial cortical cultures. *Neuropharmacology, 33*(11), 1425–1430.

Dawson, T. M., Bredt, D. S., Fotuhi, M., Hwang, P. M., & Snyder, S. H. (1991). Nitric oxide synthase and neuronal NADPH diaphorase are identical in brain and peripheral tissues. *Proceedings of the National Academy of Sciences of the United States of America, 88*(17), 7797–7801.

Dawson, V. L., & Dawson, T. M. (1996). Free radicals and neuronal cell death. *Cell Death and Differentiation, 3*(1), 71–78.
Dawson, V. L., & Dawson, T. M. (1998). Nitric oxide in neurodegeneration. *Progress in Brain Research, 118*, 215–229.
Dawson, T. M., & Dawson, V. L. (2017). Mitochondrial mechanisms of neuronal cell death: Potential therapeutics. *Annual Review of Pharmacology and Toxicology, 57*, 437–454. https://doi.org/10.1146/annurev-pharmtox-010716-105001.
Dawson, V. L., Dawson, T. M., Bartley, D. A., Uhl, G. R., & Snyder, S. H. (1993). Mechanisms of nitric oxide-mediated neurotoxicity in primary brain cultures. *The Journal of Neuroscience, 13*(6), 2651–2661.
Dawson, V. L., Dawson, T. M., Filloux, F. M., & Wamsley, J. K. (1988). Evidence for dopamine D-2 receptors on cholinergic interneurons in the rat caudate-putamen. *Life Sciences, 42*(20), 1933–1939.
Dawson, V. L., Dawson, T. M., London, E. D., Bredt, D. S., & Snyder, S. H. (1991). Nitric oxide mediates glutamate neurotoxicity in primary cortical cultures. *Proceedings of the National Academy of Sciences of the United States of America, 88*(14), 6368–6371.
Dawson, V. L., Dawson, T. M., Uhl, G. R., & Snyder, S. H. (1993). Human immunodeficiency virus type 1 coat protein neurotoxicity mediated by nitric oxide in primary cortical cultures. *Proceedings of the National Academy of Sciences of the United States of America, 90*(8), 3256–3259.
Dawson, V. L., Dawson, T. M., & Wamsley, J. K. (1990). Muscarinic and dopaminergic receptor subtypes on striatal cholinergic interneurons. *Brain Research Bulletin, 25*(6), 903–912.
Dawson, T. M., Gehlert, D. R., McCabe, R. T., Barnett, A., & Wamsley, J. K. (1986). D-1 dopamine receptors in the rat brain: A quantitative autoradiographic analysis. *The Journal of Neuroscience, 6*(8), 2352–2365.
Dawson, V. L., Kizushi, V. M., Huang, P. L., Snyder, S. H., & Dawson, T. M. (1996). Resistance to neurotoxicity in cortical cultures from neuronal nitric oxide synthase-deficient mice. *The Journal of Neuroscience, 16*(8), 2479–2487.
Dawson, T. M., & Snyder, S. H. (1994). Gases as biological messengers: Nitric oxide and carbon monoxide in the brain. *The Journal of Neuroscience, 14*(9), 5147–5159.
de Murcia, G., & Menissier de Murcia, J. (1994). Poly(ADP-ribose) polymerase: A molecular nick-sensor. *Trends in Biochemical Sciences, 19*(4), 172–176.
de Murcia, G., Schreiber, V., Molinete, M., Saulier, B., Poch, O., Masson, M., et al. (1994). Structure and function of poly(ADP-ribose) polymerase. *Molecular and Cellular Biochemistry, 138*(1–2), 15–24.
Deckel, A. W. (2001). Nitric oxide and nitric oxide synthase in Huntington's disease. *Journal of Neuroscience Research, 64*(2), 99–107. https://doi.org/10.1002/jnr.1057.
Dehmer, T., Lindenau, J., Haid, S., Dichgans, J., & Schulz, J. B. (2000). Deficiency of inducible nitric oxide synthase protects against MPTP toxicity in vivo. *Journal of Neurochemistry, 74*(5), 2213–2216.
Dichter, M. A. (1978). Rat cortical neurons in cell culture: Culture methods, cell morphology, electrophysiology, and synapse formation. *Brain Research, 149*(2), 279–293.
Dorheim, M. A., Tracey, W. R., Pollock, J. S., & Grammas, P. (1994). Nitric oxide synthase activity is elevated in brain microvessels in Alzheimer's disease. *Biochemical and Biophysical Research Communications, 205*(1), 659–665. https://doi.org/10.1006/bbrc.1994.2716.
Eliasson, M. J., Sampei, K., Mandir, A. S., Hurn, P. D., Traystman, R. J., Bao, J., et al. (1997). Poly(ADP-ribose) polymerase gene disruption renders mice resistant to cerebral ischemia. *Nature Medicine, 3*(10), 1089–1095.
Fatokun, A. A., Liu, J. O., Dawson, V. L., & Dawson, T. M. (2013). Identification through high-throughput screening of 4′-methoxyflavone and 3′,4′-dimethoxyflavone as novel

neuroprotective inhibitors of parthanatos. *British Journal of Pharmacology, 169*(6), 1263–1278. https://doi.org/10.1111/bph.12201.

Feng, X., Zhou, Y., Proctor, A. M., Hopkins, M. M., Liu, M., & Koh, D. W. (2012). Silencing of apoptosis-inducing factor and poly(ADP-ribose) glycohydrolase reveals novel roles in breast cancer cell death after chemotherapy. *Molecular Cancer, 11*, 48. https://doi.org/10.1186/1476-4598-11-48.

Ferrante, R. J., Kowall, N. W., Beal, M. F., Richardson, E. P., Jr., Bird, E. D., & Martin, J. B. (1985). Selective sparing of a class of striatal neurons in Huntington's disease. *Science, 230*(4725), 561–563.

Fotuhi, M., Sharp, A. H., Glatt, C. E., Hwang, P. M., von Krosigk, M., Snyder, S. H., et al. (1993). Differential localization of phosphoinositide-linked metabotropic glutamate receptor (mGluR1) and the inositol 1,4,5-trisphosphate receptor in rat brain. *The Journal of Neuroscience, 13*(5), 2001–2012.

Fouquerel, E., Goellner, E. M., Yu, Z., Gagne, J. P., Barbi de Moura, M., Feinstein, T., et al. (2014). ARTD1/PARP1 negatively regulates glycolysis by inhibiting hexokinase 1 independent of NAD+ depletion. *Cell Reports, 8*(6), 1819–1831. https://doi.org/10.1016/j.celrep.2014.08.036.

Garthwaite, J., Charles, S. L., & Chess-Williams, R. (1988). Endothelium-derived relaxing factor release on activation of NMDA receptors suggests role as intercellular messenger in the brain. *Nature, 336*(6197), 385–388. https://doi.org/10.1038/336385a0.

Ghasemi, M., & Fatemi, A. (2014). Pathologic role of glial nitric oxide in adult and pediatric neuroinflammatory diseases. *Neuroscience and Biobehavioral Reviews, 45*, 168–182. https://doi.org/10.1016/j.neubiorev.2014.06.002.

Giasson, B. I., Duda, J. E., Murray, I. V., Chen, Q., Souza, J. M., Hurtig, H. I., et al. (2000). Oxidative damage linked to neurodegeneration by selective alpha-synuclein nitration in synucleinopathy lesions. *Science, 290*(5493), 985–989.

Gonzalez-Zulueta, M., Ensz, L. M., Mukhina, G., Lebovitz, R. M., Zwacka, R. M., Engelhardt, J. F., et al. (1998). Manganese superoxide dismutase protects nNOS neurons from NMDA and nitric oxide-mediated neurotoxicity. *The Journal of Neuroscience, 18*(6), 2040–2055.

Ha, H. C., & Snyder, S. H. (1999). Poly(ADP-ribose) polymerase is a mediator of necrotic cell death by ATP depletion. *Proceedings of the National Academy of Sciences of the United States of America, 96*(24), 13978–13982.

Hall, E. D., Wang, J. A., & Miller, D. M. (2012). Relationship of nitric oxide synthase induction to peroxynitrite-mediated oxidative damage during the first week after experimental traumatic brain injury. *Experimental Neurology, 238*(2), 176–182. https://doi.org/10.1016/j.expneurol.2012.08.024.

Hewett, S. J., Csernansky, C. A., & Choi, D. W. (1994). Selective potentiation of NMDA-induced neuronal injury following induction of astrocytic iNOS. *Neuron, 13*(2), 487–494.

Hibbs, J. B., Jr., Taintor, R. R., & Vavrin, Z. (1987). Macrophage cytotoxicity: Role for L-arginine deiminase and imino nitrogen oxidation to nitrite. *Science, 235*(4787), 473–476.

Hibbs, J. B., Jr., Taintor, R. R., Vavrin, Z., & Rachlin, E. M. (1988). Nitric oxide: A cytotoxic activated macrophage effector molecule. *Biochemical and Biophysical Research Communications, 157*(1), 87–94.

Hill, M. D., Martin, R. H., Mikulis, D., Wong, J. H., Silver, F. L., Terbrugge, K. G., et al. (2012). Safety and efficacy of NA-1 in patients with iatrogenic stroke after endovascular aneurysm repair (ENACT): A phase 2, randomised, double-blind, placebo-controlled trial. *Lancet Neurology, 11*(11), 942–950. https://doi.org/10.1016/S1474-4422(12)70225-9.

Hilton, J. F., Hadfield, M. J., Tran, M. T., & Shapiro, G. I. (2013). Poly(ADP-ribose) polymerase inhibitors as cancer therapy. *Frontiers in Bioscience, 18*, 1392–1406.

Hodara, R., Norris, E. H., Giasson, B. I., Mishizen-Eberz, A. J., Lynch, D. R., Lee, V. M., et al. (2004). Functional consequences of alpha-synuclein tyrosine nitration: Diminished binding to lipid vesicles and increased fibril formation. *The Journal of Biological Chemistry, 279*(46), 47746–47753. https://doi.org/10.1074/jbc.M408906200.

Hope, B. T., Michael, G. J., Knigge, K. M., & Vincent, S. R. (1991). Neuronal NADPH diaphorase is a nitric oxide synthase. *Proceedings of the National Academy of Sciences of the United States of America, 88*(7), 2811–2814.

Huang, Z., Huang, P. L., Ma, J., Meng, W., Ayata, C., Fishman, M. C., et al. (1996). Enlarged infarcts in endothelial nitric oxide synthase knockout mice are attenuated by nitro-L-arginine. *Journal of Cerebral Blood Flow and Metabolism, 16*(5), 981–987. https://doi.org/10.1097/00004647-199609000-00023.

Huang, Z., Huang, P. L., Panahian, N., Dalkara, T., Fishman, M. C., & Moskowitz, M. A. (1994). Effects of cerebral ischemia in mice deficient in neuronal nitric oxide synthase. *Science, 265*(5180), 1883–1885.

Hyman, B. T., Marzloff, K., Wenniger, J. J., Dawson, T. M., Bredt, D. S., & Snyder, S. H. (1992). Relative sparing of nitric oxide synthase-containing neurons in the hippocampal formation in Alzheimer's disease. *Annals of Neurology, 32*(6), 818–820. https://doi.org/10.1002/ana.410320618.

Iadecola, C., & Alexander, M. (2001). Cerebral ischemia and inflammation. *Current Opinion in Neurology, 14*(1), 89–94.

Ikeda, K., Iwasaki, Y., & Kinoshita, M. (1998). Neuronal nitric oxide synthase inhibitor, 7-nitroindazole, delays motor dysfunction and spinal motoneuron degeneration in the wobbler mouse. *Journal of the Neurological Sciences, 160*(1), 9–15.

Kang, H. C., Lee, Y. I., Shin, J. H., Andrabi, S. A., Chi, Z., Gagne, J. P., et al. (2011). Iduna is a poly(ADP-ribose) (PAR)-dependent E3 ubiquitin ligase that regulates DNA damage. *Proceedings of the National Academy of Sciences of the United States of America, 108*(34), 14103–14108. https://doi.org/10.1073/pnas.1108799108.

Khan, M., Dhammu, T. S., Matsuda, F., Annamalai, B., Dhindsa, T. S., Singh, I., et al. (2016). Targeting the nNOS/peroxynitrite/calpain system to confer neuroprotection and aid functional recovery in a mouse model of TBI. *Brain Research, 1630*, 159–170. https://doi.org/10.1016/j.brainres.2015.11.015.

Knowles, R. G., Palacios, M., Palmer, R. M., & Moncada, S. (1989). Formation of nitric oxide from L-arginine in the central nervous system: A transduction mechanism for stimulation of the soluble guanylate cyclase. *Proceedings of the National Academy of Sciences of the United States of America, 86*(13), 5159–5162.

Koh, J. Y., & Choi, D. W. (1988). Cultured striatal neurons containing NADPH-diaphorase or acetylcholinesterase are selectively resistant to injury by NMDA receptor agonists. *Brain Research, 446*(2), 374–378.

Koh, D. W., Lawler, A. M., Poitras, M. F., Sasaki, M., Wattler, S., Nehls, M. C., et al. (2004). Failure to degrade poly(ADP-ribose) causes increased sensitivity to cytotoxicity and early embryonic lethality. *Proceedings of the National Academy of Sciences of the United States of America, 101*(51), 17699–17704. https://doi.org/10.1073/pnas.0406182101.

Koh, J. Y., Peters, S., & Choi, D. W. (1986). Neurons containing NADPH-diaphorase are selectively resistant to quinolinate toxicity. *Science, 234*(4772), 73–76.

Kollegger, H., McBean, G. J., & Tipton, K. F. (1993). Reduction of striatal N-methyl-D-aspartate toxicity by inhibition of nitric oxide synthase. *Biochemical Pharmacology, 45*(1), 260–264.

Kostic, M., Zivkovic, N., & Stojanovic, I. (2013). Multiple sclerosis and glutamate excitotoxicity. *Reviews in the Neurosciences, 24*(1), 71–88. https://doi.org/10.1515/revneuro-2012-0062.

Kuhar, M. J., & Aghajanian, G. K. (1973). Selective accumulation of 3 H-serotonin by nerve terminals of raphe neurones: An autoradiographic study. *Nature: New Biology, 241*(110), 187–189.

Kuhar, M. J., & Yamamura, H. I. (1975). Light autoradiographic localisation of cholinergic muscarinic receptors in rat brain by specific binding of a potent antagonist. *Nature, 253*(5492), 560–561.

Kurosaki, R., Muramatsu, Y., Michimata, M., Matsubara, M., Kato, H., Imai, Y., et al. (2002). Role of nitric oxide synthase against MPTP neurotoxicity in mice. *Neurological Research, 24*(7), 655–662. https://doi.org/10.1179/016164102101200717.

Kusama, T., Spivak, C. E., Whiting, P., Dawson, V. L., Schaeffer, J. C., & Uhl, G. R. (1993). Pharmacology of GABA rho 1 and GABA alpha/beta receptors expressed in Xenopus oocytes and COS cells. *British Journal of Pharmacology, 109*(1), 200–206.

Lai, T. W., Zhang, S., & Wang, Y. T. (2014). Excitotoxicity and stroke: Identifying novel targets for neuroprotection. *Progress in Neurobiology, 115*, 157–188. https://doi.org/10.1016/j.pneurobio.2013.11.006.

Lee, Y., Karuppagounder, S. S., Shin, J. H., Lee, Y. I., Ko, H. S., Swing, D., et al. (2013). Parthanatos mediates AIMP2-activated age-dependent dopaminergic neuronal loss. *Nature Neuroscience, 16*(10), 1392–1400. https://doi.org/10.1038/nn.3500.

Liberatore, G. T., Jackson-Lewis, V., Vukosavic, S., Mandir, A. S., Vila, M., McAuliffe, W. G., et al. (1999). Inducible nitric oxide synthase stimulates dopaminergic neurodegeneration in the MPTP model of Parkinson disease. *Nature Medicine, 5*(12), 1403–1409. https://doi.org/10.1038/70978.

Libikova, H., Pogady, J., Wiedermann, V., & Breier, S. (1975). Search for herpetic antibodies in the cerebrospinal fluid in senile dementia and mental retardation. *Acta Virologica, 19*(6), 493–495.

Lipton, S. A., Choi, Y. B., Pan, Z. H., Lei, S. Z., Chen, H. S., Sucher, N. J., et al. (1993). A redox-based mechanism for the neuroprotective and neurodestructive effects of nitric oxide and related nitroso-compounds. *Nature, 364*(6438), 626–632. https://doi.org/10.1038/364626a0.

Lustig, H. S., von Brauchitsch, K. L., Chan, J., & Greenberg, D. A. (1992). Cyclic GMP modulators and excitotoxic injury in cerebral cortical cultures. *Brain Research, 577*(2), 343–346.

Martin, L. J. (2007). Transgenic mice with human mutant genes causing Parkinson's disease and amyotrophic lateral sclerosis provide common insight into mechanisms of motor neuron selective vulnerability to degeneration. *Reviews in the Neurosciences, 18*(2), 115–136.

Mashimo, M., Kato, J., & Moss, J. (2013). ADP-ribosyl-acceptor hydrolase 3 regulates poly (ADP-ribose) degradation and cell death during oxidative stress. *Proceedings of the National Academy of Sciences of the United States of America, 110*(47), 18964–18969. https://doi.org/10.1073/pnas.1312783110.

Mattson, M. P. (2003). Excitotoxic and excitoprotective mechanisms: Abundant targets for the prevention and treatment of neurodegenerative disorders. *Neuromolecular Medicine, 3*(2), 65–94. https://doi.org/10.1385/NMM:3:2:65.

Mehta, A., Prabhakar, M., Kumar, P., Deshmukh, R., & Sharma, P. L. (2013). Excitotoxicity: Bridge to various triggers in neurodegenerative disorders. *European Journal of Pharmacology, 698*(1–3), 6–18. https://doi.org/10.1016/j.ejphar.2012.10.032.

Meldrum, B. (1990). Protection against ischaemic neuronal damage by drugs acting on excitatory neurotransmission. *Cerebrovascular and Brain Metabolism Reviews, 2*(1), 27–57.

Meldrum, B. S. (1992). Excitatory amino acid receptors and disease. *Current Opinion in Neurology and Neurosurgery, 5*(4), 508–513.

Meldrum, B., & Garthwaite, J. (1990). Excitatory amino acid neurotoxicity and neurodegenerative disease. *Trends in Pharmacological Sciences, 11*(9), 379–387.

Moncada, C., Lekieffre, D., Arvin, B., & Meldrum, B. (1992). Effect of NO synthase inhibition on NMDA- and ischaemia-induced hippocampal lesions. *Neuroreport, 3*(6), 530–532.

Moroni, F. (2008). Poly(ADP-ribose)polymerase 1 (PARP-1) and postischemic brain damage. *Current Opinion in Pharmacology*, *8*(1), 96–103. https://doi.org/10.1016/j.coph.2007.10.005.

Mourey, R. J., Dawson, T. M., Barrow, R. K., Enna, A. E., & Snyder, S. H. (1992). [3H] noscapine binding sites in brain: Relationship to indoleamines and the phosphoinositide and adenylyl cyclase messenger systems. *Molecular Pharmacology*, *42*(4), 619–626.

Mukherjee, P., Cinelli, M. A., Kang, S., & Silverman, R. B. (2014). Development of nitric oxide synthase inhibitors for neurodegeneration and neuropathic pain. *Chemical Society Reviews*, *43*(19), 6814–6838. https://doi.org/10.1039/c3cs60467e.

Murphy, S. (2000). Production of nitric oxide by glial cells: Regulation and potential roles in the CNS. *Glia*, *29*(1), 1–13.

Nakanishi, S. (1992). Molecular diversity of glutamate receptors and implications for brain function. *Science*, *258*(5082), 597–603.

Nathan, C., & Xie, Q. W. (1994). Nitric oxide synthases: Roles, tolls, and controls. *Cell*, *78*(6), 915–918.

Oury, T. D., Ho, Y. S., Piantadosi, C. A., & Crapo, J. D. (1992). Extracellular superoxide dismutase, nitric oxide, and central nervous system O2 toxicity. *Proceedings of the National Academy of Sciences of the United States of America*, *89*(20), 9715–9719.

Pacher, P., & Szabo, C. (2008). Role of the peroxynitrite-poly(ADP-ribose) polymerase pathway in human disease. *The American Journal of Pathology*, *173*(1), 2–13. https://doi.org/10.2353/ajpath.2008.080019.

Pert, C. B., & Snyder, S. H. (1973). Opiate receptor: Demonstration in nervous tissue. *Science*, *179*(4077), 1011–1014.

Przedborski, S., Jackson-Lewis, V., Yokoyama, R., Shibata, T., Dawson, V. L., & Dawson, T. M. (1996). Role of neuronal nitric oxide in 1-methyl-4-phenyl-1,2,3,6-tetrahydropyridine (MPTP)-induced dopaminergic neurotoxicity. *Proceedings of the National Academy of Sciences of the United States of America*, *93*(10), 4565–4571.

Rostasy, K., Monti, L., Yiannoutsos, C., Kneissl, M., Bell, J., Kemper, T. L., et al. (1999). Human immunodeficiency virus infection, inducible nitric oxide synthase expression, and microglial activation: Pathogenetic relationship to the acquired immunodeficiency syndrome dementia complex. *Annals of Neurology*, *46*(2), 207–216.

Saez, T. E., Pehar, M., Vargas, M., Barbeito, L., & Maccioni, R. B. (2004). Astrocytic nitric oxide triggers tau hyperphosphorylation in hippocampal neurons. *In Vivo*, *18*(3), 275–280.

Samdani, A. F., Dawson, T. M., & Dawson, V. L. (1997). Nitric oxide synthase in models of focal ischemia. *Stroke*, *28*(6), 1283–1288.

Samdani, A. F., Newcamp, C., Resink, A., Facchinetti, F., Hoffman, B. E., Dawson, V. L., et al. (1997). Differential susceptibility to neurotoxicity mediated by neurotrophins and neuronal nitric oxide synthase. *The Journal of Neuroscience*, *17*(12), 4633–4641.

Santiago, E., Perez-Mediavilla, L. A., & Lopez-Moratalla, N. (1998). The role of nitric oxide in the pathogenesis of multiple sclerosis. *Journal of Physiology and Biochemistry*, *54*(4), 229–237.

Sattler, R., Xiong, Z., Lu, W. Y., Hafner, M., MacDonald, J. F., & Tymianski, M. (1999). Specific coupling of NMDA receptor activation to nitric oxide neurotoxicity by PSD-95 protein. *Science*, *284*(5421), 1845–1848.

Sen, N., Hara, M. R., Ahmad, A. S., Cascio, M. B., Kamiya, A., Ehmsen, J. T., et al. (2009). GOSPEL: A neuroprotective protein that binds to GAPDH upon S-nitrosylation. *Neuron*, *63*(1), 81–91. https://doi.org/10.1016/j.neuron.2009.05.024.

Sen, N., Hara, M. R., Kornberg, M. D., Cascio, M. B., Bae, B. I., Shahani, N., et al. (2008). Nitric oxide-induced nuclear GAPDH activates p300/CBP and mediates apoptosis. *Nature Cell Biology*, *10*(7), 866–873. https://doi.org/10.1038/ncb1747.

Sepers, M. D., & Raymond, L. A. (2014). Mechanisms of synaptic dysfunction and excitotoxicity in Huntington's disease. *Drug Discovery Today*, *19*, 990–996. https://doi.org/10.1016/j.drudis.2014.02.006.

Sharp, A. H., Dawson, T. M., Ross, C. A., Fotuhi, M., Mourey, R. J., & Snyder, S. H. (1993). Inositol 1,4,5-trisphosphate receptors: Immunohistochemical localization to discrete areas of rat central nervous system. *Neuroscience, 53*(4), 927–942.

Soriano, F. X., Martel, M. A., Papadia, S., Vaslin, A., Baxter, P., Rickman, C., et al. (2008). Specific targeting of pro-death NMDA receptor signals with differing reliance on the NR2B PDZ ligand. *The Journal of Neuroscience, 28*(42), 10696–10710. https://doi.org/10.1523/JNEUROSCI.1207-08.2008.

Steiner, J. P., Dawson, T. M., Fotuhi, M., Glatt, C. E., Snowman, A. M., Cohen, N., et al. (1992). High brain densities of the immunophilin FKBP colocalized with calcineurin. *Nature, 358*(6387), 584–587. https://doi.org/10.1038/358584a0.

Sugimoto, K., & Iadecola, C. (2002). Effects of aminoguanidine on cerebral ischemia in mice: Comparison between mice with and without inducible nitric oxide synthase gene. *Neuroscience Letters, 331*(1), 25–28.

Sultana, R., Poon, H. F., Cai, J., Pierce, W. M., Merchant, M., Klein, J. B., et al. (2006). Identification of nitrated proteins in Alzheimer's disease brain using a redox proteomics approach. *Neurobiology of Disease, 22*(1), 76–87. https://doi.org/10.1016/j.nbd.2005.10.004.

Sun, H. S., Doucette, T. A., Liu, Y., Fang, Y., Teves, L., Aarts, M., et al. (2008). Effectiveness of PSD95 inhibitors in permanent and transient focal ischemia in the rat. *Stroke, 39*(9), 2544–2553. https://doi.org/10.1161/STROKEAHA.107.506048.

Szabo, C., & Dawson, V. L. (1998). Role of poly(ADP-ribose) synthetase in inflammation and ischaemia-reperfusion. *Trends in Pharmacological Sciences, 19*(7), 287–298.

Thomas, E., & Pearse, A. G. (1961). The fine localization of dehydrogenases in the nervous system. *Zeitschrift für Zellforschung und Mikroskopische Anatomie Abteilung Histochemie, 2*, 266–282.

Thomas, E., & Pearse, A. G. (1964). The solitary active cells. Histochemical demonstration of damage-resistant nerve cells with a Tpn-diaphorase reaction. *Acta Neuropathologica, 3*, 238–249.

Tinker, A. C., & Wallace, A. V. (2006). Selective inhibitors of inducible nitric oxide synthase: Potential agents for the treatment of inflammatory diseases? *Current Topics in Medicinal Chemistry, 6*(2), 77–92.

Uemura, Y., Kowall, N. W., & Beal, M. F. (1990). Selective sparing of NADPH-diaphorase-somatostatin-neuropeptide Y neurons in ischemic gerbil striatum. *Annals of Neurology, 27*(6), 620–625. https://doi.org/10.1002/ana.410270606.

Virag, L., & Szabo, C. (2002). The therapeutic potential of poly(ADP-ribose) polymerase inhibitors. *Pharmacological Reviews, 54*(3), 375–429.

Wamsley, J. K., Zarbin, M. A., Birdsall, N. J., & Kuhar, M. J. (1980). Muscarinic cholinergic receptors: Autoradiographic localization of high and low affinity agonist binding sites. *Brain Research, 200*(1), 1–12.

Wang, Y., An, R., Umanah, G. K., Park, H., Nambiar, K., Eacker, S. M., et al. (2016). A nuclease that mediates cell death induced by DNA damage and poly(ADP-ribose) polymerase-1. *Science, 354*(6308). https://doi.org/10.1126/science.aad6872.

Wang, Y., Kim, N. S., Haince, J. F., Kang, H. C., David, K. K., Andrabi, S. A., et al. (2011). Poly(ADP-ribose) (PAR) binding to apoptosis-inducing factor is critical for PAR polymerase-1-dependent cell death (parthanatos). *Science Signaling, 4*(167), ra20. https://doi.org/10.1126/scisignal.2000902.

Williams, K., Dawson, V. L., Romano, C., Dichter, M. A., & Molinoff, P. B. (1990). Characterization of polyamines having agonist, antagonist, and inverse agonist effects at the polyamine recognition site of the NMDA receptor. *Neuron, 5*(2), 199–208.

Xia, Y., Dawson, V. L., Dawson, T. M., Snyder, S. H., & Zweier, J. L. (1996). Nitric oxide synthase generates superoxide and nitric oxide in arginine-depleted cells leading to peroxynitrite-mediated cellular injury. *Proceedings of the National Academy of Sciences of the United States of America*, *93*(13), 6770–6774.

Xu, J. C., Fan, J., Wang, X., Eacker, S. M., Kam, T. I., Chen, L., et al. (2016). Cultured networks of excitatory projection neurons and inhibitory interneurons for studying human cortical neurotoxicity. *Science Translational Medicine*, *8*(333), 333ra48. https://doi.org/10.1126/scitranslmed.aad0623.

Yao, D., Gu, Z., Nakamura, T., Shi, Z. Q., Ma, Y., Gaston, B., et al. (2004). Nitrosative stress linked to sporadic Parkinson's disease: S-nitrosylation of parkin regulates its E3 ubiquitin ligase activity. *Proceedings of the National Academy of Sciences of the United States of America*, *101*(29), 10810–10814. https://doi.org/10.1073/pnas.0404161101.

Young, W. S., 3rd., Wamsley, J. K., Zarbin, M. A., & Kuhar, M. J. (1980). Opioid receptors undergo axonal flow. *Science*, *210*(4465), 76–78.

Yu, S. W., Andrabi, S. A., Wang, H., Kim, N. S., Poirier, G. G., Dawson, T. M., et al. (2006). Apoptosis-inducing factor mediates poly(ADP-ribose) (PAR) polymer-induced cell death. *Proceedings of the National Academy of Sciences of the United States of America*, *103*(48), 18314–18319. https://doi.org/10.1073/pnas.0606528103.

Yu, S. W., Wang, H., Dawson, T. M., & Dawson, V. L. (2003). Poly(ADP-ribose) polymerase-1 and apoptosis inducing factor in neurotoxicity. *Neurobiology of Disease*, *14*(3), 303–317.

Yu, S. W., Wang, H., Poitras, M. F., Coombs, C., Bowers, W. J., Federoff, H. J., et al. (2002). Mediation of poly(ADP-ribose) polymerase-1-dependent cell death by apoptosis-inducing factor. *Science*, *297*(5579), 259–263. https://doi.org/10.1126/science.1072221.

Yun, H. Y., Dawson, V. L., & Dawson, T. M. (1996). Neurobiology of nitric oxide. *Critical Reviews in Neurobiology*, *10*(3–4), 291–316.

Zhang, J., Dawson, V. L., Dawson, T. M., & Snyder, S. H. (1994). Nitric oxide activation of poly(ADP-ribose) synthetase in neurotoxicity. *Science*, *263*(5147), 687–689.

Zhang, Y., Liu, S., Mickanin, C., Feng, Y., Charlat, O., Michaud, G. A., et al. (2011). RNF146 is a poly(ADP-ribose)-directed E3 ligase that regulates axin degradation and Wnt signalling. *Nature Cell Biology*, *13*(5), 623–629. https://doi.org/10.1038/ncb2222.

Zhao, X., Haensel, C., Araki, E., Ross, M. E., & Iadecola, C. (2000). Gene-dosing effect and persistence of reduction in ischemic brain injury in mice lacking inducible nitric oxide synthase. *Brain Research*, *872*(1–2), 215–218.

CHAPTER FIVE

Carboxypeptidase E and the Identification of Novel Neuropeptides as Potential Therapeutic Targets

Lloyd D. Fricker[1]
Albert Einstein College of Medicine, Bronx, NY, United States
[1]Corresponding author: e-mail address: lloyd.fricker@einstein.yu.edu

Contents

Abstract

Peptides and small molecules that bind to peptide receptors are important classes of drugs that are used for a wide variety of different applications. The search for novel neuropeptides traditionally involved a time-consuming approach to purify each peptide to homogeneity and determine its amino acid sequence. The discovery in the 1980s of enkephalin convertase/carboxypeptidase E (CPE), and the observation that this enzyme was involved in the production of nearly every known neuropeptide led to the idea for a one-step affinity purification of CPE substrates. This approach was successfully used to isolate hundreds of known neuropeptides in mouse brain, as well as over a dozen novel peptides. Some of the novel peptides found using this approach are among the most abundant peptides present in brain, but had not been previously identified by traditional approaches. Recently, receptors for two of the novel peptides have been identified, confirming their role as neuropeptides that function in cell–cell signaling. Small

Advances in Pharmacology, Volume 82
ISSN 1054-3589
https://doi.org/10.1016/bs.apha.2017.09.001

molecules that bind to one of these receptors have been developed and found to significantly reduce food intake and anxiety-like behavior in an animal model. This review describes the entire project, from discovery of CPE to the novel peptides and their receptors.

ABBREVIATIONS

CPE carboxypeptidase E
GPCRs G protein-coupled receptors
PC prohormone convertase
PTM posttranslational modification
NPY neuropeptide Y
POMC proopiomelanocortin

1. INTRODUCTION

1.1 Peptides and Peptide Receptors as Pharmacological Targets

Peptides have many diverse functions and are found in virtually all organisms (Chung & Civelli, 2006; Fricker, 2012; Husson, Mertens, Janssen, Lindemans, & Schoofs, 2007; Sobrino Crespo, Perianes Cachero, Puebla Jimenez, Barrios, & Arilla Ferreiro, 2014; Strand, 2003). In multicellular organisms, a large number of peptides are known to signal between cells, either between tissues as peptide hormones or between neurons as neuropeptides. Because of their important roles in signaling, peptides are used as drugs (Fosgerau & Hoffmann, 2015; Kaspar & Reichert, 2013). In some cases, the peptides used as therapeutics are identical in sequence and posttranslational modification (PTM) as the endogenous neuropeptides or peptide hormone; examples include insulin and vasopressin. In other cases, the peptides used as therapeutic agents are modified to enhance their stability; such modifications include the introduction of D-amino acids or PTMs that block the action of peptidases. There are currently more than 60 peptides that have been approved by the Food and Drug Administration and marketed as therapeutic agents, and many more peptides are in clinical testing (Fosgerau & Hoffmann, 2015; Kaspar & Reichert, 2013).

In addition to peptides themselves, small molecules that bind to peptide receptors are important drugs for many diverse applications. Examples include drugs for treatment of pain (mu opioid receptor agonists such as morphine, oxycodone, and many others), nausea and vomiting (aprepitant, a neurokinin receptor antagonist), and narcolepsy (suvorexant, an orexin receptor antagonist) (Levy, 2001; Preskorn, 2014). Additional drugs targeting other peptide receptors are in various stages of the development pipeline (Fosgerau & Hoffmann, 2015; Kaspar & Reichert, 2013).

Hundreds of bioactive peptides have been identified since the first peptide hormone was discovered and characterized in the early 1900s (Bayliss & Starling, 1902; Fricker, 2012; Strand, 2003). In addition to the known neuropeptides and peptide hormones, there are many peptides of unknown function—these are termed "orphan peptides" (Chung & Civelli, 2006; Fricker, 2010, 2012; Ozawa, Lindberg, Roth, & Kroeze, 2010). It is possible that some of these orphan peptides bind to receptors and function as neurotransmitters or peptide hormones. There are dozens of orphan G protein-coupled receptors (GPCRs) and it is likely that some of these bind peptides (Chung & Civelli, 2006; Civelli, 2008; Civelli et al., 2013; Ozawa et al., 2010). Thus, the identification of novel peptides and "deorphanization" of their receptors is an area with potential therapeutic applications.

2. BIOSYNTHESIS OF NEUROPEPTIDES: DISCOVERY OF ENKEPHALIN CONVERTASE/CARBOXYPEPTIDASE E

In the mid-1970s, endogenous peptides with opiate-like properties were discovered in mammalian tissue extracts, including Met- and Leu-enkephalin, beta-endorphin, and various dynorphin peptides (Goldstein, Tachibana, Lowney, Hunkapiller, & Hood, 1979; Hughes et al., 1975; Lazarus, Ling, & Guillemin, 1976; Li, Chung, & Doneen, 1976; Roberts & Herbert, 1977; Stern et al., 1979). Precursors of these peptides were identified and in most cases, the precursors contained lysine and/or arginine residues on either side of the bioactive peptides (Kimura et al., 1980; Lewis et al., 1980). This led to the hypothesis that a trypsin-like endopeptidase initially cleaved the neuropeptide precursor protein into intermediates that contained C-terminal Lys/Arg residues, and these were subsequently removed by a carboxypeptidase B-like enzyme (Roberts, Phillips, Rosa, Budarf, & Herbert, 1979). Because trypsin and carboxypeptidase B were produced in the exocrine pancreas and not known to be produced in brain or other endocrine tissues, it was likely that novel enzymes were involved in neuropeptides production. When I joined Dr. Solomon Snyder's laboratory as a student in 1980, he proposed that I identify the unknown carboxypeptidase that produced enkephalin, the so-called enkephalin convertase.

If enkephalin convertase was specific for producing enkephalin, it would recognize more than the C-terminal basic residues (i.e., Lys or Arg). Because the existing assays for pancreatic carboxypeptidase B used very short peptides such as hippuryl-Arg (Folk, Piez, Carroll, & Gladner, 1960), these substrates were not likely to be useful to detect an enzyme with specificity for a longer peptide. A new assay was developed that used the C-terminal sequence of an enkephalin precursor: Phe-Leu-Arg (Fricker & Snyder, 1982). A fluorescent group was attached to the N-terminus of this peptide so that it could be readily detected, and enzymatic conversion of substrate (dansyl-Phe-Leu-Arg) into product (dansyl-Phe-Leu) monitored by extraction of the product into chloroform. Using this assay, enkephalin convertase was detected in bovine adrenal chromaffin granules (Fricker & Snyder, 1982). Chromaffin granules were previously reported to contain enkephalin as well as enkephalin precursors, implying that they contain the carboxypeptidase that generates enkephalin (Lewis, Stern, Rossier, Stein, & Udenfriend, 1979; Stern et al., 1979). The enzyme detected in the chromaffin granules was a metallopeptidase with pH optimum around 5.5 (Fricker & Snyder, 1982). These properties were similar to those of an enzyme associated with pancreatic beta cells (Zuhlke et al., 1977; Zuhlke, Steiner, Lernmark, & Lipsey, 1976), but distinct from an enzyme that was claimed to be the enkephalin-producing carboxypeptidase (Hook, Eiden, & Brownstein, 1982). The chromaffin granule metallopeptidase was purified to homogeneity from adrenal, brain, and pituitary (Fricker & Snyder, 1983). Upon characterization, the enzyme was shown to convert enkephalin precursors into enkephalin and was named enkephalin convertase in the initial publication (Fricker & Snyder, 1982). However, enkephalin convertase was not specific for enkephalin precursors, cleaving basic residues from a wide range of peptides containing C-terminal Lys or Arg, although not from dipeptides such as hippuryl-Arg which are too short to be efficient substrates of this enzyme (Fricker & Snyder, 1983; Supattapone, Fricker, & Snyder, 1984). The finding that enkephalin convertase was not specific for the sequence of the enkephalin precursor matched the broad distribution of the enzyme in all neuroendocrine tissues, with no correlation with the distribution of enkephalin. Taken together, it appeared that enkephalin convertase was a common enzyme for the production of all neuropeptides that were produced from precursors that required removal of basic amino acids, including the synthesis of insulin and other peptide hormones (Davidson & Hutton, 1987; Docherty & Hutton, 1983; Mains & Eipper, 1984). Therefore, the name enkephalin convertase was considered inaccurate and the enzyme was renamed carboxypeptidase E (CPE) (Fricker, 1985, 1988). Other names have been used for this enzyme, such as carboxypeptidase H, but CPE is most commonly used.

3. CPE AND THE DISCOVERY OF NOVEL NEUROPEPTIDES

If CPE functions in the biosynthesis of a large number of known neuropeptides, then it was predicted that this enzyme would also function in the production of novel neuropeptides. At the time of the discovery of CPE in the early 1980s, novel neuropeptides were being discovered every year or two, and it was assumed that many unknown neuropeptides awaited discovery (Tatemoto, Carlquist, & Mutt, 1982; Tatemoto et al., 1986; Tatemoto, Jornvall, McDonald, et al., 1984; Tatemoto, Jornvall, Siimesmaa, et al., 1984; Tatemoto, Lundberg, Jornvall, & Mutt, 1985; Tatemoto & Mutt, 1980; Tatemoto, Rokaeus, Jornvall, McDonald, & Mutt, 1983). One major limitation to the discovery of neuropeptides was the purification approach, which usually started with many kilograms of tissue and took years to separate the bioactive neuropeptide from all other proteins and peptides present in the extracts (Burgus & Guillemin, 1970; Hughes et al., 1975; Tatemoto et al., 1982; Tatemoto & Mutt, 1980).

Because CPE seemed to be specific for neuropeptide production, based on the enzyme's neuroendocrine distribution and localization to peptide-containing secretory vesicles, CPE could be used to rapidly identify novel neuropeptides. The idea was to use affinity chromatography to isolate CPE substrates in a single step, instead of using conventional chromatography that only afforded a 5- to 10-fold purification in each step and therefore required multiple steps to achieve sufficient purity for sequence determination. This idea consisted of two steps (Fig. 1). The first involved inhibition of CPE to accumulate the Lys/Arg-extended CPE substrates—these are normally present at extremely low levels within brain and other neuroendocrine tissues. The second step involved purification on an affinity column, using an inactive enzyme that could bind substrates but not cleave them.

For step 1 of the scheme, potent inhibitors of CPE were identified from a screen of compounds previously developed as inhibitors of carboxypeptidase B and related enzymes (Fricker, Plummer, & Snyder, 1983; McKay & Plummer, 1978; Plummer & Ryan, 1981). However, none of these compounds was able to penetrate the secretory vesicles where the production of neuropeptides occurred, presumably due to the highly charged nature

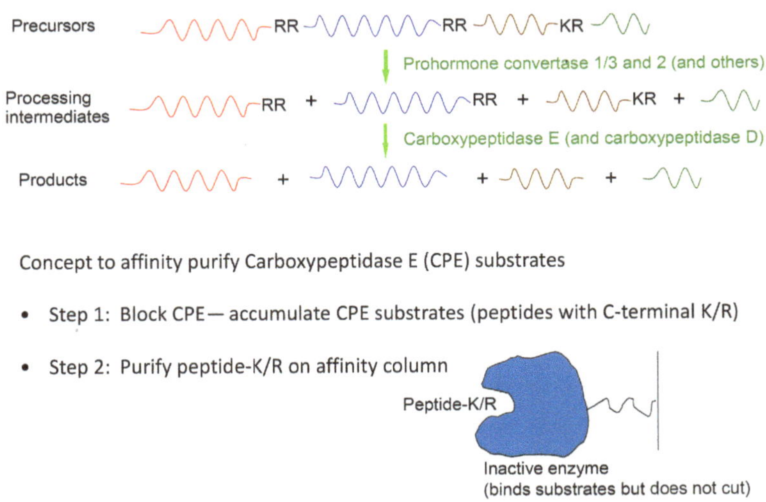

Fig. 1 Neuropeptide processing scheme and concept for the affinity purification of CPE substrates. *Top*: Neuropeptides are produced from precursors by selective cleavages at sites that usually contain basic amino acids lysine (K) and arginine (R). Initially, an endopeptidase cleaves the precursor to generate intermediates that contain basic residues on their C-terminus except for the C-terminal peptide, which does not require additional processing to generate the mature form. Endopeptidases include prohormone convertase 1 (PC1, also known as PC3) and prohormone convertase 2 (PC2). For some neuropeptides, the processing of their precursors starts in the late Golgi and is mediated by endopeptidases in this compartment such as furin and other furin-like enzymes. Following the endopeptidase, a carboxypeptidase removes the C-terminal basic residue. Carboxypeptidase E (CPE) is the major neuropeptide-processing carboxypeptidase that is present within secretory vesicles. For neuropeptide precursors initially cleaved in the Golgi by furin or furin-like enzymes, carboxypeptidase D is present in this compartment and is able to remove the basic residues from the intermediates to produce the mature peptides. For some peptides, additional posttranslational modifications are required, such as C-terminal amidation, N-terminal acetylation, or phosphorylation of Ser or Thr residues (not shown). *Bottom*: The general concept for the affinity purification of CPE substrates. Step 1 requires inhibition of CPE to enrich for CPE substrates—otherwise the peptides containing C-terminal lysine or arginine are present at extremely low levels in brain and other tissues. As the scheme was originally envisioned, step 2 required purification on a column of inactive CPE, which could bind substrates but not cleave them. In practice, anhydrotrypsin has the required specificity for peptides with C-terminal basic residues and does not bind with high affinity to peptides with internal basic residues. Following purification of the CPE substrates, the column eluate contains a mixture of hundreds of peptides. These are fractionated on reverse phase liquid chromatography columns and analyzed by on-line electrospray ionization mass spectrometry, which can often determine the sequence of peptides in complex mixtures.

of the compounds. Without the essential first step of in vivo inhibition of CPE activity, it was not possible to pursue the idea of affinity purification of neuropeptides precursors.

In the late-1980s, techniques to generate mice with a targeted disruption of a specific gene (termed "knock-out" mice) were developed (Capecchi, 1989, 2001; Evans, 2001; Smithies, 2001). Knock-out of the *Cpe* gene would lead to elevated levels of CPE substrates, a requirement for the peptide purification scheme to succeed (Fig. 1). However, it was assumed that the knockout would completely eliminate the mature forms of most bioactive peptides and this would be embryonic lethal. At the time, CPE was incorrectly thought to be the only neuropeptide-producing carboxypeptidase in the secretory pathway (Fricker, 1988, 1993; Fricker & Devi, 1994). Fortunately, mice lacking CPE activity were viable. In fact, such mice already existed—a spontaneous mutation in the *Cpe* gene occurred in the early 1970s at The Jackson Laboratory in a colony of inbred mice, and because the mutant mouse was notably overweight, the mutation was named *fat* (Coleman & Eicher, 1990). Mice homozygous for the *fat* mutation (i.e., *fat/fat* mice) were extremely overweight and also sterile, but mice heterozygous for the *fat* mutation were fertile and had normal body weights. Geneticists mapped the location of the *fat* mutation to chromosome 8 near the *Cpe* gene, and my laboratory helped determine that these mice had a mutation in the protein-coding region of the gene that caused CPE to be completely inactive (Naggert et al., 1995). The mutation was renamed Cpe^{fat} to reflect the altered gene.

Analysis of peptides in brain and neuroendocrine tissues of Cpe^{fat}/Cpe^{fat} mice revealed that mature fully processed neuropeptides were present, albeit at extremely low levels for most peptides (Cain, Wang, & Beinfeld, 1997; Fricker, Berman, Leiter, & Devi, 1996; Naggert et al., 1995; Rovere, Viale, Nahon, & Kitabgi, 1996). This led to the discovery of carboxypeptidase D, a CPE-like enzyme that is mainly present in the trans Golgi network of the secretory pathway where it primarily functions in the processing of proteins and peptides that transit to the cell surface via the constitutive secretory pathway (Song & Fricker, 1995; Varlamov & Fricker, 1998; Xin et al., 1997). Although carboxypeptidase D appears to be excluded from the mature secretory vesicles where CPE is enriched and the majority of the neuropeptide processing occurs, the presence of carboxypeptidase D in the trans Golgi network and immature secretory vesicles is sufficient to produce enough of the mature bioactive forms of neuropeptides to permit the animals to live a fairly normal lifespan (Varlamov, Eng, Novikova, & Fricker, 1999; Varlamov, Wu, Shields, & Fricker, 1999).

As predicted from earlier studies on the substrate specificity and distribution of CPE, studies on *Cpe^fat^/Cpe^fat^* mice confirmed that CPE is the major carboxypeptidase involved in the production of nearly every neuropeptide (Che, Biswas, & Fricker, 2005; Che & Fricker, 2002; Zhang et al., 2008). The only exceptions are secretory pathway peptides that do not require removal of C-terminal basic residues, and peptides that are not produced within the secretory pathway. For example, secretory pathway peptides that are present in the Cpe^{fat}/Cpe^{fat} mice include peptides located on the C-terminus of their precursor such as beta-endorphin which only require endopeptidase cleavage, or peptides in which the C-terminal basic residues are not removed such as alpha-neoendorphin which terminates in Pro-Arg and is not an efficient substrate of CPE (Zhang et al., 2008).

In addition to the secretory pathway peptides, a large number of other peptides are detected in brains of both wild-type and Cpe^{fat}/Cpe^{fat} mice as well as all other genotypes of mice that have been studied (Fricker, 2010; Zhang et al., 2008). These other peptides are mainly derived from proteins known to be localized to the cell cytoplasm, mitochondria, and/or nucleus; these are termed "intracellular peptides" to distinguish them from neuropeptides derived from secretory pathway proteins (Ferro, Rioli, Castro, & Fricker, 2014; Fricker, 2010). Quantitative peptidomics studies indicated that the intracellular peptides are present at comparable levels in wild-type and Cpe^{fat}/Cpe^{fat} mice brains, and therefore are not substrates of CPE, consistent with their intracellular location as well as the absence of basic amino acid cleavage sites (Zhang et al., 2008). Some of these intracellular peptides have been found to be secreted via an unknown mechanism from brain slices and these secreted peptides may function as nonclassical neuropeptides (Gelman, Dasgupta, Berezniuk, & Fricker, 2013). For example, the peptide RVD-hemopressin is secreted from mouse brain slices and binds to cannabinoid CB1 receptors (Gomes et al., 2009; Heimann et al., 2007). Intracellular peptides that are not secreted from cells may bind to intracellular proteins and alter their folding and/or interactions with other proteins (Ferro et al., 2014). However, these potential functions of peptides are difficult to identify and the targets are not easily druggable because of their intracellular location, as opposed to the cell surface location of neuropeptide receptors.

3.1 Using Mice Lacking CPE to Identify Novel Neuropeptides: Discovery of proSAAS-Derived Peptides

Once the Cpe^{fat}/Cpe^{fat} mutation was found to inactivate CPE activity and lead to the accumulation of neuropeptides, which is step 1 of the scheme shown in Fig. 1, my laboratory began working on step 2; the affinity column to purify peptides with C-terminal Lys/Arg residues in a single step. Mutagenesis of a critical active site residue in CPE ($Glu^{300}Gln$) rendered the enzyme inactive but still able to bind substrates (Qian, Varlamov, & Fricker, 1999). (This is not the same point mutation as found in the Cpe^{fat}/Cpe^{fat} mice, which is $Ser^{202}Pro$ and causes the protein to be unstable and rapidly degraded.) Alternatively, treatment of the wild-type enzyme with chelating agents to remove the active site zinc ion also eliminated enzyme activity without compromising substrate binding. Either of these approaches were able to produce the intended result; a protein that bound CPE substrates without cleaving them. However, it was difficult to produce large amounts of CPE and couple it to a solid-phase matrix (e.g., agarose) in high yield. Instead, the commercially available anhydrotrypsin-agarose was found to be comparable in terms of binding specificity (Che et al., 2001; Fricker et al., 2000). This was unexpected, in that trypsin typically cleaves peptides with internal Lys/Arg residues, and peptides with these residues on the C-terminus represent trypsin products, not substrates. Usually, enzymes bind substrates with much higher affinity than products. However, in testing it was found that the anhydrotrypsin-agarose bound poorly to peptides with internal Lys/Arg residues and with high affinity to peptides with C-terminal Lys/Arg residues (Che et al., 2001; Fricker et al., 2000). Thus, the commercially available resin was an ideal resource for step 2 of the scheme to purify neuropeptide precursors from brains of Cpe^{fat}/Cpe^{fat} mice.

Using the anhydrotrypsin affinity column, hundreds of peptide were purified from Cpe^{fat}/Cpe^{fat} mouse brains and identified using mass spectrometry (Che et al., 2001; Fricker et al., 2000). Many of these peptides corresponded to known neuropeptides with C-terminal Lys/Arg, as predicted. This finding confirmed that CPE is involved in the production of the vast majority of neuropeptides. In addition to the predicted peptides from known neuropeptide precursors, several novel peptides were found from a new precursor (Che et al., 2001; Fricker et al., 2000). Because the functions of the peptides were not known at the time, and there was no amino acid sequence homology to known peptides, it was impossible to name the novel peptides with a functional name. Thus, the peptides were named based on amino acid sequence motifs found within the peptides. The first peptide identified had a Ser-Ala-Ala-Ser sequence in the middle of the peptide, and so the peptide was named SAAS based on the single letter amino acid nomenclature (Fricker et al., 2000). Because two forms of this peptide were found, the larger was named Big SAAS and the smaller was named Little SAAS. The precursor was therefore named proSAAS, using the tradition of naming neuropeptide precursors. Other peptides identified in the affinity column eluate that were subsequently found to arise from different regions of proSAAS include peptides named GAV (Big and Little), PEN, and LEN (Big and Little). The big and little forms of the proSAAS-derived peptides arose from partial cleavage by the prohormone convertases (PCs) at basic amino acid-containing sites that are not efficiently cleaved (e.g., single basic residues)—this is also found with many other neuropeptide precursors that undergo differential processing into big and little forms (Fricker, 2012).

The initial report on the discovery of proSAAS raised the possibility that the proSAAS-derived peptides functioned as neuropeptides but did not directly test this, which can take years to prove (Fricker et al., 2000). Another function for proSAAS was found and described in the initial report—that of PC1/3 inhibition (Fricker et al., 2000). The enzyme PC2 has an endogenous inhibitor, named 7B2, but 7B2 is specific for PC2 and does not inhibit PC1/3 (Braks & Martens, 1994; Martens, Braks, Eib, Zhou, & Lindberg, 1994). Because the distribution of proSAAS in mouse neuroendocrine tissue was very broad and overlapped with the distribution of PC1/3, it was logical to test proSAAS as a PC1/3 inhibitor (Fricker et al., 2000). While proSAAS is a potent inhibitor of PC1/3, further studies mapped the inhibitory region to the junction of PEN and LEN and not the mature peptides, raising the possibility that the mature forms of these peptides had additional functions as neuropeptides (Basak et al., 2001; Cameron, Fortenberry, & Lindberg, 2000; Qian et al., 2000).

To explore functions of proSAAS and/or proSAAS-derived peptides, transgenic mice that overexpress proSAAS, and knock-out mice lacking proSAAS were generated (Morgan et al., 2010; Wei et al., 2004). The transgenic mice were slightly overweight, and the knock-out mice were leaner than wild-type littermates, suggesting a role of proSAAS-derived peptides in body weight regulation. ProSAAS-derived peptides may also contribute to rewarding behavior and anxiety, based on the behavior of transgenic and/or knock-out mice (Morgan et al., 2010; Wei et al., 2004). Although proSAAS is present in most neuroendocrine cells, levels in some cell types are much higher than in others; very high levels of proSAAS expression are found in the amygdala and the hypothalamus, especially the arcuate nucleus (Fricker et al., 2000). Within the arcuate nucleus, proSAAS peptides are most abundant in neurons that express neuropeptide Y (NPY), and are not abundant in neurons that express peptides derived from proopiomelanocortin (POMC) (Wardman, Berezniuk, Di, Tasker, & Fricker, 2011). NPY neurons are orexigenic while POMC neurons are anorexigenic (Crown, Clifton, & Steiner, 2007). The colocalization of proSAAS peptides and NPY is consistent with a role for these peptides in body weight regulation, possibly as neuropeptides.

Evidence that a proSAAS-derived peptide functioned in cell–cell signaling was provided from whole-cell patch clamp recordings of parvocellular neurons in the hypothalamic paraventricular nucleus (Wardman et al., 2011). Application of the peptide Big LEN to these cells produced a rapid and reversible inhibition of synaptic glutamate release that was spike independent and dependent on postsynaptic G protein activity (Wardman et al., 2011). This result strongly suggested that Big LEN is a neuropeptide that activates a GPCR expressed in the hypothalamus.

3.2 Matching "Orphan" Peptides and Receptors

Direct evidence that proSAAS-derived peptides function as neuropeptides was recently provided from studies that sought to match these peptides with receptors. Rather than take a high-throughput approach, the Devi laboratory took a targeted approach and focused on orphan GPCRs that were expressed at relatively high levels in brain regions that matched the distribution of proSAAS and its peptides. Using this targeted approach, Gomes et al. screened a dozen receptors and found that Big LEN activated the orphan GPCR named GPR171 (Gomes et al., 2013). The shorter form of this peptide, Little LEN, did not bind to the receptor, but the C-terminal tetrapeptide of Big LEN that is cleaved to generate little LEN (i.e., Leu-Leu-Pro-Pro) was a weak agonist at GPR171 (Gomes et al., 2013). Thus, binding of Big LEN to GPR171 is mediated through the C-terminal portion of this peptide, and the processing step that generates Little LEN and the tetrapeptide affects its biological activity.

Using a similar approach, Devi and colleagues found that PEN activates the orphan GPCR named GPR83 (Gomes et al., 2016). GPR83 is also known as the Glucocorticoid-Induced Receptor, JP05, and GPR72, and was previously implicated in body weight regulation and other functions

(Adams, Grassie, Shahid, Hill, & Henry, 2003; Muller et al., 2013; Wang et al., 2001). GPR83 knock-out mice are resistant to diet-induced obesity when placed on a high-fat diet and have normal body weight on a regular chow diet (Muller et al., 2013). Interestingly, GPR83 and GPR171 are colocalized in some brain regions, as are their peptide ligands; PEN and Big LEN. Coexpression of GPR83 and GPR171 in cultured cell lines alters the signaling properties of each receptor, suggesting functional interactions of these receptors (Gomes et al., 2016).

Recently, a small molecule GPR171 agonist was identified and tested in mice (Wardman et al., 2016). As predicted from the previous studies on proSAAS, this agonist elevated food intake and body weight (Wardman et al., 2016). This effect was attenuated in mice in which GPR171 expression was reduced using short hairpin RNA-mediated knockdown, indicating that the effect was mediated by GPR171 (Wardman et al., 2016). While there is a limited commercial market for pharmaceuticals that elevate food intake (e.g., to treat anorexia), if GPR171 antagonists have the opposite effect and reduce feeding and body weight, this would be a novel therapeutic approach for a multibillion dollar market. Very recently, a small molecule GPR171 antagonist was identified (Bobeck et al., 2017). This compound significantly reduced food intake in an animal model in which NPY/AgRP neurons were stimulated, but did not affect baseline feeding in unstimulated mice (Bobeck et al., 2017). In addition, injection of the GPR171 antagonist into the basolateral amygdala reduced anxiety-like behavior (Bobeck et al., 2017). Taken together, these results are a promising new direction in the development of pharmaceuticals for treatment of disorders that have a large global market.

4. CONCLUSION

An important step in pharmacology is target identification. As a class, peptide receptors are a validated target, with numerous small molecules and peptide-based drugs on the market and more in development. There are dozens of orphan GPCRs that have defied attempts at deorphanization, potentially because their peptide ligands are novel and were not tested with the orphan GPCR. This appears to have been the case for GPR171 and GPR83, which bind peptides that are not commonly studied even though they are among the most abundant peptides in brain (Fricker, 2012).

Decades ago, the slow step in the discovery of new neuropeptides was the purification and identification of peptides using bioassays. Now, with mass spectrometry-based peptidomic approaches, peptide discovery is relatively easy and the hard part is finding functions for all of the novel peptides.

Based on the phenotype of mice lacking CPE activity, it is clear that peptides play important roles in many processes for which there is a major therapeutic demand. In addition to obesity and infertility, mice lacking CPE activity are anxious, depressed, and have memory problems (Rodriguiz et al., 2013; Woronowicz et al., 2008). Some of these same problems have been reported in a human patient lacking CPE activity due to a point mutation within the *Cpe* gene that caused a frameshift and truncation of the protein (Alsters et al., 2015). Thus, further studies to identify the peptide(s) responsible for each of these behaviors in mice may be translatable to novel therapeutic approaches for major clinical problems. Studies on conditional CPE knock-out mice in which the *Cpe* gene is disrupted in specific cell types may reveal novel roles for peptides in anxiety, depression, memory, fertility, and body weight regulation; such studies are currently in progress.

CONFLICT OF INTEREST STATEMENT

The author has no conflicts of interest to declare.

ACKNOWLEDGMENTS

The US National Institute of Drug Abuse (DA-004494) supported much of the work described in this review that was performed in the author's laboratory. The author wishes to thank Prof. Lakshmi Devi for helpful discussions, and all collaborators on the publications cited in the references for their contributions to the project.

REFERENCES

Adams, F., Grassie, M., Shahid, M., Hill, D. R., & Henry, B. (2003). Acute oral dexamethasone administration reduces levels of orphan GPCR glucocorticoid-induced receptor (GIR) mRNA in rodent brain: Potential role in HPA-axis function. *Brain Research. Molecular Brain Research, 117*, 39.

Alsters, S. I., Goldstone, A. P., Buxton, J. L., Zekavati, A., Sosinsky, A., Yiorkas, A. M., et al. (2015). Truncating homozygous mutation of carboxypeptidase E (CPE) in a morbidly obese female with type 2 diabetes mellitus, intellectual disability and hypogonadotrophic hypogonadism. *PLoS One, 10*. e0131417.

Basak, A., Koch, P., Dupelle, M., Fricker, L. D., Devi, L. A., Chretien, M., et al. (2001). Inhibitory specificity and potency of proSAAS-derived peptides toward proprotein convertase 1. *The Journal of Biological Chemistry, 276*. 32720.

Bayliss, W. M., & Starling, E. H. (1902). The mechanism of pancreatic secretion. *The Journal of Physiology, 28*, 325.

Bobeck, E. N., Gomes, I., Pena, D., Cummings, K. A., Clem, R. L., Mezei, M., et al. (2017). The BigLEN-GPR171 peptide receptor system within the basolateral amygdala regulates anxiety-like behavior and contextual fear conditioning. *Neuropsychopharmacology: Official Publication of the American College of Neuropsychopharmacology*. https://doi.org/10.1038/npp.2017.79. [Epub ahead of print].

Braks, J. A. M., & Martens, G. J. M. (1994). 7B2 is a neuroendocrine chaperone that transiently interacts with prohormone convertase PC2 in the secretory pathway. *Cell, 78*, 263.
Burgus, R., & Guillemin, R. (1970). Hypothalamic releasing factors. *Annual Review of Biochemistry, 39*, 499.
Cain, B. M., Wang, W., & Beinfeld, M. C. (1997). Cholecystokinin (CCK) levels are greatly reduced in the brains but not the duodenums of Cpe fat/Cpe fat mice: A regional difference in the involvement of carboxypeptidase E (Cpe) in pro-CCK processing. *Endocrinology, 138*, 4034.
Cameron, A., Fortenberry, Y., & Lindberg, I. (2000). The SAAS granin exhibits structural and functional homology to 7B2 and contains a highly potent hexapeptide inhibitor of PC1. *FEBS Letters, 473*, 135.
Capecchi, M. R. (1989). Altering the genome by homologous recombination. *Science, 244*, 1288.
Capecchi, M. R. (2001). Generating mice with targeted mutations. *Nature Medicine, 7*, 1086.
Che, F. Y., Biswas, R., & Fricker, L. D. (2005). Relative quantitation of peptides in wild type and Cpe(fat/fat) mouse pituitary using stable isotopic tags and mass spectrometry. *Journal of Mass Spectrometry, 40*, 227.
Che, F. Y., & Fricker, L. D. (2002). Quantitation of neuropeptides in Cpe^{fat}/Cpe^{fat} mice using differential isotopic tags and mass spectrometry. *Analytical Chemistry, 74*, 3190.
Che, F. Y., Yan, L., Li, H., Mzhavia, N., Devi, L., & Fricker, L. D. (2001). Identification of peptides from brain and pituitary of Cpe^{fat}/Cpe^{fat} mice. *Proceedings of the National Academy of Sciences of the United States of America, 98*, 9971.
Chung, S., & Civelli, O. (2006). Orphan neuropeptides. Novel neuropeptides modulating sleep or feeding. *Neuropeptides, 40*, 233.
Civelli, O. (2008). The orphanin FQ/nociceptin (OFQ/N) system. *Results and Problems in Cell Differentiation, 46*, 1.
Civelli, O., Reinscheid, R. K., Zhang, Y., Wang, Z., Fredriksson, R., & Schioth, H. B. (2013). G protein-coupled receptor deorphanizations. *Annual Review of Pharmacology and Toxicology, 53*, 127.
Coleman, D. L., & Eicher, E. M. (1990). Fat (fat) and tubby (tub), two autosomal recessive mutations causing obesity syndromes in the mouse. *The Journal of Heredity, 81*, 424.
Crown, A., Clifton, D. K., & Steiner, R. A. (2007). Neuropeptide signaling in the integration of metabolism and reproduction. *Neuroendocrinology, 86*, 175.
Davidson, H. W., & Hutton, J. C. (1987). The insulin secretory granule carboxypeptidase H: Purification and demonstration of involvement in proinsulin processing. *The Biochemical Journal, 245*, 575.
Docherty, K., & Hutton, J. C. (1983). Carboxypeptidase activity in the insulin secretory granule. *FEBS Letters, 162*, 137.
Evans, M. J. (2001). The cultural mouse. *Nature Medicine, 7*, 1081.
Ferro, E. S., Rioli, V., Castro, L. M., & Fricker, L. D. (2014). Intracellular peptides: From discovery to function. *EuPA Open Proteomics, 3*, 143.
Folk, J. E., Piez, K. A., Carroll, W. R., & Gladner, J. A. (1960). Carboxypeptidase B: Purification and characterization of the porcine enzyme. *The Journal of Biological Chemistry, 235*, 2272.
Fosgerau, K., & Hoffmann, T. (2015). Peptide therapeutics: Current status and future directions. *Drug Discovery Today, 20*, 122.
Fricker, L. D. (1985). Neuropeptide biosynthesis: Focus on the carboxypeptidase processing enzyme. *Trends in Neurosciences, 8*, 210.
Fricker, L. D. (1988). Carboxypeptidase E. *Annual Review of Physiology, 50*, 309.

Fricker, L. D. (1993). Opioid peptide processing enzymes. In A. Herz (Ed.), *Opioids: Vol 104/I. Handbook of experimental pharmacology (p. 529). Berlin: Springer-Verlag.*

Fricker, L. D. (2010). Analysis of mouse brain peptides using mass spectrometry-based peptidomics: Implications for novel functions ranging from non-classical neuropeptides to microproteins. *Molecular BioSystems, 6*, 1355.

Fricker, L. D. (2012). *Neuropeptides and other bioactive peptides.* Charleston, S.C: Morgan & Claypool Life Sciences.

Fricker, L. D., Berman, Y. L., Leiter, E. H., & Devi, L. A. (1996). Carboxypeptidase E activity is deficient in mice with the fat mutation: Effect on peptide processing. *The Journal of Biological Chemistry, 271*. 30619.

Fricker, L. D., & Devi, L. (1994). Enzymes involved in opioid peptide biosynthesis. In L. Tseng (Ed.), *Pharmacology of opioid peptides* (p. 87). Switzerland: Harwood Academic Publishers.

Fricker, L. D., McKinzie, A. A., Sun, J., Curran, E., Qian, Y., Yan, L., et al. (2000). Identification and characterization of proSAAS, a granin-like neuroendocrine peptide precursor that inhibits prohormone processing. *The Journal of Neuroscience, 20*, 639.

Fricker, L. D., Plummer, T. H. J., & Snyder, S. H. (1983). Enkephalin convertase: Potent, selective, and irreversible inhibitors. *Biochemical and Biophysical Research Communications, 111*, 994.

Fricker, L. D., & Snyder, S. H. (1982). Enkephalin convertase: Purification and characterization of a specific enkephalin-synthesizing carboxypeptidase localized to adrenal chromaffin granules. *Proceedings of the National Academy of Sciences of the United States of America, 79*, 3886.

Fricker, L. D., & Snyder, S. H. (1983). Purification and characterization of enkephalin convertase, an enkephalin-synthesizing carboxypeptidase. *The Journal of Biological Chemistry, 258*. 10950.

Gelman, J. S., Dasgupta, S., Berezniuk, I., & Fricker, L. D. (2013). Analysis of peptides secreted from cultured mouse brain tissue. *Biochimica et Biophysica Acta, 1834*, 2408.

Goldstein, A., Tachibana, S., Lowney, L. I., Hunkapiller, M., & Hood, L. (1979). Dynorphin-(1-13), an extraordinarily potent opioid peptide. *Proceedings of the National Academy of Sciences of the United States of America, 76*, 6666.

Gomes, I., Aryal, D. K., Wardman, J. H., Gupta, A., Gagnidze, K., Rodriguiz, R. M., et al. (2013). GPR171 is a hypothalamic G protein-coupled receptor for BigLEN, a neuropeptide involved in feeding. *Proceedings of the National Academy of Sciences of the United States of America, 110*, 16211–16216.

Gomes, I., Bobeck, E. N., Margolis, E. B., Gupta, A., Sierra, S., Fakira, A. K., et al. (2016). Identification of GPR83 as the receptor for the neuroendocrine peptide PEN. *Science Signaling, 9*, ra43.

Gomes, I., Grushko, J. S., Golebiewska, U., Hoogendoorn, S., Gupta, A., Heimann, A. S., et al. (2009). Novel endogenous peptide agonists of cannabinoid receptors. *The FASEB Journal, 23*, 3020.

Heimann, A. S., Gomes, I., Dale, C. S., Pagano, R. L., Gupta, A., de Souza, L. L., et al. (2007). Hemopressin is an inverse agonist of CB1 cannabinoid receptors. *Proceedings of the National Academy of Sciences of the United States of America, 104*. 20588.

Hook, V. Y. H., Eiden, L. E., & Brownstein, M. J. (1982). A carboxypeptidase processing enzyme for enkephalin precursors. *Nature, 295*, 341.

Hughes, J., Smith, T. W., Kosterlitz, H. W., Fothergill, L. A., Morgan, B. A., & Morris, H. R. (1975). Identification of two related pentapeptides from the brain with potent opiate agonist activity. *Nature, 258*, 577.

Husson, S. J., Mertens, I., Janssen, T., Lindemans, M., & Schoofs, L. (2007). Neuropeptidergic signaling in the nematode *Caenorhabditis elegans*. *Progress in Neurobiology, 82*, 33.

Kaspar, A. A., & Reichert, J. M. (2013). Future directions for peptide therapeutics development. *Drug Discovery Today, 18*, 807.

Kimura, S., Lewis, R. V., Stern, A. S., Rossier, J., Stein, S., & Udenfriend, S. (1980). Probable precursors of [Leu]enkephalin and [Met]enkephalin in adrenal medulla: Peptides of 3-5 kilodaltons. *Proceedings of the National Academy of Sciences of the United States of America, 77*, 1681.

Lazarus, L. H., Ling, N., & Guillemin, R. (1976). Beta-Lipotropin as a prohormone for the morphinomimetic peptides endorphins and enkephalins. *Proceedings of the National Academy of Sciences of the United States of America, 73*, 2156.

Levy, M. H. (2001). Advancement of opioid analgesia with controlled-release oxycodone. *European Journal of Pain, 5*(Suppl. A), 113.

Lewis, R. V., Stern, A. S., Kimura, S., Rossier, J., Brink, L., Gerber, L. D., et al. (1980). Opioid peptides and precursors in the adrenal medulla. *Advances in Biochemical Psychopharmacology, 22*, 167.

Lewis, R. V., Stern, A. S., Rossier, J., Stein, S., & Udenfriend, S. (1979). Putative enkephalin precursors in bovine adrenal medulla. *Biochemical and Biophysical Research Communications, 89*, 822.

Li, C. H., Chung, D., & Doneen, B. A. (1976). Isolation, characterization and opiate activity of beta-endorphin from human pituitary glands. *Biochemical and Biophysical Research Communications, 72*, 1542.

Mains, R. E., & Eipper, B. A. (1984). Secretion and regulation of two biosynthetic enzyme activities, peptidyl-glycine alpha-amidating monooxygenase and a carboxypeptidase, by mouse pituitary corticotropic tumor cells. *Endocrinology, 115*, 1683.

Martens, G. J., Braks, J. A., Eib, D. W., Zhou, Y., & Lindberg, I. (1994). The neuroendocrine polypeptide 7B2 is an endogenous inhibitor of prohormone convertase PC2. *Proceedings of the National Academy of Sciences of the United States of America, 91*, 5784.

McKay, T. J., & Plummer, T. H. J. (1978). By-product analogues for bovine carboxypeptidase B. *The Biochemist, 17*, 401.

Morgan, D. J., Wei, S., Gomes, I., Czyzyk, T., Mzhavia, N., Pan, H., et al. (2010). The propeptide precursor proSAAS is involved in fetal neuropeptide processing and body weight regulation. *Journal of Neurochemistry, 113*, 1275.

Muller, T. D., Muller, A., Yi, C. X., Habegger, K. M., Meyer, C. W., Gaylinn, B. D., et al. (2013). The orphan receptor Gpr83 regulates systemic energy metabolism via ghrelin-dependent and ghrelin-independent mechanisms. *Nature Communications, 4*, 1968.

Naggert, J. K., Fricker, L. D., Varlamov, O., Nishina, P. M., Rouille, Y., Steiner, D. F., et al. (1995). Hyperproinsulinemia in obese fat/fat mice associated with a point mutation in the carboxypeptidase E gene and reduced carboxypeptidase E activity in the pancreatic islets. *Nature Genetics, 10*, 135.

Ozawa, A., Lindberg, I., Roth, B., & Kroeze, W. K. (2010). Deorphanization of novel peptides and their receptors. *The AAPS Journal, 12*, 378.

Plummer, T. H. J., & Ryan, T. J. (1981). A potent mercapto bi-product analogue inhibitor for human carboxypeptidase N. *Biochemical and Biophysical Research Communications, 98*, 448.

Preskorn, S. H. (2014). CNS drug development: Lessons from the development of ondansetron, aprepitant, ramelteon, varenicline, lorcaserin, and suvorexant. Part I. *Journal of Psychiatric Practice, 20*, 460.

Qian, Y., Devi, L. A., Mzhavia, N., Munzer, S., Seidah, N. G., & Fricker, L. D. (2000). The C-terminal region of proSAAS is a potent inhibitor of prohormone convertase 1. *The Journal of Biological Chemistry, 275*. 23596.

Qian, Y., Varlamov, O., & Fricker, L. D. (1999). Glu300 of rat carboxypeptidase E is essential for enzymatic activity but not substrate binding or routing to the regulated secretory pathway. *The Journal of Biological Chemistry, 274*. 11582.

Roberts, J. L., & Herbert, E. (1977). Characterization of a common precursor to corticotropin and beta-lipotropin: Identification of beta-lipotropin peptides and their arrangement relative to corticotropin in the precursor synthesized in a cell-free system. *Proceedings of the National Academy of Sciences of the United States of America, 74*, 5300.
Roberts, J. L., Phillips, M., Rosa, P. A., Budarf, M., & Herbert, E. (1979). Processing of common precursor forms of adrenocorticotropin and endorphins in cultures of mouse pituitary cells and in mouse pituitary. *Progress in Clinical and Biological Research, 31*, 761.
Rodriguiz, R. M., Wilkins, J. J., Creson, T. K., Biswas, R., Berezniuk, I., Fricker, A. D., et al. (2013). Emergence of anxiety-like behaviours in depressive-like Cpe(fat/fat) mice. *The International Journal of Neuropsychopharmacology, 16*, 1623.
Rovere, C., Viale, A., Nahon, J., & Kitabgi, P. (1996). Impaired processing of brain proneurotensin and promelanin-concentrating hormone in obese fat/fat mice. *Endocrinology, 137*, 2954.
Smithies, O. (2001). Forty years with homologous recombination. *Nature Medicine, 7*, 1083.
Sobrino Crespo, C., Perianes Cachero, A., Puebla Jimenez, L., Barrios, V., & Arilla Ferreiro, E. (2014). Peptides and food intake. *Frontiers in Endocrinology, 5*, 58.
Song, L., & Fricker, L. D. (1995). Purification and characterization of carboxypeptidase D, a novel carboxypeptidase E-like enzyme, from bovine pituitary. *The Journal of Biological Chemistry, 270*. 25007.
Stern, A. S., Lewis, R. V., Kimura, S., Rossier, J., Gerber, L. D., Brink, L., et al. (1979). Isolation of the opioid heptapeptide Met-enkephalin [Arg6,Phe7] from bovine adrenal medullary granules and striatum. *Proceedings of the National Academy of Sciences of the United States of America, 76*, 6680.
Strand, F. L. (2003). Neuropeptides: General characteristics and neuropharmaceutical potential in treating CNS disorders. *Progress in Drug Research, 61*, 1.
Supattapone, S., Fricker, L. D., & Snyder, S. H. (1984). Purification and characterization of a membrane-bound enkephalin-forming carboxypeptidase, "enkephalin convertase" *Journal of Neurochemistry, 42*, 1017.
Tatemoto, K., Carlquist, M., & Mutt, V. (1982). Neuropeptide Y—A novel brain peptide with structural similarities to peptide YY and pancreatic polypeptide. *Nature, 296*, 659.
Tatemoto, K., Efendic, S., Mutt, V., Makk, G., Feistner, G. J., & Barchas, J. D. (1986). Pancreastatin, a novel pancreatic peptide that inhibits insulin secretion. *Nature, 324*, 476.
Tatemoto, K., Jornvall, H., McDonald, T. J., Carlquist, M., Go, V. L., Johansson, C., et al. (1984). Isolation and primary structure of human PHI (peptide HI). *FEBS Letters, 174*, 258.
Tatemoto, K., Jornvall, H., Siimesmaa, S., Hallden, G., & Mutt, V. (1984). Isolation and characterization of cholecystokinin-58 (CCK-58) from porcine brain. *FEBS Letters, 174*, 289.
Tatemoto, K., Lundberg, J. M., Jornvall, H., & Mutt, V. (1985). Neuropeptide K: Isolation, structure and biological activities of a novel brain tachykinin. *Biochemical and Biophysical Research Communications, 128*, 947.
Tatemoto, K., & Mutt, V. (1980). Isolation of two novel candidate hormones using a chemical method for finding naturally occurring polypeptides. *Nature, 285*, 417.
Tatemoto, K., Rokaeus, A., Jornvall, H., McDonald, T. J., & Mutt, V. (1983). Galanin—A novel biologically active peptide from porcine intestine. *FEBS Letters, 164*, 124.
Varlamov, O., Eng, F. J., Novikova, E. G., & Fricker, L. D. (1999). Localization of metallocarboxypeptidase D in AtT-20 cells: Potential role in prohormone processing. *The Journal of Biological Chemistry, 274*. 14759.
Varlamov, O., & Fricker, L. D. (1998). Intracellular trafficking of metallocarboxypeptidase D in AtT-20 cells: Localization to the trans-Golgi network and recycling from the cell surface. *Journal of Cell Science, 111*, 877.

Varlamov, O., Wu, F., Shields, D., & Fricker, L. D. (1999). Biosynthesis and packaging of carboxypeptidase D into nascent secretory vesicles in pituitary cell lines. *The Journal of Biological Chemistry*, *274*. 14040.
Wang, D., Herman, J. P., Pritchard, L. M., Spitzer, R. H., Ahlbrand, R. L., Kramer, G. L., et al. (2001). Cloning, expression, and regulation of a glucocorticoid-induced receptor in rat brain: Effect of repetitive amphetamine. *The Journal of Neuroscience*, *21*, 9027.
Wardman, J. H., Berezniuk, I., Di, S., Tasker, J. G., & Fricker, L. D. (2011). ProSAAS-derived peptides are colocalized with neuropeptide Y and function as neuropeptides in the regulation of food intake. *PloS One*, *6*. e28152.
Wardman, J. H., Gomes, I., Bobeck, E. N., Stockert, J. A., Kapoor, A., Bisignano, P., et al. (2016). Identification of a small-molecule ligand that activates the neuropeptide receptor GPR171 and increases food intake. *Science Signaling*, *9*, ra55.
Wei, S., Feng, Y., Che, F. Y., Pan, H., Mzhavia, N., Devi, L., et al. (2004). Obesity and diabetes in transgenic mice expressing proSAAS. *The Journal of Endocrinology*, *180*, 357.
Woronowicz, A., Koshimizu, H., Chang, S. Y., Cawley, N. X., Hill, J. M., Rodriguiz, R. M., et al. (2008). Absence of carboxypeptidase E leads to adult hippocampal neuronal degeneration and memory deficits. *Hippocampus*, *18*, 1051.
Xin, X., Varlamov, O., Day, R., Dong, W., Bridgett, M. M., Leiter, E. H., et al. (1997). Cloning and sequence analysis of cDNA encoding rat carboxypeptidase D. *DNA and Cell Biology*, *16*, 897.
Zhang, X., Che, F. Y., Berezniuk, I., Sonmez, K., Toll, L., & Fricker, L. D. (2008). Peptidomics of Cpe(fat/fat) mouse brain regions: Implications for neuropeptide processing. *Journal of Neurochemistry*, *107*, 1596.
Zuhlke, H., Kohnert, K. D., Jahr, H., Schmidt, S., Kirscke, H., & Steiner, D. F. (1977). Proteolytic and transhydrogenolytic activities in isolated pancreatic islets of rats. *Acta Biologica et Medica Germanica*, *36*, 1695.
Zuhlke, H., Steiner, D. F., Lernmark, A., & Lipsey, C. (1976). Carboxypeptidase B-like and trypsin-like activities in isolated rat pancreatic islets. *Ciba Foundation Symposium*, *41*, 183.

CHAPTER SIX

Regulation of Mitochondrial, Cellular, and Organismal Functions by TSPO

Moshe Gavish[1], **Leo Veenman**
Faculty of Medicine, Rappaport Institute, Technion—Israel Institute of Technology, Haifa, Israel
[1]Corresponding author: e-mail address: mgavish@technion.ac.il

Contents

Advances in Pharmacology, Volume 82
ISSN 1054-3589
https://doi.org/10.1016/bs.apha.2017.09.004

Abstract

In 1999, the enigma of the 18 kDa mitochondrial translocator protein (TSPO), also known as the peripheral-type benzodiazepine receptor, was the seeming disparity of the many functions attributed to TSPO, ranging from the potential of TSPO acting as a housekeeping gene at molecular biological levels to adaptations to stress, and even involvement in higher emotional and cognitive functioning, such as anxiety and depression. In the years since then, knowledge regarding the many functions modulated by TSPO has expanded, and understanding has deepened. In addition, new functions could be firmly associated with TSPO, such as regulation of programmed cell death and modulation of gene expression. Interestingly, control by the mitochondrial TSPO over both of these life and death functions appears to include Ca^{++} homeostasis, generation of reactive oxygen species (ROS), and ATP production. Other mitochondrial functions under TSPO control are considered to be steroidogenesis and tetrapyrrole metabolism. As TSPO effects on gene expression and on programmed cell death can be related to the wide range of functions that can be associated with TSPO, several of these five elements of Ca^{++}, ROS, ATP, steroids, and tetrapyrroles may indeed form the basis of TSPO's capability to operate as a multifunctional housekeeping gene to maintain homeostasis of the cell and of the whole multicellular organism.

ABBREVIATIONS

ΔΨm	mitochondrial membrane potential
2-Cl-MGV-1	2-(2-chlorophenyl)quinazolin-4-yl dimethylcarbamate
Complex V	F(o)F(1)-ATP(synth)ase
FGIN-1-27	2-[2-(4-fluorophenyl)-1H-indol-3-yl]-*N,N*-dihexylacetamide
G0	Gap0 quiescence phase of the cell cycle
G1	Gap1 DNA synthesis phase of the cell cycle
G2	Gap2 cell growth phase of the cell cycle
GFAP	glial fibrillary acidic protein
M	mitotic phase of the cell cycle
MGV-1	2-phenylquinazolin-4-yl dimethylcarbamate
NMR	nuclear magnetic resonance
NO	nitric oxide
pDCs	plasmacytoid dendritic cells
PET	positron emission tomography
PK 11195	*N*-butan-2-yl-1-(2-chlorophenyl)-*N*-methylisoquinoline-3-carboxamide
PPIX	protoporphyrin IX
Ro5 4864	7-chloro-5-(4-chlorophenyl)-1-methyl-3*H*-1,4-benzodiazepin-2-one

ROS	reactive oxygen species
RT-PCR	real-time polymerase chain reaction
S	DNA synthesis phase of the cell cycle
siRNA	short interfering RNA
TBI	traumatic brain injury
TSPO	18 kDa translocator protein
TSPO(−/−)	TSPO knockout (mice in this study)

1. INTRODUCTION

The 18 kDa translocator protein (TSPO) was discovered in 1977 (Braestrup & Squires, 1977). TSPO is a widely distributed transmembrane protein that is located mainly in the outer mitochondrial membrane (Anholt, Pedersen, De Souza, & Snyder, 1986; Gavish et al., 1999). TSPO binds to specific synthetic TSPO ligands, including, for example, PK 11195 (IUPAC name: *N*-butan-2-yl-1-(2-chlorophenyl)-*N*-methylisoquinoline-3-carboxamide), Ro5 4864 (IUPAC name: 7-chloro-5-(4-chlorophenyl)-1-methyl-3*H*-1,4-benzodiazepin-2-one), and FGIN-1-27 (IUPAC name: 2-[2-(4-fluorophenyl)-1*H*-indol-3-yl]-*N*,*N*-dihexylacetamide), as well as various endogenous molecules, including, for example, protoporphyrin IX (PPIX) and cholesterol, and several others (Jaipuria et al., 2017; Verma, Nye, & Snyder, 1987; for reviews, see Veenman & Gavish, 2006; Veenman, Vainshtein, Yasin, Azrad, & Gavish, 2016). Many functions are associated directly or indirectly with TSPO, for example, regulation of cholesterol transport, synthesis of steroid hormones, and programmed cell death (for a review, see Papadopoulos et al., 2006). Early on, based on the variety of these functions, it was recognized that there are many potential clinical applications of TSPO modulation, including treatment and diagnosis of cancer, as well as traumatic brain injury (TBI) and neurodegeneration (for a review, see Gavish et al., 1999). As targeting TSPO for therapeutic or diagnostic purposes is typically pharmaceutical, the development of adequate TSPO ligands is of paramount importance (Kim & Pae, 2016a, 2016b). Nonetheless, it should be kept in mind that even the most advanced synthetic ligands also bind to non-TSPO sites, which typically are not well defined (Eberl et al., 2017; Liu et al., 2015; Middleton, Liu, & Banati, 2015; Vicidomini et al., 2015). This caveat always has to be kept in mind when interpreting data from TSPO ligand studies. Having said this, each and every approach may have its own caveats. We ourselves typically applied

TSPO ligands as well as TSPO knockdown by genetic manipulation to validate their effects mutually. We have detailed various findings of these dual studies of these applications of TSPO ligands and TSPO knockdown throughout this review.

Twenty-two years after the discovery of TSPO, the knowledge generated regarding this enigmatic mitochondrial protein and the ensuing questions were formulated concisely in the conclusions of the review of Gavish et al. (1999). We shall shortly recapitulate these points as they gave direction to much of the research regarding TSPO at the beginning of the 21st century, even up to now, and will probably do so for many more years to come. In this review, we hope to show several successful approaches to these questions, including some only established within the last few years. The list of subjects and questions put forward by Gavish et al. (1999) included the following: (1) TSPO as a housekeeping gene; (2) regulation of its own gene expression; (3) TSPO in evolution; (4) its cellular location; and (5) its structure. The (6) primary mechanisms for TSPO's many functions include but are not restricted to: (7) cellular functions; (8) mitochondrial cholesterol transport; (9) steroidogenesis; (10) cell proliferation; (11) immune response; and (12) tumorigenicity. The influence of TSPO on (13) whole organisms includes effects on: (14) stress disorders; (15) anxiety disorders; (16) neurodegenerative disorders; (17) neurotoxic effects; and (18) traumatic–ischemic brain damage. TSPO is a target for (19) diagnosis and (20) medical interventions. (21) New functions are related to TSPO. In this review we hope to deal with a few of these subjects and questions.

2. TSPO AS A HOUSEKEEPING GENE

It has been pointed out previously that the *TSPO* gene appears to have the hallmarks of a typical housekeeping gene, suggesting that TSPO has a basic cellular function (Gavish et al., 1999; Weisinger et al., 2004). In molecular biology, housekeeping genes are typically constitutive genes that are required for the maintenance of basic cellular function and are expressed in all cells of an organism under normal and pathophysiological conditions. Such functions can include programmed cell death and regulation of gene expression (e.g., Kusumawidjaja et al., 2007; Morrow & Tanguay, 2012). One novel basic cellular function of TSPO was recently found to be mitochondrial signaling for the regulation of cell nuclear gene expression (Bode et al., 2014; Veenman et al., 2012; Yasin et al., 2017). Another basic TSPO function is regulation of programmed cell death, now well established

(Caballero, Veenman, & Gavish, 2013; Veenman, Gavish, & Kugler, 2014). It can be safely assumed that Ca^{++} transport over the mitochondrial membrane, mitochondrial reactive oxygen species (ROS) generation, and mitochondrial ATP production all present core mechanisms that are part of TSPO functions related to modulation of gene expression and programmed cell death (Gomes et al., 2013; Li et al., 2011; Parikh, Morgan, Scott, Clements, & Butow, 1987; Veenman et al., 2010; Yasin et al., 2017; Zeno, Zaaroor, Leschiner, Veenman, & Gavish, 2009). We postulate that these housekeeping characteristics of the TSPO gene and protein serve to maintain homeostasis of the cell and the organism. See Section 8 for discussion of this maintenance of homeostasis, and the other sections for the description of the various conditions where such maintenance of homeostasis is relevant. In the appropriate sections, we discuss these TSPO functions of modulation of gene expression and programmed cell death underlying TSPO's postulated function as a housekeeping gene and protein.

2.1 TSPO and Gene Expression

To study the ability of TSPO to regulate gene expression, especially regarding known TSPO functions, we applied microarray analysis of gene expression to U118MG glioblastoma cells. In particular, we exposed U118MG cells to the classical TSPO ligand PK 11195 at a concentration of 25 μM (Yasin et al., 2017), and the novel TSPO ligand 2-Cl-MGV-1 (2-(2-chlorophenyl)quinazolin-4-yl dimethylcarbamate) at the concentrations of 50 and 100 μM (Gavish et al., 2017; Yasin et al., 2017). In this time response study, within 15 min we observed changes in expression of immediate early genes and transcription factors. At later time points up to 24 h of PK 11195 exposure, the changes in gene expression related to well-known TSPO functions, including cell viability, proliferation, differentiation, adhesion, migration, tumorigenesis, and angiogenesis (Yasin et al., 2017). At even later time points (48 h of PK 11195 exposure), and also with TSPO knockdown application, our observations included changes in gene expression similar to those within 24 h of PK 11195 exposure, in addition to numerous others (Bode et al., 2014; Veenman et al., 2012; Yasin et al., 2017). Recent studies by others also suggested changes in gene expression effected by TSPO ligands. For example, data from Feng et al. (2017) showed that the TSPO ligand vinpocetine significantly downregulated the expression of CD40, CD80, and CD86, and increased the expression of TSPO in plasmacytoid dendritic cells (pDCs). In 2017 it was reported that the TSPO ligands

FGIN-1-27 and Ro5 4864 suppressed cytokine and interferon γ production in a dose-dependent manner by purified human $CD4^+$ T-cells from peripheral blood mononuclear cells (PBMCs) (Zhang, Yu, Li, Yang, & Wu, 2017). Thus, apart from its relation to differentiation, TSPO also appear to be able to regulate gene expression in relation to inflammation and immune response (Feng et al., 2017; Yasin et al., 2017; Zhang et al., 2017). As mentioned earlier we postulated that ROS, generation, ATP production, and Ca^{++} levels were important factors underlying the regulation of cell nuclear gene expression by mitochondrial TSPO (Yasin et al., 2017). It would be worthwhile to intensify studies regarding ROS generation, ATP production, and Ca^{++} levels, including measuring levels of calcium-binding proteins such as calmodulin and calcineurin, as these appear to be intermediaries between TSPO and its ability to regulate homeostasis.

2.2 Programmed Cell Death

In studies published in 2004 and 2005 we showed that TSPO knockdown and TSPO ligands could reduce programmed cell death rates (Levin et al., 2005; Veenman et al., 2004). While such findings were not uncommon (Bono, Lamarche, Prabonnaud, Le Fur, & Herbert, 1999; Obame, Zini, Souktani, Berdeaux, & Morin, 2007), the prevailing assumption was that TSPO ligands would commonly induce programmed cell death, instead of preventing cell death (Papadopoulos et al., 2006, 1999; Santidrián et al., 2007). In 2007, with an extensive overview of TSPO research focusing on cell death, we showed that programmed cell death induced by TSPO ligands was concentration-dependent. The same study showed that the effectiveness of TSPO knockdown appeared to predict resulting changes in programmed cell death rates (Veenman, Papadopoulos, & Gavish, 2007). In particular, at nM concentrations, the TSPO-specific ligands, PK 11195 and Ro5 4864, appear to be antiapoptotic. At concentrations in the μM range, in general >50 μM of PK 11195 and Ro5 4864 were proapoptotic. Knockdown of TSPO by genetic manipulation, giving a reduction by more than 50% in [^{3}H]PK 11195 binding, resulted in antiapoptotic effects, suggesting a potential proapoptotic function of TSPO (Veenman et al., 2007). Finally, in this overview of TSPO research up to 2007, a reduction of more than 70% of TSPO abundance was found to cause cell death (Veenman et al., 2007). Studying the effects of TSPO ligands, in particular PK 11195, Ro5 4864, and FGIN-1-27, on cell death of U118MG cells induced by ammonium chloride, we found that at nM concentrations, these TSPO ligands were antiapoptotic and at μM concentrations, they were proapoptotic (Caballero, Veenman, Bode, Leschiner, & Gavish, 2014). It is plausible that apoptotic effects at relatively high concentrations are due to other "nonspecific" TSPO receptors that bind to even the most sophisticated TSPO ligands, as discussed in Section 1. Nowadays, it is also more and more realized that relatively low-affinity TSPO ligands (e.g., curcumin, Etifoxine, 2-Cl-MGV-1, 7e) [7e is a 2-(2-aryloxyphenyl)-1,4-dihydroisoquinolin-3(2*H*)-one derivative] are more effective at inducing a beneficial physiological effect than high-affinity ligands are (Costa et al., 2017; Eckert et al., 2013; Elkamhawy et al., 2017; Vainshtein et al., 2015; Veenman, Vainshtein, & Gavish, 2015). As it was realized that concentration-dependent TSPO ligands could prevent programmed cell death, we undertook a research project to investigate the molecular biological mechanisms that may underlie TSPO's initiation of programmed cell death. Basically, first of all we further established that TSPO knockdown as well as TSPO ligands indeed reduced apoptotic rates (Kugler et al., 2008; Levin et al., 2005; Shoukrun et al., 2008; Veenman et al., 2004, 2007). After establishing the consistency of the effect of TSPO knockdown and TSPO ligands on the reduction of programmed cell death rates, we investigated and revealed that TSPO regulated the mitochondrial membrane potential ($\Delta\Psi m$) (Shoukrun et al., 2008; Veenman, Shandalov, & Gavish, 2008), mitochondrial ROS generation (Shargorodsky et al., 2012; Zeno et al., 2009), ATP production (Rosenberg et al., 2011; Rosenberg, Rosenberg, Weizman, Veenman, & Gavish, 2013; Rosenberg, Rosenberg, Weizman, Veenman, & Gavish, 2014; Veenman et al., 2010), mitochondrial cardiolipin oxidation (Zeno et al., 2009), release of cytochrome *c* from peroxidized cardiolipins out of the mitochondria into the cytosol and caspase activation (Kugler et al., 2008), and DNA fragmentation and cell morphological signs of apoptosis (Levin et al., 2005; Veenman et al., 2004; Zeno et al., 2009). We also found that TSPO could regulate expression of genes coding for proteins associated with apoptotic processes (Yasin et al., 2017). With the last study it was also realized that: (1) exchange of Ca^{++} across the outer mitochondrial membrane; (2) mitochondrial ROS generation; and (3) mitochondrial ATP production were processes driving both initiation of programmed cell death and modulation of gene expression. By searching through the available information regarding this subject, it can be postulated that substantial enhancement of exchange of Ca^{++}, mitochondrial ROS generation, and mitochondrial ATP production can lead to programmed cell death, while less intensive effects can lead to changes in gene expression (Gomes et al., 2013; Parikh et al., 1987; Wu, Kazumura, Maruyama, Osawa, & Naoi, 2015). Indeed, it is worthwhile to invest in research concerning the subjects of ROS, ATP, and Ca^{++} in this respect. A number of recent reviews have summarized and systemized the findings in the field of TSPO—programmed cell death research (Caballero et al., 2013; Gatliff & Campanella, 2016; Morin, Musman, Pons, Berdeaux, & Ghaleh, 2016; Repalli, 2014; Veenman et al., 2014). TSPO's capacity to regulate programmed cell death, in association with modulation of components of the mitochondrial respiratory chain, appears to be one of TSPO's most basic functions. This is also suggested by the evolutionary development of TSPO's interactions with its host cells (Veenman, Denora, Rosenberg, & Gavish, 2017; Veenman et al., 2016), as will be described later in this chapter.

3. TSPO IN EVOLUTION

TSPO gene is conserved throughout evolution from prokaryotes to eukaryotes, including in humans (Busch & Montgomery, 2017; Gavish et al., 1999; Veenman et al., 2017, 2016). The oldest remnants of eukaryotes, which are spheroidal and cupshaped, carbonaceous alga-like bodies, occur in sedimentary rocks of the Onverwacht Series (Swaziland System) in South Africa (Engel et al., 1968). The basal Onverwacht sediments lie approximately 10,000 m stratigraphically below the Fig Tree sedimentary rocks of South Africa (>3.100 million years old) where spheroidal microfossils (*Archaeosphaeroides barbertonensis*) present unicellular alga-like photosynthetic organisms (Schopf & Barghoorn, 1967). These alga-like spheroids of the Fig Tree and Onverwacht sediments are among the oldest fossil organisms now known (Engel et al., 1968; Leister, 2016). This indicates that the endosymbiosis between eukaryotes and prokaryotes was already established in the Mesoarchean eon.

4. TSPO AND MITOCHONDRIAL AND CELLULAR FUNCTIONS

4.1 TSPO–Tetrapyrrole Interaction

TSPO and tetrapyrroles regulate each other (Veenman et al., 2016). For example, by exposing cells of the U118MG glioblastoma cell line to PPIX in culture, we found that TSPO knockdown by stable transfection of TSPO silencing siRNA vectors into U118MG cells leads to mitochondrial PPIX accumulation (Zeno et al., 2012). The prevention of PPIX accumulation by TSPO was not due to conversion of PPIX to heme in the sham control cells (Zeno et al., 2012). We assumed that ROS generation under control of

TSPO could serve to metabolize PPIX in mitochondria. As in mitochondria, in bacteria TSPO is located in the outer membrane. It was reported that *Bacillus cereus* TSPO-mediated PPIX reactions included catalytic degradation of PPIX to a previously undescribed heme derivative (Guo et al., 2015). These authors concluded that the catalytic activity in PPIX degradation suggests physiological importance for TSPOs in protection against oxidative stress. Furthermore, PPIX can act as a TSPO ligand and modulate various cellular functions (Rosenberg et al., 2013). It has been suggested that TSPO may transport tetrapyrroles (Balsemão-Pires et al., 2011). TSPO–tetrapyrrole interactions may be part of the establishment of the bacterial–eukaryote relationships, i.e., mitochondrial–eukaryote and plastid–plant endosymbiotic relationships (Veenman et al., 2017, 2016).

4.2 Metabolism

Recent studies have reported changes in glucose homeostasis and cellular energy production when TSPO function is modulated by selective ligands (Gut, 2015; Veenman et al., 2016). For example, in a series of studies (Rosenberg et al., 2011, 2013, 2014), we found in cultured primary human osteoblasts, following exposure to 10 μM of PPIX, that cellular fludeoxyglucose (^{18}F) (INN) (^{18}F-FDG) incorporation, mitochondrial mass, and ATP content were suppressed, which was indicative of reduced metabolism (Rosenberg et al., 2013). We also found that the TSPO ligands PK 11195, Ro5 4864, and FGIN-1-27 when applied at a concentration of 10 μM did not exert the exact same effects as PPIX in the primary osteoblast cell culture (Rosenberg et al., 2011, 2013, 2014). For example, PK 11195 did not significantly affect ^{18}F-FDG incorporation. There was also an increase in mitochondrial mass and mitochondrial ATP content. It is considered that the functional differences may be due to the structural differences between PPIX, Ro5 4864, PK 11195, and FGIN-1-27, as well as the different binding sites for PPIX and the synthetic TSPO ligands Ro5 4864, PK 11195, and FGIN-1-27 (as concluded from an overview by Veenman et al., 2016). In a more recent study, it was demonstrated that TSPO gene insertion causes increased transcription of genes involved in the mitochondrial electron transport chain, as well as increased mitochondrial ATP production (Liu et al., 2017).

4.3 Generation of ROS and Oxidative Stress

One of the functions mentioned above (ROS generation/oxidative stress), first of all, is the effects on free radical generation by TSPO ligands as, for example, studied in cultured neural cells, including primary cultures of rat brain astrocytes and neurons as well as cells of the murine BV-2 microglial cell line (Jayakumar, Panickar, & Norenberg, 2002). In this study, free radical production was measured at the time points of 2, 30, 60, and 120 min of treatment with the TSPO ligands PK 11195, Ro5 4864, and PPIX, all at a concentration of 10 nM. For example, in astrocytes, all ligands showed a significant increase in free radical production at 2 min. Later TSPO knockdown studies including comparisons with PK 11195 treatment further elucidated the functional implications of this ROS generation via TSPO (Zeno et al., 2009). In this study, we demonstrated that this TSPO function was essential for programmed cell death induction by $CoCl_2$ (Zeno et al., 2009). Subsequently, we found this also to be true, for example, for nitric oxide (NO) and glutamate (Shargorodsky et al., 2012; Vainshtein et al., 2015). In short, our various studies showed that TSPO ligands and TSPO knockdown attenuated ROS generation, cardiolipin oxidation, collapse of the $\Delta\Psi m$, and induction of programmed cell death by these otherwise lethal agents (reviewed by Caballero et al., 2013; Veenman et al., 2014).

4.4 The Mitochondrial Respiratory Chain

As it is well known that TSPO modulates ROS generation, it is important to know how TSPO can affect the mitochondrial respiratory chain. It was found that TSPO mediates inhibition of mitochondrial respiratory control (Hirsch, Beyer, Malkowitz, Beer, & Blume, 1989). In this context, Krestinina et al. (2009) found in isolated rat brain mitochondria that TSPO ligands and TSPO antibodies appeared to affect the structure and function of the mitochondrial F(o)F(1)-ATP(synth)ase (complex V of the mitochondrial respiration chain) (see Section 4.5). At the same time, we investigated the role of the mitochondrial F(o)F(1)-ATP(synth)ase in association with TSPO in U87MG and U118MG human glioblastoma cell lines (Veenman et al., 2010). For example, oligomycin and piceatannol were studied as inhibitors of the F(o) and F(1) subunits of F(o)F(1)-ATP (synth)ase, respectively. Oligomycin attenuated reductions in cellular ATP levels otherwise induced via TSPO, while piceatannol did not. Thus, our findings strongly pointed to a role for the F(o) subunit of the mitochondrial F(o)F(1)-ATP(synth)ase in interactions between TSPO and complex V (Veenman et al., 2010). Later, our findings were corroborated in dissociated brain cells isolated from SAMP8 mice showing significantly reduced levels of matrix metalloproteinases (MMP) and ATP, probably due to significantly diminished complex V protein expression, and increased expression of TSPO (Eckert et al., 2013). Treatment of SAMP8 mice with curcumin enhanced MMP and ATP levels and restored mitochondrial fusion, probably by upregulating nuclear factor PGC1α protein expression (Eckert et al., 2013). Curcumin binds to the TSPO dimer with low μM affinity (Li, Xia, Meiler, & Ferguson-Miller, 2013).

4.5 Phosphorylation and Nitrosylation

Phosphorylation of proteins via TSPO modulation may be one mechanism whereby TSPO can affect cellular function. We emphasize here one study that implicates phosphorylation of subunit c of F(o)F(1)-ATPase via TSPO (Krestinina et al., 2009). We assume that this is one essential factor for the initiation of various downstream functions such as modulation of programmed cell death and regulation of nuclear gene expression (Veenman et al., 2010; Yasin et al., 2017; Zhang & Moye-Rowley, 2001). In particular, Krestinina et al. (2009) found that 100 nM of the synthetic TSPO ligand Ro5 4864 and 1 μM of the endogenous TSPO ligand PPIX promoted reduction of the $\Delta\Psi m$, while 100 nM of PK 11195 suppressed this reduction of the $\Delta\Psi m$. In mitochondria from an intact brain, incorporation of [γ-^{32}P]ATP into a specific 3.5 kDa peptide (subunit c of F(o)F(1)-ATPase) was decreased in the presence of Ro5 4864 and PPIX, and increased in the presence of PK 11195. At threshold Ca^{++} concentrations leading to $\Delta\Psi m$ reductions, TSPO ligands were found to stimulate dephosphorylation of this 3.5 kDa peptide (Krestinina et al., 2009). For more general functions, subject to TSPO-dependent phosphorylation/dephosphorylation such as inflammatory and immune response, the TSPO ligands PK 11195, Ro5 4864, and FGIN-1-27 can downregulate phosphorylation of STAT1, STAT4, and STAT5 (Zhang et al., 2017). Regarding S-nitrosylation of proteins, we found that the nitric oxide donor, sodium nitroprusside, requires TSPO to induce cell death, but although various proteins were found to be S-nitrosylated in this study, TSPO itself was not nitrosylated (Shargorodsky et al., 2012).

4.6 Steroidogenesis

One of TSPO's well-studied putative functions is its rate-limiting effect on steroidogenesis (Krueger & Papadopoulos, 1992). This rate-limiting step is considered to be based on regulation of cholesterol transport by TSPO from the cytoplasm to the mitochondrial matrix (Krueger & Papadopoulos, 1990).

It appears that binding of cholesterol to TSPO's cholesterol-recognition motif leads to structural changes across the protein that shift the dynamic equilibrium toward the translocator monomer (Jaipuria et al., 2017).

Several proteins interacting with TSPO have been hypothesized to play a role in steroidogenesis (Papadopoulos et al., 2015). These proteins include: (1) VDAC (McEnery, Snowman, Trifiletti, & Snyder, 1992); (2) DBI (Besman et al., 1989); (3) acyl-CoA-binding domain 3 (ACBD3) protein (Li et al., 2001); (4) a protein kinase A (PKA) anchor protein; and (5) two members of the 14-3-3 protein family of cellular. Interestingly, steroidogenic acute regulatory protein (StAR) and VDAC interaction have also been demonstrated, suggesting a role of VDAC in mediating mitochondrial cholesterol (Bose, Whittal, Miller, & Bose, 2008). Intermolecular interactions of all these proteins remain an open area of research, with TSPO–VDAC interactions independently corroborated several times (Anholt et al., 1986; Garnier et al., 1994). However, investigations of TSPO–StAR molecular interactions yielded mixed results (Bogan, Davis, & Niswender, 2007; West et al., 2001). In general, controversies regarding TSPO involvement in steroidogenesis remain (Selvaraj, Tu, & Stocco, 2016). For example, it was found that TSPO knockout TSPO(−/−) mice survived, and examination of adrenal and gonadal steroidogenesis showed no defects in TSPO(−/−) mice (Tu et al., 2014). In another study, in an attempt to reconcile discrepancies between physiological and pharmacological interpretations of TSPO function, TSPO knockout MA-10 mouse Leydig tumor cells (MA-10:TspoΔ/Δ) were generated, and their steroidogenic potential after exposure to either dibutyryl-cAMP or PK 11195 was determined (Tu, Zhao, Stocco, & Selvaraj, 2015). In these cells, progesterone production after dibutyryl-cAMP was not different from control MA-10:Tspo +/+ cells, giving a further indication that TSPO function is not essential for steroidogenesis. Interestingly, when treated with increasing concentrations of PK 11195, both control MA-10:Tspo +/+ cells and MA-10:TspoΔ/Δ cells responded in a similar dose-dependent manner, showing increases in progesterone production. Tu et al. (2015) concluded that PK 11195 effect on steroidogenesis is not mediated via TSPO. Nonetheless, as redundancy and degeneracy are typical for biological systems, compensatory mechanisms cannot be excluded, i.e., when TSPO is intact, we do not exclude the possibility that TSPO may very well be involved in steroidogenesis (Middleton et al., 2015; Yasin et al., 2017).

Interestingly, in addition to TSPO's intensively studied putative role in the modulation of steroid production (Liere, Pianos, Oudinet, Schumacher, & Akwa, 2017), our studies showed that steroids affect TSPO expression

(Bar-Ami, Fares, & Gavish, 1989; Gavish, 1995; Veenman & Gavish, 2012). In general, steroid–TSPO interactions are thought to be part of adaptations to stress, and responses to injury, including brain injury (Lehmann et al., 1999; Wolf et al., 2015). It is thought that modulation of neurosteroidogenesis via TSPO ligands may be neuroprotective, neurotrophic, and antiapoptotic in relation to neurodegenerative diseases (Porcu et al., 2016). Steroid–TSPO interactions may also be essential for reproductive events (Lassance, Haghiac, Minium, Catalano, & Hauguel-de Mouzon, 2015).

5. TSPO AND DEVELOPMENTAL PROCESSES

5.1 Cell Cycle

The TSPO ligand PK 11195 induces apoptosis and cell cycle arrest in pre- and postrelapse neuroblastoma cell lines (Mendonça-Torres & Roberts, 2013). In the MCF-7 breast carcinoma cell line, we found that at concentrations of 10–100 μM, PK 11195 and Ro5 4864 induced an accumulation of MCF-7 cells in the G0/G1 and G2/M phases of the cell cycle (Carmel et al., 1999). In other studies by us, knockdown of TSPO and TSPO ligands enhanced tumorigenicity in the C6 glioma cell lines, including reduced programmed cell death rates and increased proliferation (Levin et al., 2005; Veenman et al., 2004). Later we found that induction of apoptosis by TSPO ligands is concentration-dependent (Caballero et al., 2014; Kugler et al., 2008; Veenman et al., 2007). We studied this in detail in the U118MG cell line, applying PK 11195, Ro5 4864, and FGIN-1-27 as TSPO ligands, showing that at nM concentrations these TSPO ligands were antiapoptotic and at μM concentrations they were proapoptotic (Caballero et al., 2014). In one of our projects, to study gene expression, we exposed U118MG glioblastoma cells to PK 11195 at a concentration of 25 μM (for 24 and 48 h) and we also subjected U118MG glioblastoma cells to permanent TSPO silencing by siRNA (TSPO knockdown). In this project, we applied microarray analysis of gene expression, followed up by validation with real-time polymerase chain reaction (RT-PCR), and showed effects on gene expression related to the cell cycle, including programmed cell death (Bode et al., 2014). Applying a twofold cutoff to microarray analysis, followed up by RT-PCR analysis, revealed five genes related to the cell cycle under TSPO control in this study (Bode et al., 2014). Interestingly, taking a 2.5-fold cutoff, only gene expression of v-FOS was found to be modulated by both of the PK 11195 exposures and also the TSPO knockdown. Focusing further on the cell cycle: (1) TSPO silencing increased numbers of cells in the S (to 321%) and G2/M (to 131%) phases, and caused a decrease in the G0/G1 phase (to 69%); (2) 24 h of PK 11195 exposure caused decreases in the S (to 81%) and G2/M (to 94%) phases, and an increase in the G0/G1 (to 112%) phase; and (3) 48 h of PK 11195 exposure caused decreases in the S (to 70%) and G0/G1 (to 96%) phases, and an increase in the G2/M (to 124%) phase (Bode et al., 2014; Veenman et al., 2012). Thus, TSPO appeared to provide regulation of the cell cycle via specific modulation of gene expression for key gene products in these glioblastoma cells (Bode et al., 2014). In a follow-up study regarding the cell cycle and immediate early genes, we thoroughly investigated gene expression modulation via TSPO in a time response fashion (Yasin et al., 2017). This showed that TSPO can indeed regulate the cell cycle by modulating gene expression, including modulation of expression of immediately early genes and of genes coding for proteins regulating the cell cycle.

5.2 TSPO and Cell Proliferation

In a study of TSPO expression in different glioblastoma cell lines, we showed that relatively high expression of TSPO correlated with high proliferation rates (Veenman et al., 2004). We also applied TSPO ligands and TSPO knockdown to C6 cells, and found that this increased proliferation rates, as assessed by anchorage-independent growth (Levin et al., 2005; Veenman et al., 2004). In the MCF-7 breast carcinoma cell line, we found that at concentrations of 10–100 μM, PK 11195 and Ro5 4864 inhibited cell proliferation (Carmel et al., 1999). In implant models of mouse brain and chicken embryo chorioallantois, TSPO knockdown as well as TSPO ligands could promote proliferation and migration of glioblastoma cells (Bode et al., 2012). Regarding immune response, TSPO ligands suppressed cell proliferation and activation of $CD4^+$ T-cells by the inhibition of T-cell receptor signal transduction including membrane proteins: Zap, Lck, Src; cytoplasm proteins: Plcγ1, Slp-76, ERK, JNK; and the nucleoproteins: c-Jun and c-Fos (Zhang et al., 2017). Furthermore, it was found recently that insertion of the TSPO gene in Jurkat cells (the immortalized line of human T lymphocyte cells) resulted in increases in cell proliferation and motility, which were inhibited by PK 11195 (Liu et al., 2017). Regarding the different outcomes of the studies presented earlier; on the one hand the different findings between the various studies may be due to use of different cell strains and/or different research models; on the other hand it is becoming more and more recognized that TSPO exerts homeostatic functions, implying it can upregulate as well as downregulate specific mechanisms and functions, depending on the context (Caballero et al., 2014; Nagler et al., 2010; Veenman et al., 2007; Yasin et al., 2017). In the study of Nagler et al. (2010) we found that tumors and their healthy tissue environments display different TSPO responses to particular challenges, such as cigarette smoke exposure. For a more detailed discussion of homeostatic TSPO functions, see Section 8.

5.3 TSPO and Differentiation

In addition to proliferation, we found that classical and novel TSPO ligands induced neuronal differentiation of cells of the PC12 cell line, which is of pheochromocytoma origin, presenting cells with neuronal characteristics (Vainshtein et al., 2015; Veenman et al., 2015; Yasin et al., 2017). This included outgrowth of neurites, tubulin expression, and NeuN expression. However, in relation to immune response, the TSPO ligands, FGIN-1-27, and Ro5 4864 can inhibit differentiation of naïve $CD4^+$ T-cells into Th1 cells by suppressing the activity of the corresponding transcription factors (Zhang et al., 2017). This contrast between cells of the immune system and other types of cells is reminiscent of similarly contrasting observations presented in the previous section.

5.4 TSPO and Adhesion, Migration, and Angiogenesis

We have found that TSPO ligands as well as TSPO knockdown could modulate processes such as adhesion, migration, and angiogenesis that may contribute to differentiation of cells and tissue (Bode et al., 2012). In another study, to elucidate the functional role of TSPO on vascular endothelial cell activation, it was found that adenoviral TSPO overexpression [10–100 MOI (multiplicities of infection)] inhibited phorbol 12-myristate 13-acetate (PMA)-induced vascular cell adhesion molecule-1 (VCAM-1) and intracellular cell adhesion molecule-1 (ICAM-1) expression in a dose-dependent manner (Joo et al., 2015). It was concluded that mitochondrial TSPO can inhibit PMA-induced endothelial inflammation via suppression of VCAM-1 and mitochondrial ROS production in endothelial cells. A recent gene expression study by us suggested that PK 11195 can modulate adhesion, migration, and angiogenesis by regulation of gene expression via mitochondria to cell nucleus signaling (Yasin et al., 2017).

5.5 TSPO in Reproductive Processes and Embryonic Development

Elevated TSPO mRNA and protein expression can be detected at specific steps of germ cell development in rats (Manku, Wang, Thuillier, Rhodes, & Culty, 2012). For example, in fetal and neonatal gonocytes, TSPO appears to be mainly nuclear. TSPO is present in pachytene spermatocytes and dividing spermatogonia in prepubertal testes, and in adult testes in pachytene spermatocyte, round spermatid nuclei, and mitotic spermatogonia. This TSPO expression suggests that TSPO might play a role in spermatogonial mitosis (Manku et al., 2012). We found that testosterone levels serve to maintain TSPO levels in Cowper's gland of the male reproductive tract (Weizman, Amiri, Katz, Snyder, & Gavish, 1992). In female rats, TSPO expression increases in the ovaries and uterus of pregnant rats (Weizman, Dagan, Snyder, & Gavish, 1997). In another study, in pseudopregnant rats we found a twofold increase in ovarian TSPO-binding capacity and a threefold increase in TSPO-binding capacity in the uterus (Bar-Ami et al., 2006).

Surprisingly, after all of this being said in the preceding sections, TSPO knockout does not appear to have major effects on embryonic development. For example, Tu et al. (2014) and Zhao et al. (2016) reported that TSPO (−/−) mice survived with no apparent phenotypic abnormalities and were fertile. The same was true for subsequent TSPO knockout mouse studies, although here in adult-aged mice, changes in phenotype could be detected. For example, the GuwiyangWurra mouse showed that microglia of this knockout produced significantly less ATP (Banati et al., 2014; Liu et al., 2017; Middleton et al., 2015). In a study of Daugherty, Chechneva, Mayrhofer, and Deng (2016) their TSPO −/− mouse showed a decrease in GFAP expression, correlating with a decrease in astrogliosis in response to neural injury during experimental autoimmune encephalomyelitis. In one study it was argued that TSPO knockout impaired preimplantation embryo development and ACTH-stimulated steroid biosynthesis (Fan, Campioli, Midzak, Culty, & Papadopoulos, 2015). However, in a similar TSPO knockout model, the outcomes were more similar to those of Tu et al. (2014) and Zhao et al. (2016), but not to those of Fan et al. (2015), as reported by Wang et al. (2016). Thus, it appears that TSPO is more important for responses to various phenomena in adulthood (as studied in mice so far) than it is needed for embryonic development.

6. PRIMARY MECHANISMS UNDERLYING TSPO's VARIOUS FUNCTIONS

While many functions have been attributed to TSPO, the underlying primary mechanisms were an enigma (Gavish et al., 1999). Subsequent research elucidated several of the questions.

6.1 TSPO Structure

To understand TSPO function better, the structure of TSPO was presented as a major subject in need of thorough research (Gavish et al., 1999). In 2014, a three-dimensional high-resolution structure of mammalian TSPO was presented in a complex with its high-affinity ligand PK 11195 for the first time (Jaremko, Jaremko, Giller, Becker, & Zweckstetter, 2014). This TSPO-PK 11195 structure is described as a tight bundle of five transmembrane α helices that form a hydrophobic pocket accepting PK 11195. Ligand-induced stabilization of the structure of TSPO suggested a molecular mechanism for modulation of TSPO function (Jaremko et al., 2014). The new structural evidence of various studies reviewed by Li et al. (2016) implies that cholesterol and porphyrin are bound at two distinct binding sites. Yet it should be noted that cholesterol synthesis and further conversion to steroid hormones depend on heme-containing enzymes, suggesting a possible interplay between the development of cholesterol-binding and porphyrin-binding capacities in TSPO (Li et al., 2016). Residue-specific analysis of TSPO by solid-state NMR spectroscopy revealed a dynamic monomer–dimer equilibrium of TSPO in the membrane (Jaipuria et al., 2017). It was found in this study that binding of cholesterol to TSPO's cholesterol-recognition motif leads to structural changes that shift the dynamic equilibrium toward the translocator monomer.

6.2 Cellular Location

Questions regarding TSBO's cellular location ranged from mitochondrial to nuclear. While TSPO's primary location is mitochondria (Anholt et al., 1986), other locations are not uncommon. For example, in fetal and neonatal gonocytes, TSPO appears to be mainly nuclear (Manku et al., 2012). Recently, a novel finding was that under the influence of ligands, the location of TSPO together with its mitochondria can change from evenly spread throughout the cytosol to more perinuclear locations (Yasin et al., 2017).

6.3 Regulation of TSPO Gene Expression

To understand the molecular mechanisms that regulate TSPO expression in human breast cancer cells, the TSPO promoter was identified, cloned, and functionally characterized, including its transcriptional regulation in: (1) poor-in-TSPO hormone-dependent, nonaggressive MCF-7 cells; and (2) rich-in-TSPO hormone-independent, aggressive, and metastatic MDA-MB-231 breast cancer cells (Batarseh, Barlow, Martinez-Arguelles, & Papadopoulos, 2012). Nonetheless, regulation of TSPO gene transcription is still in need of further research (Fan & Papadopoulos, 2012).

7. RESPONSE TO INJURY AND DISEASE

7.1 TSPO as a Target for Diagnosis and Medical Interventions

It is now well recognized that TSPO presents a primary target for diagnosis and medical interventions for various injuries and diseases (Kim & Pae, 2016a, 2016b; Taliani, Da Settimo, Da Pozzo, Chelli, & Martini, 2009). Already in 1996 PK 11195 was proposed as a potential drug for neurodegenerative diseases (Gee, 1996). It is considered that TSPO ligands may be effective against malaria, as they can kill *Plasmodium falciparum* and *Toxoplasma gondii* in vitro (Dzierszinski et al., 2002). By applying Ro5 4864 to rats, it was suggested that TSPO is involved in the development and maintenance of inflammatory pain behaviors (Hernstadt, Wang, Lim, & Mao, 2009). It was also recognized that TSPO qualifies as a target for innovative diagnostic and therapeutic approaches for cancer treatment (Maaser et al., 2005). For example, in Unio Internationale Contra Cancrum (UICC) III colorectal cancers, a high level of TSPO overexpression correlated with poor prognosis (Maaser et al., 2005). In 2006, positron emission tomography (PET) scans were applied to patients with hepatic encephalopathy (HE) (Iversen, Hansen, Bender, Rodell, & Munk, 2006). However, at that time the results could not confirm the hypothesis of increased TSPO in patients with HE. Nonetheless, over the years the usefulness of TSPO-PET imaging and its clinical impact in neurodegenerative diseases has improved considerably (Dupont et al., 2017). The review by Dupont and colleagues discusses the application of TSPO PET to patients with Parkinson's disease, Huntington's disease, dementia, amyotrophic lateral sclerosis, multiple sclerosis, and psychiatric disorders (Dupont et al., 2017). The usefulness of TSPO-PET imaging appeared self-evident over the years, offering better understanding of neuroinflammation in CNS disorders. TSPO-PET imaging can also be applied to arthritis (Gent et al., 2014). Nonetheless, it has not yet found its way into the clinic as a routine tool for diagnosis, development of therapeutic strategies, and posttreatment assessments (Dupont et al., 2017).

7.2 TSPO and Inflammatory and Immune Response

In several studies on the cardiovascular system it could be seen that TSPO ligands can affect inflammatory and immune responses (for a review, see Veenman & Gavish, 2006). More recent studies give some more details regarding the involvement of TSPO in inflammatory and immune responses. Data from Feng et al. (2017) showed that the TSPO ligand vinpocetine significantly downregulated the expression of CD40, CD80, and CD86 in pDCs and increased the expression of TSPO in these cells. Vinpocetine significantly inhibited the Toll-like receptor 9 signaling pathway and reduced the secretion of related cytokines in pDCs. Furthermore, the viability of pDCs was significantly promoted by vinpocetine (Feng et al., 2017). As mentioned earlier, Zhang et al. (2017) found that the TSPO ligands, FGIN-1-27 and Ro5 4864, suppressed inflammatory and immune responses of human $CD4^+$ T-cells from PBMCs. Thus, TSPO ligands can apparently be applied to reduce inflammatory and immune responses.

7.3 TSPO and Pathological Cardiovascular Conditions

Our recent studies suggested that the TSPO ligand 2-Cl-MGV-1 could postpone the incidence of cardiac arrest in a transgenic mouse model for Huntington's disease (Vainshtein et al., 2015), the same being true for PK 11195 and MGV-1 (2-phenylquinazolin-4-yl dimethylcarbamate) in kainic acid-injected rats (Vainshtein et al., 2015; Veenman et al., 2002). Others have intensively studied the mechanisms whereby TSPO and its ligands can exert myocardial protection (Obame et al., 2007; Tsamatsoulis et al., 2016). Obame et al. (2007) investigated the mechanisms by which Ro5 4864 protected the myocardium against ischemia–reperfusion in rats. Ro5 4864 reduced infarct size in a dose-dependent manner. Furthermore, Ro5 4864 at a dose of 10 mg/kg reduced apoptosis, restored mitochondrial recovery, improved oxidative phosphorylation parameters, and reduced $\Delta\Psi m$ transition, including inhibition of cytochrome *c* and apoptosis-inducing factor releases (Obame et al., 2007). Furthermore, Ro5 4864 increased the resistance of mitochondria to Ca^{++}-induced $\Delta\Psi m$ transition (Obame et al., 2007). These effects are now all well known to be under TSPO control (Caballero et al., 2013; Veenman et al., 2014). In rat aortas and livers, in association with atherosclerosis, we found that chronic high fat, high cholesterol supplementation decreases TSPO-binding capacity in association with increased oxidative stress, further implicating TSPO in cardiovascular disorders (Dimitrova-Shumkovska, Veenman, Ristoski, Leschiner, & Gavish, 2010).

7.4 TSPO and Cancer

In early studies we found that TSPO density was increased in various types of cancer, including ovarian cancer and colonic adenocarcinoma (Katz, Ben-Baruch, Kloog, Menczer, & Gavish, 1990; Katz, Eitan, & Gavish, 1990). We then continued to study TSPO involvement in tumorigenesis, in particular glioblastoma. These studies uncovered that the parameters apparently regulated by TSPO include proliferation, programmed cell death, glutamate metabolism, the cell cycle, adhesion, migration, angiogenesis, intracellular TSPO location, and gene expression (Bode et al., 2012, 2014; Kugler et al., 2008; Levin et al., 2005; Veenman et al., 2012, 2004; Yasin et al., 2017). Finally, the typical high expression of TSPO that can be seen in various glioblastomas (Veenman et al., 2004) continues to generate intensive research activities to improve imaging techniques for application to cancer diagnosis (Werry, Barron, & Kassiou, 2015). For example, TSPO brain imaging in glioblastoma multiforme (GBM) may be a useful tool for predicting tumor progression at follow-up and may be less susceptible to changes in blood–brain barrier permeability than other imaging agents are (Jensen et al., 2015).

7.5 TSPO and Anxiety and Stress

We have reviewed TSPO's apparent involvement in the biological coping with stress and anxiety disorders (Gavish et al., 1999), which may be a core phenotypical TSPO function (Li et al., 2016; Wang et al., 2017). Drugan, Basile, Crawley, Paul, and Skolnick (1986) found that inescapable shock reduces [^{3}H]Ro5 4864 binding to TSPO in the rat. Our research on blood cells and the brain suggests that TSPO density changes due to acute and chronic stress are different in that acute stress often results in enhanced TSPO density, and chronic stress in decreased TSPO density (Karp, Weizman, Tyano, & Gavish, 1989; Weizman et al., 1994, 1987).

In general it is thought that TSPO–steroid interactions form the basis for this general TSPO "stress response" function (Veenman & Gavish, 2012). In more detail, it was found that anxiolytic-like effects of the TSPO ligand AC-5216 were inhibited by trilostane and finasteride, both inhibitors of steroidogenic enzymes (Kita & Furukawa, 2008). These results demonstrated that the anxiolytic-like effects of AC-5216 are due to newly synthesized neurosteroids that enhance $GABA_A$ receptor function. In another model, single prolonged stress (SPS) rats received daily midazolam during exposure to SPS and behavioral assessments, which included the open field test, the contextual fear paradigm, and the elevated plus-maze. Midazolam significantly reversed the behavioral deficiencies of the SPS rats, including post-traumatic stress disorder (PTSD)-associated freezing and anxiety-like behavior, but not the effects on spontaneous locomotor activity. In addition, the anti-PTSD effects of midazolam were antagonized by PK 11195, the central benzodiazepine receptor (CBR) antagonist flumazenil, and the inhibitor of steroidogenic enzymes finasteride, which by themselves had no effect on PTSD-associated freezing and anxiety-like behavior. Thus, midazolam ameliorates the behavioral deficits of a rat PTSD model via TSPO, neurosteroidogenesis, and the CBR (Miao et al., 2014). In principle, interactions between TSPO, steroidogenesis, and the CBR are considered the basis for TSPO's potential to be targeted for treatment of stress disorders.

7.6 TSPO, Brain Injury, and Neurodegeneration

Traumatic brain injury (TBI) is a multifaceted condition with a broad spectrum of symptoms and disabilities (Ghajar, 2000; Quatman-Yates et al., 2016). TBI and its sequelae represent the leading cause of death among people aged $\leq$45 years. It is estimated that 2% of the US population lives with disabilities directly attributable to TBI (Centers for Disease Control and Prevention web page, http://www.cdc.gov/traumaticbraininjury, accessed June 28, 2013). Mild TBI, also referred to as concussion, typically affects orientation and memory, and may involve loss of consciousness (Giza et al., 2013). To date, there is no effective curative treatment applicable in the clinic. Fortunately, various types of TSPO ligands appear to be effective for neurodegenerative disease as well as TBI in various animal and cell culture models, e.g., curcumin prevents mitochondrial dysfunction in the brain of the senescence-accelerated mouse-prone 8 (Eckert et al., 2013). It was also shown that the TSPO ligand Etifoxine improves sensorimotor deficits and reduces glial activation, neuronal degeneration, and neuroinflammation in a rat model of TBI (Simon-O'Brien, Gauthier, Riban, & Verleye, 2016). A novel TSPO ligand named compound 7e was shown to prevent amyloid-β-induced ΔΨm transition (Elkamhawy et al., 2017). These TSPO ligands have in common that they present low affinity for TSPO. It was pointed out in studies by us on programmed cell death and neurodifferentiation that this was a most favorable attribute of TSPO ligands for curative effects in TBI and neurodegenerative diseases (Vainshtein et al., 2015; Veenman et al., 2015). This was also observed by Kim and Pae in their reviews of patents from 2010 to 2015, including ours (Kim & Pae, 2016a, 2016b).

However, regulation of programmed cell death is not sufficient to establish brain repair. Animal studies, using a retina model, have shown that TSPO ligands can mitigate degeneration and reduce the number of activated microglia, together with a reduction of proinflammatory gene expression of Ccl2 and IL-6 (Scholz et al., 2015). It also appears that mitochondrial TSPO, including its classical and novel ligands, appears to be able to stimulate the mitochondria to cell nucleus pathway for regulation of cell nuclear gene expression, including in gene expression related to cell migration and neurodifferentiation, potentially beneficial attributes for tissue repair and regeneration (Yasin et al., 2017). Our studies have further shown that TSPO ligands actually promote neurodifferentiation, adhesion, and migration, which are aspects conducive to neurorepair (Bode et al., 2012; Vainshtein et al., 2015; Veenman et al., 2015).

The generality of these TSPO attributes is illustrated by a study of Lin et al. (2014), in a nonmammalian species. They showed that inactivation of CG2789/dTSPO in *Drosophila*, by P-element insertion, RNAi knockdown, and inhibition by the TSPO ligands PK 11195 and Ro5 4864, inhibited wing disk apoptosis in response to γ-irradiation or H_2O_2 exposure, and also increased male fly lifespan, and inhibited Aβ42-induced neurodegeneration in association with decreased caspase activation. These findings in *Drosophila* are similar to those found by us in rats and mice (Vainshtein et al., 2015; Veenman et al., 2015). A broader overview of comparisons between mammals and other species is provided by our study focusing on TSPO–tetrapyrrole interactions (Veenman et al., 2016).

It would be worthwhile to apply TSPO knockout mice to studies of stress, injury, disease, etc. to see if TSPO actually plays a functional role under these conditions. In general, as the conclusion of this section, it can safely be said that TSPO responds to injury and disease, and can also be targeted to treat injury and disease.

8. MAINTENANCE OF HOMEOSTASIS BY TSPO AT CELLULAR AND WHOLE ORGANISM LEVELS

Studies of TSPO knockout mice did not appear to show critical effects, as discussed in the various sections above. This suggested that TSPO has no function, or at least no essential function. However, various studies, including applications of molecular biological methods, pharmaceutical methods, genetic manipulation, and straightforward empiric observations related to stress, injury, and disease discussed in the sections above, suggest various functions for TSPO, including involvement in responses to challenges. Often, the TSPO involvement/response appears to be beneficial. For example, early on, the various studies on the subjects summarized in this review led to the postulation of a possible general role for TSPO in "adaptations" to stress, in its various forms, as originally reviewed by Gavish et al. (1999). As this may be the actual general function of TSPO, we add some more details here. In this century, various refinements to this hypothesis presented by Gavish et al. (1999) were added, such "a role in the host defense response" (Veenman & Gavish, 2006; Veenman et al., 2007) and "maintenance of homeostasis." To our knowledge, the term "maintenance of homeostasis" was first explicitly stated by Li et al. (2011), in relation to intracellular calcium levels. Subsequently, homeostasis as regulated by mitochondrial TSPO was discussed in more encompassing terms by Gatliff and Campanella (2012). The generation of transgenic mice with TSPO knockout then generated more attention regarding the general "homeostasis" function of TSPO, and the potential to research the homeostatic function of TSPO at whole-organism levels (Banati et al., 2014). As additional information, the question can be raised of whether TSPO present in intestinal flora may contribute to the normal functioning of the host (Banati et al., 2014). A more recent study considers TSPO's homeostatic function associated with neurodegeneration and neuroinflammatory responses (Cerami, Iaccarino, & Perani, 2017). Fan et al. (2015) genetically engineered two distinct TSPO knockout mice to induce gonadal and steroidogenic cell-specific TSPO deletion. In particular for steroidogenic tissues, the authors reported a role for TSPO in cellular cholesterol and lipid homeostasis. The authors (Fan et al., 2015) proposed that this relates to stress adaption. It was also found that TSPO expression is essential to safeguard healthy adipocyte functions, and that TSPO activation in adipocytes improves their metabolic status in regulating glucose homeostasis (Li & Papadopoulos,

2015). While this concept is well recognized in mammals, it is most pertinently described and approached in studies in prokaryotes. For example, in a study of cyanobacterium *Fremyella diplosiphon*, it is expressly stated that TSPO is a membrane protein implicated in stress responses across a range of organisms from bacteria to humans (Busch & Montgomery, 2017). These authors propose that these proteins regulate tetrapyrrole homeostasis and/or tetrapyrrole-modulated functions in *F. diplosiphon* in response to multiple environmental stresses. This phenomenon was also recognized for eukaryotes, including mammals (Veenman et al., 2016). Thus, it is relevant to study TSPO in comparative studies over a wide range of species.

9. CONCLUSION

Various studies reviewed here suggest that *TSPO* indeed presents a housekeeping gene, as suggested in 1999 (Gavish et al., 1999). We have postulated that ROS generation, ATP production, and Ca^{++} levels are important factors underlying regulation by mitochondrial TSPO of cell nuclear gene expression as well as programmed cell death (Veenman et al., 2014; Yasin et al., 2017). We believe that it would be worthwhile to intensify studies regarding ROS generation, ATP production, and mitochondrial and cellular Ca^{++} levels, including measuring levels of calcium-binding proteins such as calmodulin and calcineurin, as these appear to be intermediaries between TSPO and its ability to regulate homeostasis via gene expression modulation. It would also be worthwhile to expand research regarding association of ROS generation, ATP production, and cellular and mitochondrial Ca^{++} levels with TSPO activation in relation to programmed cell death. It is all the more relevant as these processes appear to be important for wide-ranging diseases and disorders, including cardiovascular disorders and brain disease and injury, tumorigenicity, inflammation, and immune response. It also remains interesting to resolve the controversies regarding interactions between TSPO, tetrapyrroles, and cholesterol to understand better the relevance of these interactions for the diseases and disorders that are associated with TSPO. As TSPO is a receptor displaying various functional effects when subjected to ligand exposure, it is indeed worthwhile to test various TSPO ligands as potential agents to various diseases.

CONFLICT OF INTEREST

Both authors declare no conflict of interest.

ACKNOWLEDGMENTS

This work is supported by a joint grant from the Center for Absorption in Science of the Ministry of Immigrant Absorption and the Committee for Planning and Budgeting of the Council of Higher Education under the framework of the KAMEA program. We also acknowledge the support by the KAMIN and MAGNETON programs of the Israel Ministry of Trade and Industry.

REFERENCES

Anholt, R. R., Pedersen, P. L., De Souza, E. B., & Snyder, S. H. (1986). The peripheral-type benzodiazepine receptor. Localization to the mitochondrial outer membrane. *The Journal of Biological Chemistry*, *261*, 576–583.

Balsemão-Pires, E., Jaillais, Y., Olson, B. J., Andrade, L. R., Umen, J. G., Chory, J., et al. (2011). The Arabidopsis translocator protein (AtTSPO) is regulated at multiple levels in response to salt stress and perturbations in tetrapyrrole metabolism. *BMC Plant Biology*, *11*, 108.

Banati, R. B., Middleton, R. J., Chan, R., Hatty, C. R., Kam, W. W., Quin, C., et al. (2014). Positron emission tomography and functional characterization of a complete PBR/TSPO knockout. *Nature Communications*, *5*, 5452.

Bar-Ami, S., Bendel, N., Leschiner, S., Levin, E., Veenman, L., & Gavish, M. (2006). The effects of prostaglandin F2alpha treatment on peripheral-type benzodiazepine receptors in the ovary and uterus during pseudopregnancy of rats. *Biochemical Pharmacology*, *71*, 472–478.

Bar-Ami, S., Fares, F., & Gavish, M. (1989). Effect of hypophysectomy and hormone treatment on the induction of peripheral-type benzodiazepine binding sites in female rat genital axis. *Hormone and Metabolic Research*, *21*, 106–107.

Batarseh, A., Barlow, K. D., Martinez-Arguelles, D. B., & Papadopoulos, V. (2012). Functional characterization of the human translocator protein (18kDa) gene promoter in human breast cancer cell lines. *Biochimica et Biophysica Acta*, *1819*, 38–56.

Besman, M. J., Yanagibashi, K., Lee, T. D., Kawamura, M., Hall, P. F., & Shively, J. E. (1989). Identification of des-(Gly-Ile)-endozepine as an effector of corticotropin-dependent adrenal steroidogenesis: Stimulation of cholesterol delivery is mediated by the peripheral benzodiazepine receptor. *Proceedings of the National Academy of Sciences of the United States of America*, *86*, 4897–4901.

Bode, J., Veenman, L., Caballero, B., Lakomek, M., Kugler, W., & Gavish, M. (2012). The 18 kDa translocator protein influences angiogenesis, as well as aggressiveness, adhesion, migration, and proliferation of glioblastoma cells. *Pharmacogenetics and Genomics*, *22*, 538–550.

Bode, J., Veenman, L., Vainshtein, A., Kugler, W., Rosenberg, N., & Gavish, M. (2014). Modulation of gene expression associated with the cell cycle and tumorigenicity of glioblastoma cells by the 18 kDa translocator protein (TSPO). *Austin Journal of Pharmacolology and Therapeutics*, *2*, 1053.

Bogan, R. L., Davis, T. L., & Niswender, G. D. (2007). Peripheral-type benzodiazepine receptor (PBR) aggregation and absence of steroidogenic acute regulatory protein (StAR)/PBR association in the mitochondrial membrane as determined by bioluminescence resonance energy transfer (BRET). *The Journal of Steroid Biochemistry and Molecular Biology*, *104*, 61–67.

Bono, F., Lamarche, I., Prabonnaud, V., Le Fur, G., & Herbert, J. M. (1999). Peripheral benzodiazepine receptor agonists exhibit potent antiapoptotic activities. *Biochemical and Biophysical Research Communications*, *265*, 457–461.

Bose, M., Whittal, R. M., Miller, W. L., & Bose, H. S. (2008). Steroidogenic activity of StAR requires contact with mitochondrial VDAC1 and phosphate carrier protein. *The Journal of Biological Chemistry*, *283*, 8837–8845.

Braestrup, C., & Squires, R. F. (1977). Specific benzodiazepine receptors in rat brain characterized by high-affinity (3H)diazepam binding. *Proceedings of the National Academy of Sciences of the United States of America*, *74*, 3805–3809.

Busch, A. W., & Montgomery, B. L. (2017). Distinct light-, stress-, and nutrient-dependent regulation of multiple tryptophan-rich sensory protein (TSPO) genes in the cyanobacterium Fremyella diplosiphon. *Plant Signaling & Behavior*, *12*, e1293221.

Caballero, B., Veenman, L., Bode, J., Leschiner, S., & Gavish, M. (2014). Concentration-dependent bimodal effect of specific 18 kDa translocator protein (TSPO) ligands on cell death processes induced by ammonium chloride: Potential implications for neuropathological effects due to hyperammonemia. *CNS & Neurological Disorders Drug Targets*, *13*, 574–592.

Caballero, B., Veenman, L., & Gavish, M. (2013). Role of mitochondrial translocator protein (18 kDa) on mitochondrial-related cell death processes. *Recent Patents on Endocrine, Metabolic & Immune Drug Discovery*, 7, 86–101.

Carmel, I., Fares, F. A., Leschiner, S., Scherübl, H., Weisinger, G., & Gavish, M. (1999). Peripheral-type benzodiazepine receptors in the regulation of proliferation of MCF-7 human breast carcinoma cell line. *Biochemical Pharmacology*, *58*, 273–278.

Cerami, C., Iaccarino, L., & Perani, D. (2017). Molecular imaging of neuroinflammation in neurodegenerative dementias: The role of in vivo PET imaging. *International Journal of Molecular Science*, *18*. pii: E993.

Costa, B., Cavallini, C., Da Pozzo, E., Taliani S, Da Settimo F., Martini, C. (2017). The anxiolytic etifoxine binds to TSPO Ro5-4864 binding site with long residence time showing a high neurosteroidogenic activity. ACS Chemical Neuroscience, 8:1448-1454. https://doi.org/10.1021/acschemneuro.7b00027. [Epub 2017 Apr 4].

Daugherty, D. J., Chechneva, O., Mayrhofer, F., & Deng, W. (2016). The hGFAP-driven conditional TSPO knockout is protective in a mouse model of multiple sclerosis. *Scientific Reports*, *6*, 22556.

Dimitrova-Shumkovska, J., Veenman, L., Ristoski, T., Leschiner, S., & Gavish, M. (2010). Chronic high fat, high cholesterol supplementation decreases 18 kDa translocator protein binding capacity in association with increased oxidative stress in rat liver and aorta. *Food and Chemical Toxicology*, *48*, 910–921.

Drugan, R. C., Basile, A. S., Crawley, J. N., Paul, S. M., & Skolnick, P. (1986). Inescapable shock reduces [3H]Ro 5-4864 binding to "peripheral-type" benzodiazepine receptors in the rat. *Pharmacology, Biochemistry, and Behavior*, *24*, 1673–1677.

Dupont, A. C., Largeau, B., Santiago Ribeiro, M. J., Guilloteau, D., Tronel, C., & Arlicot, N. (2017). Translocator protein-18 kDa (TSPO) positron emission tomography (PET) imaging and its clinical impact in neurodegenerative diseases. *International Journal of Molecular Science*, *18*. pii: E785.

Dzierszinski, F., Coppin, A., Mortuaire, M., Dewailly, E., Slomianny, C., Ameisen, J. C., et al. (2002). Ligands of the peripheral benzodiazepine receptor are potent inhibitors of Plasmodium falciparum and Toxoplasma gondii in vitro. *Antimicrobial Agents and Chemotherapy*, *46*, 3197–3207.

Eberl, S., Katsifis, A., Peyronneau, M. A., Wen, L., Henderson, D., Loc'h, C., et al. (2017). Preclinical in vivo and in vitro comparison of the translocator protein PET ligands [(18) F]PBR102 and [(18)F]PBR111. *European Journal of Nuclear Medicine and Molecular Imaging*, *44*, 296–307.

Eckert, G. P., Schiborr, C., Hagl, S., Abdel-Kader, R., Müller, W. E., Rimbach, G., et al. (2013). Curcumin prevents mitochondrial dysfunction in the brain of the senescence-accelerated mouse-prone 8. *Neurochemistry International*, *62*, 595–602.

Elkamhawy, A., Park, J. E., Hassan, A. H. E., Pae, A. N., Lee, J., & Park, B. G. (2017). Design, synthesis, biological evaluation and molecular modelling of 2-(2-aryloxyphenyl)-1,4-dihydroisoquinolin-3(2H)-ones: A novel class of TSPO ligands modulating amyloid-β-induced mPTP opening. *European Journal of Pharmaceutical Sciences, 104*, 366–381.

Engel, A. E., Nagy, B., Nagy, L. A., Engel, C. G., Kremp, G. O., & Drew, C. M. (1968). Alga-like forms in onverwacht series, South Africa: Oldest recognized lifelike forms on earth. *Science, 16*, 1005–1008.

Fan, J., Campioli, E., Midzak, A., Culty, M., & Papadopoulos, V. (2015). Conditional steroidogenic cell-targeted deletion of TSPO unveils a crucial role in viability and hormone-dependent steroid formation. *Proceedings of the National Academy of Sciences of the United States of America, 112*, 7261–7266.

Fan, J., & Papadopoulos, V. (2012). Transcriptional regulation of translocator protein (Tspo) via a SINE B2-mediated natural antisense transcript in MA-10 Leydig cells. *Biology of Reproduction, 86*(147), 1–15.

Feng, X., Wang, Y., Hao, Y., Ma, Q., Dai, J., Liang, Z., et al. (2017). Vinpocetine inhibited the CpG oligodeoxynucleotide-induced immune response in plasmacytoid dendritic cells. *Immunological Investigations, 46*, 263–273.

Garnier, M., Dimchev, A. B., Boujrad, N., Price, J. M., Musto, N. A., & Papadopoulos, V. (1994). In vitro reconstitution of a functional peripheral-type benzodiazepine receptor from mouse Leydig tumor cells. *Molecular Pharmacology, 45*, 201–211.

Gatliff, J., & Campanella, M. (2012). The 18 kDa translocator protein (TSPO): A new perspective in mitochondrial biology. *Current Molecular Medicine, 12*, 356–368.

Gatliff, J., & Campanella, M. (2016). TSPO: Kaleidoscopic 18-kDa amid biochemical pharmacology, control and targeting of mitochondria. *The Biochemical Journal, 473*(2), 107–121.

Gavish, M. (1995). Hormonal regulation of peripheral-type benzodiazepine receptors. *The Journal of Steroid Biochemistry and Molecular Biology, 53*, 57–59.

Gavish, M., Bachman, I., Shoukrun, R., Katz, Y., Veenman, L., Weisinger, G., et al. (1999). Enigma of the peripheral benzodiazepine receptor. *Pharmacological Reviews, 51*, 629–650.

Gavish, M., Veenman, L., Shterenberg, A., Marek, M., Vainshtein, A., Avital, A. (2017). Quinazoline scaffold based compounds, pharmaceutical compositions and methods of use thereof. Patent application: EP 3134389 A1, also published as WO2015162615A1.

Gee, K.W. (1996). Use of peripheral-type benzodiazepine sites for treatments of CNS trauma or disease. US Patent 5550124.

Gent, Y. Y., Weijers, K., Molthoff, C. F., Windhorst, A. D., Huisman, M. C., & Kassiou, M. (2014). Promising potential of new generation translocator protein tracers providing enhanced contrast of arthritis imaging by positron emission tomography in a rat model of arthritis. *Arthritis Research & Therapy, 16*, R70.

Ghajar, J. (2000). Traumatic brain injury. *Lancet, 356*, 923–929.

Giza, C. C., Kutcher, J. S., Ashwal, S., Barth, J., Getchius, T. S., & Gioia, G. A. (2013). Summary of evidence-based guideline update: Evaluation and management of concussion in sports: Report of the guideline development Subcommittee of the American Academy of neurology. *Neurology, 80*, 2250–22573.

Gomes, A. P., Price, N. L., Ling, A. J., Moslehi, J. J., Montgomery, M. K., Rajman, L., et al. (2013). Declining NAD+ induces a pseudohypoxic state disrupting nuclear mitochondrial communication during aging. *Cell, 155*, 1624–1638.

Guo, Y., Kalathur, R. C., Liu, Q., Kloss, B., Bruni, R., Ginter, C., et al. (2015). Protein structure. Structure and activity of tryptophan-rich TSPO proteins. *Science, 347*, 551–555.

Gut, P. (2015). Targeting mitochondrial energy metabolism with TSPO ligands. *Biochemical Society Transactions, 43*, 537–542.

Hernstadt, H., Wang, S., Lim, G., & Mao, J. (2009). Spinal translocator protein (TSPO) modulates pain behavior in rats with CFA-induced monoarthritis. *Brain Research, 1286*, 42–52.

Hirsch, J. D., Beyer, C. F., Malkowitz, L., Beer, B., & Blume, A. J. (1989). Mitochondrial benzodiazepine receptors mediate inhibition of mitochondrial respiratory control. *Molecular Pharmacology, 35*, 157–163.

Iversen, P., Hansen, D. A., Bender, D., Rodell, A., & Munk, O. L. (2006). Peripheral benzodiazepine receptors in the brain of cirrhosis patients with manifest hepatic encephalopathy. *European Journal of Nuclear Medicine and Molecular Imaging, 33*, 810–816.

Jaipuria, G., Leonov, A., Giller, K., Vasa, S. K., Jaremko, Ł., Jaremko, M., et al. (2017). Cholesterol-mediated allosteric regulation of the mitochondrial translocator protein structure. *Nature Communications, 8*, 14893.

Jaremko, L., Jaremko, M., Giller, K., Becker, S., & Zweckstetter, M. (2014). Structure of the mitochondrial translocator protein in complex with a diagnostic ligand. *Science, 343*, 1363–1366.

Jayakumar, A. R., Panickar, K. S., & Norenberg, M. D. (2002). Effects on free radical generation by ligands of the peripheral benzodiazepine receptor in cultured neural cells. *Journal of Neurochemistry, 83*, 1226–1234.

Jensen, P., Feng, L., Law, I., Svarer, C., Knudsen, G. M., Mikkelsen, J. D., et al. (2015). TSPO imaging in glioblastoma Multiforme: A direct comparison between 123I-CLINDE SPECT, 18F-FET PET, and gadolinium-enhanced MR imaging. *Journal of Nuclear Medicine, 56*, 1386–1390.

Joo, H. K., Lee, Y. R., Kang, G., Choi, S., Kim, C. S., & Ryoo, S. (2015). The 18-kDa translocator protein inhibits vascular cell adhesion molecule-1 expression via inhibition of mitochondrial reactive oxygen species. *Molecules and Cells, 38*, 1064–1070.

Karp, L., Weizman, A., Tyano, S., & Gavish, M. (1989). Examination stress, platelet peripheral benzodiazepine binding sites, and plasma hormone levels. *Life Sciences, 44*, 1077–1082.

Katz, Y., Ben-Baruch, G., Kloog, Y., Menczer, J., & Gavish, M. (1990). Increased density of peripheral benzodiazepine-binding sites in ovarian carcinomas as compared with benign ovarian tumours and normal ovaries. *Clinical Science (London), 78*, 155–158.

Katz, Y., Eitan, A., & Gavish, M. (1990). Increase in peripheral benzodiazepine binding sites in colonic adenocarcinoma. *Oncology, 47*, 139–142.

Kim, T., & Pae, A. N. (2016a). Translocator protein (TSPO) ligands for the diagnosis or treatment of neurodegenerative diseases: A patent review (2010–2015; part 1). *Expert Opinion on Therapeutic Patents, 26*, 1325–1351.

Kim, T., & Pae, A. N. (2016b). Translocator protein (TSPO) ligands for the diagnosis or treatment of neurodegenerative diseases: A patent review (2010–2015; part 2). *Expert Opinion on Therapeutic Patents, 26*, 1353–1366.

Kita, A., & Furukawa, K. (2008). Involvement of neurosteroids in the anxiolytic-like effects of AC-5216 in mice. *Pharmacology, Biochemistry, and Behavior, 89*, 171–178.

Krestinina, O. V., Grachev, D. E., Odinokova, I. V., Reiser, G., Evtodienko, Y. V., & Azarashvili, T. S. (2009). Effect of peripheral benzodiazepine receptor (PBR/TSPO) ligands on opening of Ca^{2+}-induced pore and phosphorylation of 3.5-kDa polypeptide in rat brain mitochondria. *Biochemistry (Moscow), 74*, 421–429.

Krueger, K. E., & Papadopoulos, V. (1990). Peripheral-type benzodiazepine receptors mediate translocation of cholesterol from outer to inner mitochondrial membranes in adrenocortical cells. *The Journal of Biological Chemistry, 265*, 15015–15022.

Krueger, K. E., & Papadopoulos, V. (1992). Mitochondrial benzodiazepine receptors and the regulation of steroid biosynthesis. *Annual Reviews of Pharmacological Toxicology, 32*, 211–237.

Kugler, W., Veenman, L., Shandalov, Y., Leschiner, S., Spanier, I., Lakomek, M., et al. (2008). Ligands of the mitochondrial 18 kDa translocator protein attenuate apoptosis of human glioblastoma cells exposed to Erucylphosphohomocholine. *Cellular Oncology*, *30*, 435–450.

Kusumawidjaja, G., Kayed, H., Giese, N., Bauer, A., Erkan, M., Giese, T., et al. (2007). Basic transcription factor 3 (BTF3) regulates transcription of tumor-associated genes in pancreatic cancer cells. *Cancer Biology & Therapy*, *6*, 367–376.

Lassance, L., Haghiac, M., Minium, J., Catalano, P., & Hauguel-de Mouzon, S. (2015). Obesity-induced down-regulation of the mitochondrial translocator protein (TSPO) impairs placental steroid production. *The Journal of Clinical Endocrinology and Metabolism*, *100*, E11–18.

Lehmann, J., Weizman, R., Pryce, C. R., Leschiner, S., Allmann, I., Feldon, J., et al. (1999). Peripheral benzodiazepine receptors in cerebral cortex, but not in internal organs, are increased following inescapable stress and subsequent avoidance/escape shuttle-box testing. *Brain Research*, *85*, 141–147.

Leister, D. (2016). Towards understanding the evolution and functional diversification of DNA containing plant organelles. *F1000Research*, *5*. pii: F1000 faculty Rev-330.

Levin, E., Premkumar, A., Veenman, L., Kugler, W., Leschiner, S., Spanier, I., et al. (2005). The peripheral-type benzodiazepine receptor and tumorigenicity: Isoquinoline binding protein (IBP) antisense knockdown in the C6 glioma cell line. *Biochemistry*, *44*, 9924–9935.

Li, H., Degenhardt, B., Tobin, D., Yao, Z. X., Tasken, K., & Papadopoulos, V. (2001). Identification, localization, and function in steroidogenesis of PAP7: A peripheral-type benzodiazepine receptor- and PKA (RIalpha)-associated protein. *Molecular Endocrinology*, *15*, 2211–2228.

Li, F., Liu, J., Liu, N., Kuhn, L. A., Garavito, R. M., & Ferguson-Miller, S. (2016). Translocator protein 18 kDa (TSPO): An old protein with new functions? *Biochemistry*, *55*, 2821–2831.

Li, J., & Papadopoulos, V. (2015). Translocator protein (18 kDa) as a pharmacologicaltarget in adipocytes to regulate glucose homeostasis. *Biochemical Pharmacology*, *97*, 99–110.

Li, F., Xia, Y., Meiler, J., & Ferguson-Miller, S. (2013). Characterization and modeling of the oligomeric state and ligand binding behavior of purified translocator protein 18 kDa from Rhodobacter sphaeroides. *Biochemistry*, *52*, 5884–5899.

Li, J., Xu, J., Xiao, J., Zhang, H., Liang, D., Liu, Y., et al. (2011). Preservation of TSPO by chronic intermittent hypobaric hypoxia confers antiarrhythmic activity. *Journal of Cellular and Molecular Medicine*, *15*, 134–140.

Liere, P., Pianos, A., Oudinet, J. P., Schumacher, M., & Akwa, Y. (2017). Differential effects of the 18-kDa translocator protein (TSPO). Ligand etifoxine on steroidogenesis in rat brain, plasma and steroidogenic glands: Pharmacodynamic studies. *Psychoneuroendocrinology*, *83*, 122–134.

Lin, R., Angelin, A., Da Settimo, F., Martini, C., Taliani, S., Zhu, S., et al. (2014). Genetic analysis of dTSPO, an outer mitochondrial membrane protein, reveals its functions in apoptosis, longevity, and Ab42-induced neurodegeneration. *Aging Cell*, *13*, 507–518.

Liu, B., Le, K. X., Park, M. A., Wang, S., Belanger, A. P., Dubey, S., et al. (2015). In vivo detection of age- and disease-related increases in neuroinflammation by 18F-GE180 TSPO MicroPET imaging in wild-type and Alzheimer's transgenic mice. *Journal of Neuroscience*, *35*, 15716–15730.

Liu, G. J., Middleton, R. J., Kam, W. W., Chin, D. Y., Hatty, C. R., Chan, R. H., et al. (2017). Functional gains in energy and cell metabolism after TSPO gene insertion. *Cell Cycle*, *16*, 436–447.

Maaser, K., Grabowski, P., Oezdem, Y., Krahn, A., Heine, B., Stein, H., et al. (2005). Up-regulation of the peripheral benzodiazepine receptor during human colorectal carcinogenesis and tumor spread. *Clinical Cancer Research*, *11*, 1751–1756. Erratum (2005). in: Clinical cancer research, Vol. 11, 6408.

Manku, G., Wang, Y., Thuillier, R., Rhodes, C., & Culty, M. (2012). Developmental expression of the translocator protein 18 kDa (TSPO) in testicular germ cells. *Current Molecular Medicine*, *12*, 467–475.

McEnery, M. W., Snowman, A. M., Trifiletti, R. R., & Snyder, S. H. (1992). Isolation of the mitochondrial benzodiazepine receptor: Association with the voltage-dependent anion channel and the adenine nucleotide carrier. *Proceedings of the National Academy of Sciences of the United States of America*, *89*, 3170–3174.

Mendonça-Torres, M. C., & Roberts, S. S. (2013). The translocator protein (TSPO) ligand PK 11195 induces apoptosis and cell cycle arrest and sensitizes to chemotherapy treatment in pre- and post-relapse neuroblastoma cell lines. *Cancer Biology & Therapy*, *14*, 319–326.

Miao, Y. L., Guo, W. Z., Shi, W. Z., Fang, W. W., Liu, Y., Liu, J., et al. (2014). Midazolam ameliorates the behavior deficits of a rat posttraumatic stress disorder model through dual 18 kDa translocator protein and central benzodiazepine receptor and neurosteroidogenesis. *PLoS One*, *9*, e101450.

Middleton, R. J., Liu, G. J., & Banati, R. B. (2015). Guwiyang Wurra—'Fire Mouse': A global gene knockout model for TSPO/PBR drug development, loss-of-function and mechanisms of compensation studies. *Biochemical Society Transactions*, *43*, 553–558.

Morin, D., Musman, J., Pons, S., Berdeaux, A., & Ghaleh, B. (2016). Mitochondrial translocator protein (TSPO): From physiology to cardioprotection. *Biochemical Pharmacology*, *105*, 1–13.

Morrow, G., & Tanguay, R. M. (2012). Small heat shock protein expression and functions during development. *International Journal of Biochemistry & Cell Biology*, *44*, 1613–1621.

Nagler, R., Savulescu, D., Krayzler, E., Leschiner, S., Veenman, L., & Gavish, M. (2010). Cigarette smoke decreases salivary 18 kDa translocator protein binding affinity—In association with oxidative stress. *Current Medicinal Chemistry*, *17*, 2539–2546.

Obame, F. N., Zini, R., Souktani, R., Berdeaux, A., & Morin, D. (2007). Peripheral benzodiazepine receptor-induced myocardial protection is mediated by inhibition of mitochondrial membrane permeabilization. *Journal of Pharmacology and Experimental Therapeutics*, *323*, 336–345.

Papadopoulos, V., Aghazadeh, Y., Fan, J., Campioli, E., Zirkin, B., & Midzak, A. (2015). Translocator protein-mediated pharmacology of cholesterol transport and steroidogenesis. *Molecular and Cellular Endocrinology*, *408*, 90–98.

Papadopoulos, V., Baraldi, M., Guilarte, T. R., Knudsen, T. B., Lacapère, J. J., Lindemann, P., et al. (2006). Translocator protein (18kDa): New nomenclature for the peripheral-type benzodiazepine receptor based on its structure and molecular function. *Trends in Pharmacological Sciences*, *27*, 402–409.

Papadopoulos, V., Dharmarajan, A. M., Li, H., Culty, M., Lemay, M., et al. (1999). Mitochondrial peripheral-type benzodiazepine receptor expression. Correlation with gonadotropin-releasing hormone (GnRH) agonist-induced apoptosis in the corpus luteum. *Biochemical Pharmacology*, *58*, 1389–1393.

Parikh, V. S., Morgan, M. M., Scott, R., Clements, L. S., & Butow, R. A. (1987). The mitochondrial genotype can influence nuclear gene expression in yeast. *Science*, *235*, 576–580.

Porcu, P., Barron, A. M., Frye, C. A., Walf, A. A., Yang, S. Y., He, X. Y., et al. (2016). Neurosteroidogenesis today: Novel targets for neuroactive steroid synthesis and action and their relevance for translational research. *Journal of Neuroendocrinology*, *28*, 12351.

Quatman-Yates, C., Cupp, A., Gunsch, C., Haley, T., Vaculik, S., & Kujawa, D. (2016). Physical rehabilitation interventions for post-mTBI symptoms lasting greater than 2 weeks: Systematic review. *Physical Therapy*, *96*, 1753–1763.

Repalli, J. (2014). Translocator protein (TSPO) role in aging and Alzheimer's disease. *Current Aging Science*, *7*, 168–175.

Rosenberg, N., Rosenberg, O., Weizman, A., Leschiner, S., Sakoury, Y., Fares, F., et al. (2011). In vitro mitochondrial effects of PK 11195, a synthetic translocator protein 18 kDa (TSPO) ligand, in human osteoblast-like cells. *Journal of Bioenergetics and Biomembranes*, *43*, 739–746.

Rosenberg, N., Rosenberg, O., Weizman, A., Veenman, L., & Gavish, M. (2013). In vitro catabolic effect of protoporphyrin IX in human osteoblast-like cells: Possible role of the 18 kDa mitochondrial translocator protein. *Journal of Bioenergetics and Biomembranes*, *45*, 333–341.

Rosenberg, N., Rosenberg, O., Weizman, A., Veenman, L., & Gavish, M. (2014). In vitro effect of FGIN-1-27, a ligand to 18 kDa mitochondrial translocator protein, in human osteoblast-like cells. *Journal of Bioenergetics and Biomembranes*, *46*, 197–204.

Santidrián, A. F., Cosialls, A. M., Coll-Mulet, L., Iglesias-Serret, D., de Frias, M., González-Gironès, D. M., et al. (2007). The potential anticancer agent PK11195 induces apoptosis irrespective of p53 and ATM status in chronic lymphocytic leukemia cells. *Haematologica*, *92*, 1631–1638.

Scholz, R., Caramoy, A., Bhuckory, M. B., Rashid, K., Chen, M., Xu, H., et al. (2015). Targeting translocator protein (18 kda) (TSPO) dampens pro-inflammatory microglia reactivity in the retina and protects from degeneration. *Journal of Neuroinflammation*, *12*, 201.

Schopf, J. W., & Barghoorn, E. S. (1967). Alga-like fossils from the early precambrian of South Africa. *Science*, *156*, 508–512.

Selvaraj, V., Tu, L. N., & Stocco, D. M. (2016). Crucial role reported for TSPO in viability and steroidogenesis is a misconception. Commentary: Conditional steroidogenic cell-targeted deletion of TSPO unveils a crucial role in viability and hormone-dependent steroid formation. *Frontiers in Endocrinology (Lausanne)*, *7*, 91.

Shargorodsky, L., Veenman, L., Caballero, B., Pe'er, Y., Leschiner, S., Bode, J., et al. (2012). The nitric oxide donor sodium nitroprusside requires the 18 kDa translocator protein to induce cell death. *Apoptosis*, *17*, 647–665.

Shoukrun, R., Veenman, L., Shandalov, Y., Leschiner, S., Spanier, I., Karry, R., et al. (2008). The 18-kDa translocator protein, formerly known as the peripheral-type benzodiazepine receptor, confers proapoptotic and antineoplastic effects in a human colorectal cancer cell line. *Pharmacogenetics and Genomics*, *18*, 977–988.

Simon-O'Brien, E., Gauthier, D., Riban, V., & Verleye, M. (2016). Etifoxine improves sensorimotor deficits and reduces glial activation, neuronal degeneration, and neuroinflammation in a rat model of traumatic brain injury. *Journal of Neuroinflammation*, *13*, 203.

Taliani, S., Da Settimo, F., Da Pozzo, E., Chelli, B., & Martini, C. (2009). Translocator protein ligands as promising therapeutic tools for anxiety disorders. *Current Medicinal Chemistry*, *16*, 3359–3380.

Tsamatsoulis, M., Kapelios, C. J., Katsaros, L., Vakrou, S., Sousonis, V., Sventzouri, S., et al. (2016). Cardioprotective effects of intracoronary administration of 4-chlorodiazepam in small and large animal models of ischemia-reperfusion. *International Journal of Cardiology*, *224*, 90–95.

Tu, L. N., Morohaku, K., Manna, P. R., Pelton, S. H., Butler, W. R., Stocco, D. M., et al. (2014). Peripheral benzodiazepine receptor/translocator protein global knock-out mice are viable with no effects on steroid hormone biosynthesis. *The Journal of Biological Chemistry*, *289*, 27444–27454.

Tu, L. N., Zhao, A. H., Stocco, D. M., & Selvaraj, V. (2015). PK 11195 effect on steroidogenesis is not mediated through the translocator protein (TSPO). *Endocrinology, 156*, 1033–1039.

Vainshtein, A., Veenman, L., Shterenberg, A., Singh, S., Masarwa, A., Dutta, B., et al. (2015). Quinazoline-based tricyclic compounds that regulate programmed cell death, induce neuronal differentiation, and are curative in animal models for excitotoxicity and hereditary brain disease. *Cell Death Discovery, 1*, 15027.

Veenman, L., Alten, J., Linnemannstöns, K., Shandalov, Y., Zeno, S., Lakomek, M., et al. (2010). Potential involvement of F0F1-ATP(synth)ase and reactive oxygen species in apoptosis induction by the antineoplastic agent erucylphosphohomocholine in glioblastoma cell lines: A mechanism for induction of apoptosis via the 18 kDa mitochondrial translocator protein. *Apoptosis, 15*, 753–768.

Veenman, L., Bode, J., Gaitner, M., Caballero, B., Pe'er, Y., Zeno, S., et al. (2012). Effects of 18-kDa translocator protein knockdown on gene expression of glutamate receptors, transporters, and metabolism, and on cell viability affected by glutamate. *Pharmacogenetics and Genomics, 22*, 606–619.

Veenman, L., Denora, N., Rosenberg, N., & Gavish, M. (2017). TSPO, bond of ages. In *ATLAS of science another view on science*. www.atlasofscience.org.

Veenman, L., & Gavish, M. (2006). The peripheral-type benzodiazepine receptor and the cardiovascular system. Implications for drug development. Pharmacology *& Therapeutics, 110*, 503–524.

Veenman, L., & Gavish, M. (2012). The role of 18 kDa mitochondrial translocator protein (TSPO) in programmed cell death, and effects of steroids on TSPO expression. *Current Molecular Medicine, 12*, 398–412.

Veenman, L., Gavish, M., & Kugler, W. (2014). Apoptosis induction by erucylphosphohomocholine via the 18 kDa mitochondrial translocator protein: Implications for cancer treatment. Anti-Cancer Agents in *Medicinal Chemistry, 14*, 559–577.

Veenman, L., Leschiner, S., Spanier, I., Weisinger, G., Weizman, A., Gavish, M., et al. (2002). PK 11195 attenuates kainic acid-induced seizures and alterations in peripheral-type benzodiazepine receptor (PBR) protein components in the rat brain. *Journal of Neurochemistry, 80*, 917–927.

Veenman, L., Levin, E., Weisinger, G., Leschiner, S., Spanier, I., Snyder, S. H., et al. (2004). Peripheral-type benzodiazepine receptor density and in vitro tumorigenicity of glioma cell lines. *Biochemical Pharmacology, 68*, 689–698.

Veenman, L., Papadopoulos, V., & Gavish, M. (2007). Channel-like functions of the 18-kDa translocator protein (TSPO): Regulation of apoptosis and steroidogenesis as part of the host-defense response. *Current Pharmaceutical Design, 13*, 2385–2405.

Veenman, L., Shandalov, Y., & Gavish, M. (2008). VDAC activation by the 18 kDa translocatorprotein (TSPO), implications for apoptosis. *Journal of Bioenergetics and Biomembranes, 40*, 199–205.

Veenman, L., Vainshtein, A., & Gavish, M. (2015). TSPO as a target for treatments of diseases, including neuropathological disorders. *Cell Death & Disease, 6*, e1911.

Veenman, L., Vainshtein, A., Yasin, N., Azrad, M., & Gavish, M. (2016). Tetrapyrroles as endogenous TSPO ligands in eukaryotes and prokaryotes: Comparisons with synthetic ligands. *International Journal of Molecular Science, 17*. pii: E880.

Verma, A., Nye, J. S., & Snyder, S. H. (1987). Porphyrins are endogenous ligands for the mitochondrial (peripheral-type) benzodiazepine receptor. *Proceedings of the National Academy of Sciences of the United States of America, 84*, 2256–2260.

Vicidomini, C., Panico, M., Greco, A., Gargiulo, S., Coda, A. R., Zannetti, A., et al. (2015). In vivo imaging and characterization of [(18)F]DPA-714, a potential new TSPO ligand, in mouse brain and peripheral tissues using small-animal PET. *Nuclear Medicine and Biology, 42*, 309–316.

Wang, D. S., Han, J., Li, S., Sun, T., Guo, Y. Y., Kang, W. B., et al. (2017). Antidepressant-like and anxiolytic-like effects of ZBD-2, a novel ligand for the translocator protein (18 kDa). *Neuromolecular Medicine*, *19*, 57–68.

Wang, H., Zhai, K., Xue, Y., Yang, J., Yang, Q., Fu, Y., et al. (2016). Global deletion of TSPO does not affect the viability and gene expression profile. *PLoS One*, *11*, e0167307.

Weisinger, G., Kelly-Hershkovitz, E., Veenman, L., Spanier, I., Leschiner, S., & Gavish, M. (2004). Peripheral benzodiazepine receptor antisense knockout increases tumorigenicity of MA-10 Leydig cells *in vivo* and *in vitro*. *Biochemistry*, *43*, 12315–12321.

Weizman, A., Amiri, Z., Katz, Y., Snyder, S. H., & Gavish, M. (1992). Testosterone prevents castration-induced reduction in peripheral benzodiazepine receptors in Cowper's gland and adrenal. *Brain Research*, *572*, 72–75.

Weizman, R., Dagan, E., Snyder, S. H., & Gavish, M. (1997). Impact of pregnancy and lactation on GABAA receptor and central-type and peripheral-type benzodiazepine receptors. *Brain Research*, *752*, 7–14.

Weizman, R., Laor, N., Karp, L., Dagan, E., Reiss, A., Dar, D. E., et al. (1994). Alteration of platelet benzodiazepine receptors by stress of war. *American Journal of Psychiatry*, *151*, 766–767.

Weizman, R., Tanne, Z., Granek, M., Karp, L., Golomb, M., Tyano, S., et al. (1987). Peripheral benzodiazepine binding sites on platelet membranes are increased during diazepam treatment of anxious patients. *European Journal of Pharmacology*, *138*, 289–292.

Werry, E. L., Barron, M. L., & Kassiou, M. (2015). TSPO as a target for glioblastoma therapeutics. *Biochemical Society Transactions*, *43*, 531–536.

West, L. A., Horvat, R. D., Roess, D. A., Barisas, B. G., Juengel, J. L., & Niswender, G. D. (2001). Steroidogenic acute regulatory protein and peripheral-type benzodiazepine receptor associate at the mitochondrial membrane. *Endocrinology*, *142*, 502–505.

Wolf, L., Bauer, A., Melchner, D., Hallof-Buestrich, H., Stoertebecker, P., Haen, E., et al. (2015). Enhancing neurosteroid synthesis—Relationship to the pharmacology of translocator protein (18 kDa) (TSPO) ligands and benzodiazepines. *Pharmacopsychiatry*, *48*, 72–77.

Wu, Y., Kazumura, K., Maruyama, W., Osawa, T., & Naoi, M. (2015). Rasagiline and selegiline suppress calcium efflux from mitochondria by PK11195-induced opening of mitochondrial permeability transition pore: A novel anti-apoptotic function for neuroprotection. *Journal of Neural Transmission*, *122*, 1399–1407.

Yasin, N., Veenman, L., Singh, S., Azrad, M., Bode, J., Vainshtein, A., et al. (2017). Classical and novel TSPO ligands for the mitochondrial TSPO can modulate nuclear gene expression: Implications for mitochondrial retrograde signaling. *International Journal of Molecular Science*, *18*. pii: E786.

Zeno, S., Veenman, L., Katz, Y., Bode, J., Gavish, M., & Zaaroor, M. (2012). The 18 kDa mitochondrial translocator protein (TSPO) prevents accumulation of protoporphyrin IX. Involvement of reactive oxygen species (ROS). *Current Molecular Medicine*, *12*, 494–501.

Zeno, S., Zaaroor, M., Leschiner, S., Veenman, L., & Gavish, M. (2009). CoCl(2) induces apoptosis via the 18 kDa translocator protein in U118MG human glioblastoma cells. *Biochemistry*, *48*, 4652–4661.

Zhang, X., & Moye-Rowley, W. S. (2001). Saccharomyces cerevisiae multidrug resistance gene expression inversely correlates with the status of the F(0) component of the mitochondrial ATPase. *The Journal of Biological Chemistry*, *276*, 47844–47852.

Zhang, Y., Yu, S., Li, X., Yang, B., & Wu, C. (2017). The ligands of translocator protein inhibit human Th1 responses and the rejection of murine skin allografts. *Clinical Science (London)*, *131*, 297–308.

Zhao, A. H., Tu, L. N., Mukai, C., Sirivelu, M. P., Pillai, V. V., Morohaku, K., et al. (2016). Mitochondrial translocator protein (TSPO) function is not essential for Heme biosynthesis. *The Journal of Biological Chemistry*, *291*, 1591–1603.

FURTHER READING

Bui, E. T., Bradley, P. J., & Johnson, P. J. (1996). A common evolutionary origin for mitochondria and hydrogenosomes. *Proceedings of the National Academy of Sciences of the United States of America*, *93*, 9651–9656.

French, K. L., Hallmann, C., Hope, J. M., Schoon, P. L., Zumberge, J. A., Hoshino, Y., et al. (2015). Reappraisal of hydrocarbon biomarkers in Archean rocks. *Proceedings of the National Academy of Sciences of the United States of America*, *112*, 5915–5920.

Gavish, M., Katz, Y., Bar-Ami, S., & Weizman, R. (1992). Biochemical, physiological, and pathological aspects of the peripheral benzodiazepine receptor. *Journal of Neurochemistry*, *58*, 1589–1601.

Gavish, M., Veenman, J.A., Shterenberg, A., Marek I. (2013). Heterocyclic derivatives, pharmaceutical compositions and methods of use thereof. Patent Grant: US 8541428 B2.

Ma, L., Zhang, H., Liu, N., Wang, P. Q., Guo, W. Z., Fu, Q., et al. (2016). Tspo ligand pk11195 alleviates neuroinflammation and beta-amyloid generation induced by systemic lps administration. *Brain Research Bulletin*, *121*, 192–200.

Papadopoulos, V., & Lecanu, L. (2009). Translocator protein (18 kDa) TSPO: An emerging therapeutic target in neurotrauma. *Experimental Neurology*, *219*, 53–57.

Stowe-Evans, E. L., Ford, J., & Kehoe, D. M. (2004). Genomic DNA microarray analysis: Identification of new genes regulated by light color in the cyanobacterium *Fremyella diplosiphon*. *Journal of Bacteriology*, *186*, 4338–4349.

Veenman, L., & Gavish, M. (2000). Peripheral-type benzodiazepine receptors: Their implication in brain disease. *Drug Development Research*, *50*, 355–370.

CHAPTER SEVEN

Unique Effects of Clozapine: A Pharmacological Perspective

Jibran Y. Khokhar*,†, Angela M. Henricks*,†, Emily D.K. Sullivan*,†, Alan I. Green*,†,1

*Geisel School of Medicine at Dartmouth, Hanover, NH, United States
†Dartmouth Clinical and Translational Science Institute, Dartmouth College, Hanover, NH, United States
[1]Corresponding author: e-mail address: alan.i.green@dartmouth.edu

Contents

Abstract

Schizophrenia is a heterogenous and severe neuropsychiatric disorder that affects nearly 1% of the population worldwide. Antipsychotic drugs are the mainstay of treatment, but not all patients with schizophrenia respond to treatment with these agents. Clozapine, the first atypical antipsychotic, is a highly effective medication for patients with schizophrenia who do not respond to other antipsychotics. Although clozapine tends not to produce extrapyramidal symptoms, other side effects of the drug (e.g., agranulocytosis, myocarditis, seizures) limit its widespread use. This chapter reviews clozapine's unique clinical effects and unusual pharmacological profile. In addition to its effects in treatment-resistant schizophrenia, clozapine has been shown to decrease suicidality, which occurs at an increased rate in patients with schizophrenia. Still preliminary, but consistent data, also suggest that clozapine limits substance use in these patients, an important effect since substance use disorders are common in patients with schizophrenia and are associated with a poor outcome, including an increased risk for suicide and poor response to treatment. We have suggested, from animal studies, that clozapine's apparent ability to limit substance use may occur through its actions as a weak dopamine D2 receptor antagonist, a potent

Advances in Pharmacology, Volume 82
ISSN 1054-3589
https://doi.org/10.1016/bs.apha.2017.09.009

norepinephrine α-2 receptor antagonist and a norepinephrine reuptake inhibitor. Using animal models, we have built combinations of agents toward creation of safer clozapine-like drugs to reduce substance use in these patients. Future research into the mechanisms of action of clozapine toward the development of safe clozapine-like agents is of great public health importance.

Foreword. We are delighted to contribute this chapter in honor of Solomon H. Snyder. I (Alan I. Green) was the first medical student to work in his laboratory, just 50 years ago, in the early months of 1967. Sol was then, as he has remained, an inspirational figure, encouraging a naïve student, a history major in college, that he had a talent for scientific research. Sol's many contributions to neuropsychopharmacology, including toward an early understanding of the action of antipsychotic drugs, as noted in the following chapter, while extraordinary, are at least equaled by his unique ability to launch the careers of dozens of productive scientists. While I have tried over these many years to capture the Snyder gift for inspiration, I have learned that there is only one Sol.

1. INTRODUCTION

Schizophrenia is a heterogenous and complex neuropsychiatric disorder that affects nearly 1% of the population worldwide and includes a composite of positive, negative, and cognitive symptom domains (Andreasen, 2000). The introduction of the antipsychotic drugs, beginning with chlorpromazine in the 1950s, dramatically changed the nature of treatment for patients with this severe disorder. Moreover, the realization that effective antipsychotics blocked the dopamine D2 receptor contributed to the development of the dopamine hypothesis of schizophrenia (Snyder, 1976). The seminal paper noting a correlation between potency at the dopamine D2 receptor and clinical potency (Creese, Burt, & Snyder, 1976) further cemented the notion that search for a potent dopamine receptor antagonist was the holy grail for optimal treatment of schizophrenia. The major side effects of the antipsychotics, extrapyramidal symptoms (e.g., muscle rigidity, tremor, tardive dyskinesia), were assumed to be a necessary fellow traveler with an effective antipsychotic drug. The use of chlorpromazine and the medications that followed all potent dopamine D2 receptor antagonists allowed many patients to be discharged from asylums and led to the development of the community mental health center movement. Nonetheless, it was recognized early on that while the antipsychotics were effective, many patients had only a partial response, and for a substantial component of the population of patients with schizophrenia, these "miracle drugs" had almost no effect. This situation seemed to change with the (re)introduction of clozapine, an "atypical" antipsychotic, in 1989 (Kane & Correll, 2016; Kane, Honigfeld, Singer, & Meltzer, 1988; Meltzer, 1997). This chapter will trace the use of clozapine, discuss its unique clinical applicability, and address aspects of its pharmacology that may contribute to its unusual and striking clinical effects.

2. HISTORY OF CLOZAPINE

Clozapine was first discovered in 1959 by scientists at Wander Laboratories, who were screening tricyclic compounds for antidepressant activity and were surprised to discover drugs with a chemical structure comparable to the tricyclic antidepressants but with antipsychotic properties (Naheed & Green, 2001). Since the prevailing thought at the time was that extrapyramidal side effects were required for antipsychotic efficacy, clozapine was considered "atypical" or "defective," which limited initial interest in the compound (Burns, 2001). In the early 1970s, however, Stille and Hippius challenged the prevailing extrapyramidal symptom dogma with data derived from studies in patients given clozapine demonstrating that its antipsychotic efficacy was not dependent on the development of these symptoms (Stille, Lauener, & Eichenberger, 1971). Moreover, they noted that this atypical antipsychotic (which did not produce obvious extrapyramidal effects) had excellent clinical efficacy across multiple symptom domains.

As the use of clozapine spread in Europe, a troubling side effect began to limit its popularity. In a trial in Finland, 16 patients developed agranulocytosis, and 8 of them died from overwhelming infections (de la Chapelle, Kari, Nurminen, & Hernberg, 1977; Idanpaan-Heikkila, Alhava, Olkinuora, & Palva, 1975). Because of this report, use of clozapine was dramatically reduced and research on the drug was stopped. Although it was essentially pulled from the market, some humanitarian use of clozapine continued, especially for patients unresponsive to other drugs, with very careful blood monitoring. Moreover, reports surfaced that many patients that had been responsive to clozapine relapsed when the drug was stopped, increasing the interest in determining whether there was a safe way to use the drug while managing the risk of agranulocytosis (Naheed & Green, 2001).

The publication by Kane et al. (1988), funded by Sandoz, which now owned clozapine, dramatically changed the landscape for use of the drug.

This careful investigation of patients who were refractory to other antipsychotics demonstrated the superior efficacy of clozapine over chlorpromazine for such patients—with demonstrated superiority in terms of positive and negative symptoms of psychosis, along with the development of minimal extrapyramidal side effects. Moreover, the frequent blood monitoring within the study demonstrated a way to use clozapine safely.

Sandoz used the findings of the Kane et al. (1988) study to support an application to the FDA for use of clozapine in treatment-resistant schizophrenia, with a requirement for blood testing to monitor for the risk for agranulocytosis. With such careful use, including the cessation of use at the first sign of possible agranulocytosis, the rate of agranulocytosis has been reported to be 0.38% (Schulte, 2006).

The reintroduction of clozapine in 1989 dramatically changed the treatment approach for patients with refractory psychosis—suddenly there was a medication that for many at least seemed to decrease psychosis and allow them to be treated as outpatients. With its more widespread use, however, many other potential side effects of clozapine were noted, including weight gain, diabetes, myocarditis, and seizures, that, combined with the requirement for frequent blood monitoring, tended to limit the use of this most interesting drug to a very narrow range of patients (Flanagan, 2008; Hodge & Jespersen, 2008). To this day, clozapine is seriously underprescribed by psychiatrists, with estimates suggesting that only 5%–20% of clozapine-eligible patients receive clozapine treatment (Olfson, Gerhard, Crystal, & Stroup, 2016). After the introduction of clozapine, many other "atypical" agents were developed; nonetheless, none of them have met the standard of clozapine for efficacy. This, coupled with the limited use of clozapine, has emphasized the need for revisiting the pharmacology of clozapine, and bringing attention back to a drug that may be our best option in treating a variety of schizophrenia and schizophrenia-related disorders.

Clozapine broke the mold of the first-generation antipsychotics and displayed clinical efficacy without a potent dopamine D2 receptor blockade and thereby reduced risk for the extrapyramidal side effects (Fakra & Azorin, 2012). While clozapine still remains the most effective antipsychotic, its mechanisms of action remain elusive (Wenthur & Lindsley, 2013). Attempts to create structurally related compounds have not produced agents that match clozapine's efficacy. Clozapine is an agent that seems to serendipitously benefit from actions across various neurotransmitter systems. Imaging and pharmacological studies suggest that while typical antipsychotics show high striatal dopamine receptor binding, clozapine does not (Mamo et al., 2004) but seems to be having its effects not only through dopamine receptors, but also at serotonergic, noradrenergic, and glutamatergic receptors (Meltzer, Matsubara, & Lee, 1989; Sur et al., 2003). The effects of clozapine have considerably advanced our understanding of the mechanistic underpinnings of schizophrenia and have given rise to other atypical drugs that act, for example, at serotonin 5-HT2A as well as dopamine D2 receptors (Janssen et al., 1988). Clozapine's blockade of norepinephrine alpha 2 receptors has also been thought to contribute to its activity (Baldessarini, Huston-Lyons, Campbell, Marsh, & Cohen, 1992; Breier et al., 1994) as have its possible modulatory actions on a dysfunctional glutamatergic system (Olney, Newcomer, & Farber, 1999). In the latter half of this chapter, we will further delineate the pharmacological actions of clozapine with the goal of reconstructing clozapine-like agents for use in indications in which clozapine shows clear superiority over other antipsychotic medications. Prior to that, however, we will describe three special populations of patients with schizophrenia, in which clozapine has demonstrated a unique efficacy, those with: treatment resistance; suicidality; and cooccurring substance use disorders.

3. TREATMENT-RESISTANT SCHIZOPHRENIA

As many as 30% of patients with schizophrenia are resistant to treatment with antipsychotic medications (Conley & Kelly, 2001), meaning they show no or partial clinical response to at least two different antipsychotic medications. Treatment-resistant schizophrenia is associated with an increased risk of substance use, suicidal ideation, and a poorer quality of life (Kennedy, Altar, Taylor, Degtiar, & Hornberger, 2014), and attempts to develop therapies for treatment-resistant schizophrenia have been elusive. But clozapine is uniquely effective in its ability to improve clinical outcomes in patients with treatment-resistance schizophrenia. As mentioned earlier, Kane et al. (1988) first evaluated the efficacy of clozapine for treatment-resistant schizophrenia. In this controlled clinical trial, patients with schizophrenia (who had a history of poor response to previous trials of antipsychotics) were treated with the typical antipsychotic haloperidol for 6 weeks, and those who failed to show a significant clinical response were then randomly assigned to clozapine or chlorpromazine treatment for another 6 weeks (Kane et al., 1988). The patients treated with clozapine showed significantly greater improvements in Brief Psychiatric Rating Scale (BPRS) and Clinical Global Impressions (CGI) scale scores compared to those treated with chlorpromazine.

Since this iconic study, subsequent experiments have corroborated the findings from Kane and colleagues. For instance, in a randomized double-blind study of the efficacy of clozapine compared to haloperidol, a typical antipsychotic, treatment-resistant patients receiving clozapine had significantly lower psychotic symptoms as measured by the Positive and Negative Syndrome Scale (PANSS), as well as fewer days hospitalized for psychiatric complaints, compared to those receiving haloperidol (Rosenheck et al., 1997). A metaanalysis of 12 controlled studies also confirmed that clozapine was more efficacious in reducing psychotic symptoms in patients with treatment-resistant schizophrenia, as well as decreasing the risk of extrapyramidal side effects, compared to typical antipsychotic medications (Chakos, Lieberman, Hoffman, Bradford, & Sheitman, 2001). Moreover, two large-scale clinical trials (Clinical Antipsychotic Trials of Intervention Effectiveness [CATIE] in the United States and Cost Utility of the Latest Antipsychotic Drugs in Schizophrenia Study [CUtLASS] in the United Kingdom) both demonstrated that clozapine is the most effective antipsychotic for patients with schizophrenia unresponsive to treatment with other antipsychotic drugs (including those developed after the introduction of clozapine) (Jones et al., 2006; Lewis et al., 2006; Lieberman et al., 2005; Naber & Lambert, 2009). Thus, based on the available data, clozapine continues to be considered the "gold-standard" for patients with treatment-resistant schizophrenia, although it continues to be underutilized in general clinical practice.

There has been interest in discovering indicators of preferential response to clozapine that might allow its use prior to multiple treatment trials with other antipsychotics, thus to identify predictors of treatment resistance. Significant predictors of a favorable response to clozapine treatment include younger age, more severe symptoms (as evidence by more days hospitalized for psychiatric reasons prior to schizophrenia diagnosis), a previous suicide attempt, affective symptoms, and use of antidepressant medications (Wimberley et al., 2016). Interestingly, treatment-resistant schizophrenia has been associated with reduced cortical thickness, including areas of the frontal, parietal, temporal, and occipital lobes (Zugman et al., 2013), which may have clinical relevance as a neural indicator of treatment-resistant schizophrenia and minimize the delay between diagnosis and appropriate antipsychotic treatment. Nonetheless, these imaging data have not, to this point, been directly linked to preferential response to clozapine.

Some of the biologic characteristics of treatment-resistant schizophrenia may also hint at the possible mechanism behind the efficacy of clozapine. For instance, treatment-resistant patients have been demonstrated to have reduced dopamine synthesis (rather than hyperactivity seen in other patients) in the striatum compared to nonresistant patients (Demjaha, Murray, McGuire, Kapur, & Howes, 2012), suggesting that treatment-resistant patients may have a distinct form of schizophrenia that is mediated by dysregulated neurotransmitter systems beyond dopamine. Moreover, given the wide spectrum pharmacological action of clozapine, its relatively low affinity for the dopamine D2 receptor, as well as its actions in glutamatergic, serotonergic, and noradrenergic systems (Wenthur & Lindsley, 2013), the capacity of clozapine to treat patients with treatment-resistant schizophrenia may be linked to the ability of clozapine to alter more than just dopamine synthesis.

Nonetheless, since the precise mechanisms underlying the effectiveness of clozapine for treatment-resistant schizophrenia are still poorly understood, some research has also aimed to identify how clozapine treatment alters neurobiological functioning in these patients. Reduced frontal cortical metabolic activity has been consistently associated with an increased response to clozapine treatment (Chung & Remington, 2005), suggesting the frontal cortex may be an important region involved in clozapine's efficacy. In an attempt to determine the effects of clozapine on cortical metabolic activity, Molina et al. (2005) evaluated resting neural metabolic activity in treatment-resistant patients prior to and 6 months after clozapine treatment. Clozapine treatment was associated with reductions in prefrontal cortical metabolic activity, as well as reduced basal ganglia metabolic activity. Interestingly, reductions in basal ganglia metabolic activity were associated with reductions in negative symptoms, while reductions in positive symptoms were associated with increased in metabolic activity in the visual cortex. In a follow-up study by these authors, clozapine treatment was associated with enhanced activity in the cingulate cortex, insula, and hippocampus during a cognitive task compared to risperidone treatment (Molina et al., 2008). Thus, clozapine's ability to alter activity in cortical and limbic regions compared to other antipsychotic medications may be related to its efficacy in treatment-resistant patients, but substantially more work is required to fully understand the mechanisms underlying clozapine's effectiveness for this indication and others.

4. SUICIDALITY

Patients with schizophrenia are at a significantly high risk for suicide, as approximately 50% of patients attempt suicide, compared to only 1% in the general population, and 10% of patients with schizophrenia die from suicide (Meltzer et al., 2003; Meltzer & Baldessarini, 2003). In an early trial in treatment-resistant patients, clozapine treatment was associated with significantly fewer suicide attempts compared to patients treated with typical antipsychotics (Spivak et al., 1998). Later, in the seminal InterSePT trial (International Suicide Prevention Trial), a randomized, international study comparing suicidal behavior in patients at risk of suicide who were treated with either clozapine or olanzapine (thought to be the most effective agent secondary to clozapine), Meltzer et al. (2003) showed that suicidal behavior was significantly reduced in patients treated with clozapine compared to those treated with olanzapine. Specifically, fewer clozapine-treated patients attempted suicide and clozapine patients required fewer hospitalizations and rescue interventions related to suicide. A retrospective study looking at inpatients with schizophrenia corroborated these findings; prior to clozapine treatment the rate of suicidal behavior among these patients was 28%, which was reduced to 3% during clozapine treatment (Modestin, Dal Pian, & Agarwalla, 2005). Interestingly, in a subset of patients, discontinuation of clozapine resulted in an increase in suicidal behavior to 18%. Lastly, a small study of three patients with schizophrenia further demonstrated that the effects of clozapine discontinuation on suicidal behavior; abrupt discontinuation of clozapine treatment due to side effects in these patients were rapidly followed by suicide (Patchan, Richardson, Vyas, & Kelly, 2015). Thus, clozapine appears to be exceptionally effective in reducing the risk of suicide in patients with schizophrenia, compared to both typical and atypical antipsychotic medications.

Depression is common in patients with schizophrenia, with up to 80% of patients experiencing depressive symptoms, and is associated with a poorer quality of life, increased risk of both relapse and suicide (Nakajima et al., 2015). The CATIE trial, mentioned earlier, found that clozapine was more effective than quetiapine in reducing depressive symptoms in patients (Nakajima et al., 2015). Yet, the CATIE trial also found no significant differences between clozapine, olanzapine, and risperidone in reducing symptoms of depression in patients with schizophrenia. Thus, the unique ability of clozapine to reduce suicidal behavior in patients with schizophrenia may not be entirely due to its antidepressant effects.

Little is known regarding the mechanisms behind clozapine's efficacy in reducing suicidal behavior, but it may be related to clozapine's effects on norepinephrine, a neurotransmitter thought to be involved in the emergence of depression and commonly targeted by antidepressant medications (Delgado & Moreno, 2000). Indeed, early work by our group giving clozapine to patients with treatment refractory schizophrenia showed that clozapine dramatically and chronically enhances peripheral norepinephrine levels (Green et al., 1993), which is not observed with haloperidol (Green et al., 1993), or with other typical antipsychotic medications (Spivak et al., 1998). Moreover, other atypical agents, such as risperidone, which also block the norepinephrine α-2 receptor, do not elevate peripheral norepinephrine levels to the extent of clozapine (See, Fido, Maurice, Ibrahim, & Salama, 1999). Moreover, Breier et al. (1994) noted a relationship between elevated norepinephrine levels and overall response to clozapine. Thus, the ability of clozapine to alter neurotransmitter systems other than dopamine, especially clozapine-induced increases in norepinephrine levels, may be partly associated with clozapine's ability to reduce depression (and suicidal behavior) in patients with schizophrenia. Another potential mechanism for the reduction in suicidal behavior by clozapine may be related to clozapine's apparent ability to reduce substance use in patients with schizophrenia, since substance use in these patients is associated with a risk for suicide. Previous studies have suggested that limiting substance use in dual diagnosis patients with schizophrenia may limit suicide since suicidal ideation has been shown to be greater among patients who are currently misusing substances, compared with past or nonsubstance misusers (Hunt et al., 2006; Kamali et al., 2000). Moreover, our unpublished secondary analyses of the data from the InterSePT study, showing that clozapine was efficacious in reducing the initiation of substance use in patients with schizophrenia who were at a high risk for suicide, suggests another unique subpopulation that might benefit from clozapine.

5. SUBSTANCE USE IN SCHIZOPHRENIA

In still preliminary studies, clozapine does seem to have the unusual ability (among antipsychotics) of decreasing substance use in patients with schizophrenia and cooccurring substance use disorder. The Epidemiologic Catchment Area (ECA) study in the late 1980s made it clear that individuals with schizophrenia have a high rate of substance use disorder, particularly alcohol, cannabis, and cocaine—estimated to be 4.6 times the rate in the background population (Regier et al., 1990). Moreover, the rate of tobacco smoking is known to be 70%–90% in patients with schizophrenia, in face of the decreasing rate of tobacco smoking in the general US population (falling below 20%) (Hartz et al., 2014; Kalman, Morissette, & George, 2005). In fact, it has been estimated that 44% of all cigarettes in the United States are smoked by less than 5% of the population—mainly those with severe psychiatric disorders (Lasser et al., 2000). Use of alcohol, cannabis, and cocaine has a negative effect on the course of schizophrenia, as defined by increased rates of hospitalization, decreased compliance with medication, increased violence and suicide, and overall increased societal costs (DeQuardo, Carpenter, & Tandon, 1994; Dickey & Azeni, 1996; Henquet et al., 2010; Juckel et al., 2006; Kivlahan, Heiman, Wright, Mundt, & Shupe, 1991; Knudsen & Vilmar, 1984; Linszen, Dingemans, & Lenior, 1994; Negrete & Knapp, 1986; Peralta & Cuesta, 1992; Regier et al., 1990; Sayers et al., 2005; Smith, Barzman, & Pristach, 1997; Swendsen et al., 2012; Treffert, 1978; van Dijk, Koeter, Hijman, Kahn, & van den Brink, 2012).

While the typical antipsychotic drugs (e.g., haloperidol) have clear therapeutic efficacy in treating psychosis in patients with schizophrenia, they do not appear to reduce substance use in patients with schizophrenia and substance use disorder (Green, Noordsy, Brunette, & O'Keefe, 2008), and may even lead to further use (Bedard, Maheux, Levesque, & Samaha, 2013). Atypical antipsychotics, on the other hand, seem to have varying effects on substance use. While most atypical antipsychotics have modest efficacy toward reducing substance use, we and others have shown that clozapine, unlike typical antipsychotics, appears to substantially decrease alcohol and substance use in this population (Albanese, Khantzian, Murphy, & Green, 1994; Buckley, Thompson, Way, & Meltzer, 1994; Drake, Xie, McHugo, & Green, 2000; Marcus & Snyder, 1995; Wu, Chen, & Lee, 2013; Zimmet, Strous, Burgess, Kohnstamm, & Green, 2000) and also prevent relapse to alcohol use in those whose alcohol use has remitted (Brunette, Drake, Xie, McHugo, & Green, 2006). The observation that clozapine might decrease substance use was first reported in the mid-1990s, with a series of case reports, retrospective surveys, and one naturalistic study (Akerman, Brunette, Noordsy, & Green, 2014; Albanese et al., 1994; Buckley et al., 1994; Drake et al., 2000; Marcus & Snyder, 1995; Wu et al., 2013; Zimmet et al., 2000). The naturalistic study noted a dramatic improvement of alcohol abuse (as well as cannabis use) in patients who had been given clozapine vs those remaining on a standard (typical) antipsychotic (Drake et al., 2000). Nonetheless, only one randomized trial has been published—involving a small sample of patients with schizophrenia and cannabis use disorder, which indicated that clozapine treatment was associated with a decrease in cannabis use, as compared to treatment with other antipsychotics (Brunette et al., 2011). Thus, the data on clozapine's effects on decreasing substance use are consistent, although a definitive study has not yet been done.

Many studies have investigated whether other atypical antipsychotics share clozapine's ability to limit comorbid alcohol/substance use disorders in patients with schizophrenia (Green et al., 2008). While some data exist regarding possible effects of quetiapine, olanzapine, and aripiprazole, the overall consensus is that none of the typical or atypical agents also consistently limit substance use in these patients (Akerele & Levin, 2007; Beresford et al., 2005; Brown, Jeffress, Liggin, Garza, & Beard, 2005; Brunette, Dawson, O'Keefe, Buckley, & Green, 2009; Green et al., 2008; Warsi, Sattar, Bhatia, & Petty, 2005).

6. BASIS OF SUBSTANCE USE DISORDER IN SCHIZOPHRENIA

In the remainder of this chapter, we will focus on schizophrenia and cooccurring substance use disorder to begin to delineate the potential basis of the unusual effects of clozapine—leading to the possible development of a safer clozapine-like agent. While the story is still unfinished and much research needs to be done, the theories of the basis of the cooccurrence of schizophrenia and substance use disorder may provide some clues. The four main theories of comorbid schizophrenia and substance abuse are the self-medication hypothesis, the cumulative risk factor hypothesis, the stress diathesis theory, and the primary addiction hypothesis.

A common clinical explanation for the use of alcohol and other substances in patients with schizophrenia invokes the "self-medication hypothesis," where the alcohol/substance abuse relates to an attempt by the patient to self-medicate negative symptoms or the extrapyramidal side effects of antipsychotics (Khantzian, 1997; Siris, 1990). While the self-medication hypothesis has some intuitive appeal, the available data do not provide evidence to support this as a causal explanation for the use of alcohol/substances in patients with schizophrenia (Buchanan, Strauss, Breier, Kirkpatrick, & Carpenter, 1997; Cantwell et al., 1999; Hambrecht & Hafner, 1996; Kovasznay et al., 1997; Linszen et al., 1994; Lysaker, Bell, Beam-Goulet, & Milstein, 1994). Substance use, actually, tends to be less common in patients with primarily negative symptoms, and even first episode patients, including those not treated with antipsychotic medications, frequently use substances (Batki, Leontieva, Dimmock, & Ploutz-Snyder, 2008; Brunette et al., 2017; Buchanan et al., 1997; Tomassi et al., 2017).

The cumulative risk factor hypothesis posits that patients with schizophrenia are more likely to have a substance use problem when combined with certain environmental factors such as socioeconomic status and accessibility to drugs (Mueser et al., 1990). Rosenthal (1970) proposed a similar concept, the stress diathesis theory or the "two-hit" model. Schizophrenia is widely accepted to have an important genetic component, and Rosenthal theorized that genetic factors predicted a risk for disease, but when combined with an environmental stressor (including substance use), could manifest into schizophrenia (Fowles, 1992; Pruessner, Cullen, Aas, & Walker, 2017). Some studies support the diathesis-stress theory with interactions observed between substance (especially cannabis) use and an earlier age of onset of schizophrenia and psychosis (Green & Glausier, 2016; Linszen et al., 1994).

The fourth hypothesis is the primary addiction hypothesis (Chambers, Krystal, & Self, 2001) also known as the reward deficiency syndrome hypothesis (Green, Zimmet, Strous, & Schildkraut, 1999). Both animal and human studies (in an animal model of schizophrenia and in patients with schizophrenia) find dysfunction in the dopamine-mediated brain reward circuit (Chambers, 2007; Chambers et al., 2001, 2013; Fischer, Whitfield-Gabrieli, Roth, Brunette, & Green, 2014; Thompson et al., 2013), which could underlie both schizophrenia and substance abuse (Khokhar, Dwiel, Henricks, Doucette, & Green, 2017).

Our theoretical neurobiologic formulation (Green et al., 1999), consistent with Chambers et al. (2001) and others (Nisell, Nomikos, & Svensson, 1995), suggests that a high rate of substance use disorders in patients with schizophrenia may be secondary to biological dysfunctions within the dopamine-mediated mesocorticolimbic "brain reward" pathways. Many studies suggest that negative symptoms in patients with schizophrenia are related to reduced activity in dopamine neurons projecting from the ventral tegmental area into the prefrontal cortex (i.e., mesocortical neurons) (Grace, 1991; Moghaddam & Sesack, 1996; Weinberger, 1987). At the same time, other midbrain DA neurons projecting from the ventral tegmental area to the nucleus accumbens (i.e., mesolimbic neurons), which are themselves regulated by neural projections from the prefrontal cortex (Au-Young, Shen, & Yang, 1999; Moghaddam & Sesack, 1996; Pycock, Kerwin, &

Carter, 1980), are thought to be hyperactive, leading to the positive symptoms of psychosis (Grace, 1991). Both of these dopaminergic pathways (particularly the mesolimbic) are key elements in the brain reward circuit that is thought both to mediate pleasure, contentment, and motivation within everyday life (Fibiger & Phillips, 1988; Gardner, 1997) and to be the locus for the reward-based effects of substances of abuse (Hyman, Malenka, & Nestler, 2006). Interestingly, our group and others have shown in behavioral studies that patients with schizophrenia have impaired olfactory hedonic processing (Folley & Park, 2010; Mesholam-Gately, Gibson, Seidman, & Green, 2014) and we (Fischer et al., 2014) and others have demonstrated a brain reward circuit deficit (including decreased functional connectivity between the nucleus accumbens and the prefrontal cortex) in fMRI studies of such patients (Fischer et al., 2014; Juckel et al., 2006; Moran, Sampath, Kochunov, & Hong, 2013; Moran, Sampath, Stein, & Hong, 2012; Nielsen, Rostrup, Wulff, Bak, Broberg, et al., 2012; Nielsen, Rostrup, Wulff, Bak, Lublin, et al., 2012; Wint et al., 2005).

This theory (Green et al., 1999) also proposed that the substances themselves, due to their common action of potentiating dopamine activity, might normalize the brain reward circuit dysfunction while at the same time exacerbating symptoms in the patients. Pilot data have shown that individuals with comorbid cannabis use disorder and schizophrenia have significantly lower resting-state functional activity between the nucleus accumbens and prefrontal cortical brain reward circuit regions when compared to a control group, and that either smoked cannabis or Δ^9-tetrahydrocannabinol substantially ameliorates the abnormal connectivity (Fischer et al., 2014).

7. PHARMACOLOGY OF CLOZAPINE: BUILDING A SAFER CLOZAPINE?

Why does clozapine limit substance use in patients with schizophrenia—and does it lead to clues about building a safer clozapine-like agent? Clozapine's unique clinical effects (secondary to its broad pharmacological profile that includes a relatively weak blockade at dopamine D2 receptors) may in part involve release of dopamine in the prefrontal cortex (Devoto et al., 2003; Green et al., 1999). Moreover, because of the apparent modulation of the subcortical mesolimbic dopamine system by the prefrontal cortex (Green et al., 1999; Moghaddam & Sesack, 1996), the release of dopamine by clozapine in the prefrontal cortex may also result in a decrease of dopamine release in the mesolimbic system, which, when added to its (albeit weak) D2 receptor blocking effects, may contribute to its antipsychotic potential and its ability to reduce substance use (Green et al., 1999; Moghaddam & Sesack, 1996; Pycock et al., 1980). This combined with our original work on clozapine, where we were struck by the dramatic elevation of plasma norepinephrine in patients treated with the drug, as compared to those treated with haloperidol (Green et al., 1993), and based on the original work from Svensson (2003), we hypothesized that clozapine might improve the reward dysfunction and thereby make patients less likely to use substances (Green, Burgess, Dawson, Zimmet, & Strous, 2003; Green et al., 1999). Thus far, two sets of data seem to suggest this is the case. Machielsen and colleagues recently demonstrated that clozapine (as compared to risperidone) reduces craving for cannabis and decreases insula activation during a cannabis attentional bias task (Machielsen, Veltman, van den Brink, & de Haan, 2014, 2017). Moreover, we showed that clozapine improves olfactory hedonic tone, as compared to typical antipsychotics, in patients with schizophrenia and cooccurring substance use disorder (Mesholam-Gately et al., 2014).

Our group has attempted to deconstruct the pharmacological actions of clozapine related to its effect on substance use in patients with schizophrenia, following up on our theoretical paper suggesting the importance of the ratio of norepinephrine α-2 to dopamine D2 receptor blockade (Green et al., 1999). To do this, we developed a series of studies in rodents, primarily using the Syrian golden hamster and the alcohol preferring P rat. In these studies, we focused most directly on clozapine's weak dopamine D2 receptor blockade, its potent norepinephrine α-2 receptor blockade, and the ability of clozapine to dramatically increase norepinephrine levels in plasma and brain (Chau, Gulick, Xie, Dawson, & Green, 2010; Green et al., 1993, 2004; Khokhar, Chau, Dawson, & Green, 2015) to understand its ability to reduce alcohol drinking in patients and in our rodent models.

We first showed that like patients with schizophrenia, acute and chronic treatment with clozapine (and not haloperidol) could reduce alcohol drinking in the Syrian golden hamster (Chau et al., 2010; Green et al., 2004). These early studies established the predictive validity for this model in testing the effects of antipsychotic agents since clozapine reduced alcohol drinking whereas haloperidol did not. Moreover, discontinuation of clozapine treatment in the hamster resulted in a gradual increase in alcohol drinking toward baseline levels (Green et al., 2004). Lastly, the reductions in alcohol drinking were not accompanied by decreases of sucrose, water, or food consumption, suggesting that the effects of clozapine were specific to alcohol drinking

(Chau et al., 2010). Our subsequent work showed that it was the weak antagonism of dopamine D2 receptors by clozapine that contributed to its ability to reduce alcohol drinking in the hamster (Chau et al., 2011). This was done by adding raclopride (a potent dopamine D2 receptor antagonist) to clozapine; the addition of raclopride significantly blunted clozapine's ability to reduce alcohol drinking in the Syrian golden hamster (Chau et al., 2011).

Beyond its actions on dopamine receptors, however, it may be clozapine's actions on the noradrenergic system, which, when added to (or related to) its ability to release dopamine in the prefrontal cortex, may be of greatest importance in understanding its unique clinical profile, including its effects on alcohol/substance use in patients with schizophrenia. As noted earlier, clozapine produces striking elevations of norepinephrine in the plasma (Breier et al., 1994; Green et al., 1993) and CSF (Leiberman et al., 1991) in patients, and our findings suggest that this may be explained both by its α-2 receptor antagonism (Ashby & Wang, 1996) as well as its ability to block the reuptake of norepinephrine following synaptic release (Khokhar et al., 2015; Yoshimura et al., 2000). Clozapine's actions on norepinephrine may be particularly relevant given the suggestions that norepinephrine may potentiate functioning of the dopamine-mediated "reward system" by decreasing the "noise" of basal firing patterns (i.e., by slowing and deregularizing firing) in ventral tegmental area dopamine neurons (with resultant increase in signal detection) (Grenhoff & Svensson, 1989; Nisell et al., 1995). Even as we begin to understand the effects of clozapine related to its ability to reduce substance use, however, we are still not able to use this information to inform treatment. This has led to a line of translational research in our laboratory related to designing improved medications for use in this difficult to treat population.

Specifically, we have attempted to reconstruct some of the actions of clozapine, using other antipsychotics currently available on the market. In the first of these studies, we showed that the addition of the norepinephrine reuptake inhibitor desipramine to risperidone (an atypical antipsychotic that is a potent dopamine D2 receptor antagonist, as well as a potent norepinephrine α-2 receptor antagonist, but does not reduce substance use in patients or in our animal models) significantly improved risperidone's ability to reduce alcohol drinking in the Syrian golden hamster (Gulick, Chau, Khokhar, Dawson, & Green, 2014). In this study, low doses of risperidone were used to approximate the weak dopamine D2 blockade seen with clozapine. Following up on these findings with another related atypical antipsychotic, paliperidone, the primary metabolite of risperidone, with similar effects on dopamine and noradrenergic systems, we showed that the addition of desipramine to paliperidone resulted in significant decreases in alcohol drinking in the Syrian golden hamster; consistent with this, the combination of paliperidone and desipramine also markedly reduced alcohol drinking in the alcohol preferring (P) rat, resulting in almost a complete inhibition of initiation of alcohol drinking in the this animal (Chau, Khokhar, Gulick, Dawson, & Green, 2015). In these studies, neither the desipramine nor the low doses of paliperidone alone were sufficient to reduce alcohol drinking significantly, but the combination of the two drugs was able to do so, suggesting that modulation through both the dopaminergic and noradrenergic mechanisms is required for this effect. Lastly, our recently published findings with iloperidone, an antipsychotic with an α-2/D2 receptor antagonism ratio similar to that of clozapine (Kalkman & Loetscher, 2003), showed remarkable efficacy for reducing alcohol drinking in the hamster (almost to the same extent as clozapine), and that this effect could be enhanced by the addition of desipramine, but not idazoxan (an α-2 antagonist) (Khokhar & Green, 2016). The lack of additional effect of idazoxan suggests that since iloperidone acts as a potent norepinephrine α-2 receptor antagonist, the further addition of another α-2 antagonist does not enhance iloperidone's ability to reduce alcohol drinking. Lastly, this reconstruction approach has also shown that even a typical antipsychotic that lacks any ability to reduce alcohol drinking by itself, haloperidol, can be converted to an agent that does so by the addition of desipramine and idazoxan (Khokhar et al., 2015). In this study, a low dose of haloperidol was combined with norepinephrine reuptake inhibition as well as alpha-2 antagonism, and this combination resulted in significant decreases in alcohol drinking in the hamster.

Based on these findings, we have begun to translate the theoretical clozapine reconstruction approach to clinical trials, where we have recently shown that a combination of quetiapine (a weak dopamine D2 receptor antagonist, whose primary metabolite, desalkylquetiapine, is a norepinephrine reuptake inhibitor) and mirtazapine (a norephinephrine α-2 receptor antagonist) significantly reduced alcohol in heavy drinkers (Brunette, Akerman, Dawson, O'Keefe, & Green, 2016). Planned studies by our group will test the effects of other clozapine-like combinations on alcohol and substance use in patients with schizophrenia, while further animal research is aiming to identify the exact neural underpinnings of substance use in this population toward new treatment development to improve outcomes for these patients.

8. CONCLUSION

Given the disturbing side effect profile of clozapine, however, even with its superior efficacy for treatment-resistant schizophrenia, for suicidality in patients with schizophrenia and its apparent ability to decrease substance use in these patients, its use is limited (only around 5% of patients with schizophrenia use clozapine). Many postclozapine agents that have been introduced since the mid-1990s provide little evidence that any of them are as effective as clozapine for refractory psychosis, for dealing with suicidality or for decreasing substance use in patients with schizophrenia. Our focus on the "balance" of noradrenergic and dopaminergic actions of clozapine appears to give clues to its unusual effect in decreasing substance use. Whether this research, enabled by the availability of animal models of alcohol drinking, applies as well to clozapine's unique effects on treatment refractory patients or in those at risk of suicide is not clear. Our own research program is beginning to move into study of animal models of schizophrenia to provide further clues (Khokhar & Todd, 2017). Without question, though, given the unique clinical effects of clozapine, as well as its continued underutilization, future research aimed at creating clozapine-like agents as well as studying the neurobiological underpinnings of clozapine's efficacy are of great public health importance.

CONFLICT OF INTEREST

In the past 3 years, Dr. Alan Green has received grants from Alkermes, Novartis, and Janssen to support research studies, and he has served as an (uncompensated) consultant to Otsuka and Alkermes, and as a member (uncompensated) of a Data Monitoring Board for Lilly. Moreover, he is a coinventor of one patent (and another patent application) regarding treatment of substance abuse. The other authors do not have any conflicts to disclose.

ACKNOWLEDGMENTS

This work was supported in part by a Canadian Institute of Health Research Fellowship award (J.Y.K.) and by grants from the National Institute of Alcohol Abuse and Alcoholism (A.I.G.: 1R03AA014644 and 1R01AA018151), from the National Center for Advancing Translational Science (A.I.G.: NCATS UL1TR001086), and from the National Institute on Drug Abuse (A.I.G.: R01DA032533 and R01DA034699).

REFERENCES

Akerele, E., & Levin, F. R. (2007). Comparison of olanzapine to risperidone in substance-abusing individuals with schizophrenia. *The American Journal on Addictions*, *16*(4), 260–268. https://doi.org/10.1080/10550490701389658.

Akerman, S. C., Brunette, M. F., Noordsy, D. L., & Green, A. I. (2014). Pharmacotherapy of co-occurring schizophrenia and substance use disorders. *Current Addiction Reports*, *1*(4), 251–260. https://doi.org/10.1007/s40429-014-0034-7.

Albanese, M. J., Khantzian, E. J., Murphy, S. L., & Green, A. I. (1994). Decreased substance use in chronically psychotic patients treated with clozapine. *The American Journal of Psychiatry*, *151*(5), 780–781.

Andreasen, N. C. (2000). Schizophrenia: The fundamental questions. *Brain Research. Brain Research Reviews*, *31*(2–3), 106–112.

Ashby, C. R., Jr., & Wang, R. Y. (1996). Pharmacological actions of the atypical antipsychotic drug clozapine: A review. *Synapse*, *24*(4), 349–394. https://doi.org/10.1002/(SICI)1098-2396(199612)24:4<349::AID-SYN5>3.0.CO;2-D.

Au-Young, S. M., Shen, H., & Yang, C. R. (1999). Medial prefrontal cortical output neurons to the ventral tegmental area (VTA) and their responses to burst-patterned stimulation of the VTA: Neuroanatomical and in vivo electrophysiological analyses. *Synapse*, *34*(4), 245–255.

Baldessarini, R. J., Huston-Lyons, D., Campbell, A., Marsh, E., & Cohen, B. M. (1992). Do central antiadrenergic actions contribute to the atypical properties of clozapine? *The British Journal of Psychiatry. Supplement*, *17*, 12–16.

Batki, S. L., Leontieva, L., Dimmock, J. A., & Ploutz-Snyder, R. (2008). Negative symptoms are associated with less alcohol use, craving, and "high" in alcohol dependent patients with schizophrenia. *Schizophrenia Research*, *105*(1–3), 201–207. https://doi.org/10.1016/j.schres.2008.06.020.

Bedard, A. M., Maheux, J., Levesque, D., & Samaha, A. N. (2013). Prior haloperidol, but not olanzapine, exposure augments the pursuit of reward cues: Implications for substance abuse in schizophrenia. *Schizophrenia Bulletin*, *39*(3), 692–702. https://doi.org/10.1093/schbul/sbs077.

Beresford, T. P., Clapp, L., Martin, B., Wiberg, J. L., Alfers, J., & Beresford, H. F. (2005). Aripiprazole in schizophrenia with cocaine dependence: A pilot study. *Journal of Clinical Psychopharmacology*, *25*(4), 363–366.

Breier, A., Buchanan, R. W., Waltrip, R. W., 2nd, Listwak, S., Holmes, C., & Goldstein, D. S. (1994). The effect of clozapine on plasma norepinephrine: Relationship to clinical efficacy. *Neuropsychopharmacology*, *10*(1), 1–7. https://doi.org/10.1038/npp.1994.1.

Brown, E. S., Jeffress, J., Liggin, J. D., Garza, M., & Beard, L. (2005). Switching outpatients with bipolar or schizoaffective disorders and substance abuse from their current antipsychotic to aripiprazole. *The Journal of Clinical Psychiatry*, *66*(6), 756–760.

Brunette, M. F., Akerman, S. C., Dawson, R., O'Keefe, C. D., & Green, A. I. (2016). An open-label pilot study of quetiapine plus mirtazapine for heavy drinkers with alcohol use disorder. *Alcohol*, *53*, 45–50. https://doi.org/10.1016/j.alcohol.2016.02.006.

Brunette, M. F., Dawson, R., O'Keefe, C., Buckley, P., & Green, A. I. (2009). An open label study of quetiapine in patients with schizophrenia and alcohol disorders. *Mental Health and Substance Use*, *2*(3), 203–211.

Brunette, M. F., Dawson, R., O'Keefe, C. D., Narasimhan, M., Noordsy, D. L., Wojcik, J., et al. (2011). A randomized trial of clozapine vs. other antipsychotics for cannabis use disorder in patients with schizophrenia. *Journal of Dual Diagnosis*, 7(1–2), 50–63. https://doi.org/10.1080/15504263.2011.570118.

Brunette, M. F., Drake, R. E., Xie, H., McHugo, G. J., & Green, A. I. (2006). Clozapine use and relapses of substance use disorder among patients with co-occurring schizophrenia and substance use disorders. *Schizophrenia Bulletin*, *32*(4), 637–643. https://doi.org/10.1093/schbul/sbl003.

Brunette, M. F., Mueser, K. T., Babbin, S., Meyer-Kalos, P., Rosenheck, R., Correll, C. U., et al. (2017). Demographic and clinical correlates of substance use disorders in first episode psychosis. *Schizophrenia Research.* https://doi.org/10.1016/j.schres.2017.06.039 (in press).

Buchanan, R. W., Strauss, M. E., Breier, A., Kirkpatrick, B., & Carpenter, W. T., Jr. (1997). Attentional impairments in deficit and nondeficit forms of schizophrenia. *The American Journal of Psychiatry, 154*(3), 363–370. https://doi.org/10.1176/ajp.154.3.363.

Buckley, P., Thompson, P., Way, L., & Meltzer, H. Y. (1994). Substance abuse among patients with treatment-resistant schizophrenia: Characteristics and implications for clozapine therapy. *The American Journal of Psychiatry, 151*(3), 385–389.

Burns, M. J. (2001). The pharmacology and toxicology of atypical antipsychotic agents. *Journal of Toxicology. Clinical Toxicology, 39*(1), 1–14.

Cantwell, R., Brewin, J., Glazebrook, C., Dalkin, T., Fox, R., Medley, I., et al. (1999). Prevalence of substance misuse in first-episode psychosis. *The British Journal of Psychiatry, 174,* 150–153.

Chakos, M., Lieberman, J., Hoffman, E., Bradford, D., & Sheitman, B. (2001). Effectiveness of second-generation antipsychotics in patients with treatment-resistant schizophrenia: A review and meta-analysis of randomized trials. *The American Journal of Psychiatry, 158*(4), 518–526. https://doi.org/10.1176/appi.ajp.158.4.518.

Chambers, R. A. (2007). Animal modeling and neurocircuitry of dual diagnosis. *Journal of Dual Diagnosis, 3*(2), 19–29. https://doi.org/10.1300/J374v03n02_04.

Chambers, R. A., Krystal, J. H., & Self, D. W. (2001). A neurobiological basis for substance abuse comorbidity in schizophrenia. *Biological Psychiatry, 50*(2), 71–83. https://doi.org/10.1016/S0006-3223(01)01134-9.

Chambers, R. A., McClintick, J. N., Sentir, A. M., Berg, S. A., Runyan, M., Choi, K. H., et al. (2013). Cortical-striatal gene expression in neonatal hippocampal lesion (NVHL)-amplified cocaine sensitization. *Genes, Brain, and Behavior, 12*(5), 564–575. https://doi.org/10.1111/gbb.12051.

Chau, D. T., Ahmed, J., Wang, T. T., Xie, H., Dawson, R., & Green, A. I. (2011). Raclopride lessens the ability of clozapine to suppress alcohol drinking in Syrian golden hamsters. *Neuropharmacology, 61*(4), 646–652. doi:S0028-3908(11)00187-0 [pii] https://doi.org/10.1016/j.neuropharm.2011.05.007.

Chau, D. T., Gulick, D., Xie, H., Dawson, R., & Green, A. I. (2010). Clozapine chronically suppresses alcohol drinking in Syrian golden hamsters. *Neuropharmacology, 58*(2), 351–356. https://doi.org/10.1016/j.neuropharm.2009.10.006.

Chau, D. T., Khokhar, J. Y., Gulick, D., Dawson, R., & Green, A. I. (2015). Desipramine enhances the ability of paliperidone to decrease alcohol drinking. *Journal of Psychiatric Research, 69,* 9–18. https://doi.org/10.1016/j.jpsychires.2015.07.010.

Chung, C., & Remington, G. (2005). Predictors and markers of clozapine response. *Psychopharmacology, 179*(2), 317–335. https://doi.org/10.1007/s00213-005-2174-x.

Conley, R. R., & Kelly, D. L. (2001). Management of treatment resistance in schizophrenia. *Biological Psychiatry, 50*(11), 898–911.

Creese, I., Burt, D. R., & Snyder, S. H. (1976). Dopamine receptor binding predicts clinical and pharmacological potencies of antischizophrenic drugs. *Science, 192*(4238), 481–483.

de la Chapelle, A., Kari, C., Nurminen, M., & Hernberg, S. (1977). Clozapine-induced agranulocytosis. A genetic and epidemiologic study. *Human Genetics, 37*(2), 183–194.

Delgado, P. L., & Moreno, F. A. (2000). Role of norepinephrine in depression. *The Journal of Clinical Psychiatry, 61*(Suppl. 1), 5–12.

Demjaha, A., Murray, R. M., McGuire, P. K., Kapur, S., & Howes, O. D. (2012). Dopamine synthesis capacity in patients with treatment-resistant schizophrenia. *The American Journal of Psychiatry, 169*(11), 1203–1210. https://doi.org/10.1176/appi.ajp.2012.12010144.

DeQuardo, J. R., Carpenter, C. F., & Tandon, R. (1994). Patterns of substance abuse in schizophrenia: Nature and significance. *Journal of Psychiatric Research, 28*(3), 267–275.

Devoto, P., Flore, G., Vacca, G., Pira, L., Arca, A., Casu, M. A., et al. (2003). Co-release of noradrenaline and dopamine from noradrenergic neurons in the cerebral cortex induced by clozapine, the prototype atypical antipsychotic. *Psychopharmacology*, *167*(1), 79–84.

Dickey, B., & Azeni, H. (1996). Persons with dual diagnoses of substance abuse and major mental illness: Their excess costs of psychiatric care. *American Journal of Public Health*, *86*, 973–977.

Drake, R. E., Xie, H., McHugo, G. J., & Green, A. I. (2000). The effects of clozapine on alcohol and drug use disorders among patients with schizophrenia. *Schizophrenia Bulletin*, *26*(2), 441–449.

Fakra, E., & Azorin, J. M. (2012). Clozapine for the treatment of schizophrenia. *Expert Opinion on Pharmacotherapy*, *13*(13), 1923–1935. https://doi.org/10.1517/14656566.2012.709235.

Fibiger, H. C., & Phillips, A. G. (1988). Mesocorticolimbic dopamine systems and reward. *Annals of the New York Academy of Sciences*, *537*, 206–215.

Fischer, A. S., Whitfield-Gabrieli, S., Roth, R. M., Brunette, M. F., & Green, A. I. (2014). Impaired functional connectivity of brain reward circuitry in patients with schizophrenia and cannabis use disorder: Effects of cannabis and THC. *Schizophrenia Research*, *158*(1–3), 176–182. https://doi.org/10.1016/j.schres.2014.04.033.

Flanagan, R. J. (2008). Side effects of clozapine and some other psychoactive drugs. *Current Drug Safety*, *3*(2), 115–122.

Folley, B. S., & Park, S. (2010). Relative food preference and hedonic judgments in schizophrenia. *Psychiatry Research*, *175*(1–2), 33–37. https://doi.org/10.1016/j.psychres.2008.07.026.

Fowles, D. C. (1992). Schizophrenia: Diathesis-stress revisited. *Annual Review of Psychology*, *43*, 303–336. https://doi.org/10.1146/annurev.ps.43.020192.001511.

Gardner, E. L. (1997). Brain reward mechanisms. In J. Lowinson, P. Ruiz, R. Millman, & J. Langrod (Eds.), *Substance abuse: A comprehensive texbook* (pp. 61–85). Baltimore: Williams & Wilkins.

Grace, A. A. (1991). Phasic versus tonic dopamine release and the modulation of dopamine system responsivity: A hypothesis for the etiology of schizophrenia. *Neuroscience*, *41*(1), 1–24.

Green, A. I., Alam, M. Y., Sobieraj, J. T., Pappalardo, K. M., Waternaux, C., Salzman, C., et al. (1993). Clozapine response and plasma catecholamines and their metabolites. *Psychiatry Research*, *46*(2), 139–149.

Green, A. I., Burgess, E. S., Dawson, R., Zimmet, S. V., & Strous, R. D. (2003). Alcohol and cannabis use in schizophrenia: Effects of clozapine vs. risperidone. *Schizophrenia Research*, *60*(1), 81–85.

Green, A. I., Chau, D. T., Keung, W. M., Dawson, R., Mesholam, R. I., & Schildkraut, J. J. (2004). Clozapine reduces alcohol drinking in Syrian golden hamsters. *Psychiatry Research*, *128*(1), 9–20.

Green, I. W., & Glausier, J. R. (2016). Different paths to core pathology: The equifinal model of the schizophrenia syndrome. *Schizophrenia Bulletin*, *42*(3), 542–549. https://doi.org/10.1093/schbul/sbv136.

Green, A. I., Noordsy, D. L., Brunette, M. F., & O'Keefe, C. (2008). Substance abuse and schizophrenia: Pharmacotherapeutic intervention. *Journal of Substance Abuse Treatment*, *34*(1), 61–71. https://doi.org/10.1016/j.jsat.2007.01.008.

Green, A. I., Zimmet, S. V., Strous, R. D., & Schildkraut, J. J. (1999). Clozapine for comorbid substance use disorder and schizophrenia: Do patients with schizophrenia have a reward-deficiency syndrome that can be ameliorated by clozapine? *Harvard Review of Psychiatry*, *6*(6), 287–296.

Grenhoff, J., & Svensson, T. H. (1989). Clonidine modulates dopamine cell firing in rat ventral tegmental area. *European Journal of Pharmacology*, *165*, 11–18.

Gulick, D., Chau, D. T., Khokhar, J. Y., Dawson, R., & Green, A. I. (2014). Desipramine enhances the ability of risperidone to decrease alcohol intake in the Syrian golden hamster. *Psychiatry Research, 218*(3), 329–334. https://doi.org/10.1016/j.psychres.2014.04.038.

Hambrecht, M., & Hafner, H. (1996). Substance abuse and the onset of schizophrenia. *Biological Psychiatry, 40*(11), 1155–1163.

Hartz, S. M., Pato, C. N., Medeiros, H., Cavazos-Rehg, P., Sobell, J. L., Knowles, J. A., et al. (2014). Comorbidity of severe psychotic disorders with measures of substance use. *JAMA Psychiatry, 71*(3), 248–254. https://doi.org/10.1001/jamapsychiatry.2013.3726.

Henquet, C., van Os, J., Kuepper, R., Delespaul, P., Smits, M., Campo, J. A., et al. (2010). Psychosis reactivity to cannabis use in daily life: An experience sampling study. *The British Journal of Psychiatry, 196*(6), 447–453.

Hodge, K., & Jespersen, S. (2008). Side-effects and treatment with clozapine: A comparison between the views of consumers and their clinicians. *International Journal of Mental Health Nursing, 17*(1), 2–8. https://doi.org/10.1111/j.1447-0349.2007.00506.x.

Hunt, I. M., Kapur, N., Windfuhr, K., Robinson, J., Bickley, H., Flynn, S., et al. (2006). Suicide in schizophrenia: Findings from a national clinical survey. *Journal of Psychiatric Practice, 12*(3), 139–147.

Hyman, S. E., Malenka, R. C., & Nestler, E. J. (2006). Neural mechanisms of addiction: The role of reward-related learning and memory. *Annual Review of Neuroscience, 29*, 565–598.

Idanpaan-Heikkila, J., Alhava, E., Olkinuora, M., & Palva, I. (1975). Letter: Clozapine and agranulocytosis. *Lancet, 2*(7935), 611.

Janssen, P. A., Niemegeers, C. J., Awouters, F., Schellekens, K. H., Megens, A. A., & Meert, T. F. (1988). Pharmacology of risperidone (R 64 766), a new antipsychotic with serotonin-S2 and dopamine-D2 antagonistic properties. *The Journal of Pharmacology and Experimental Therapeutics, 244*(2), 685–693.

Jones, P. B., Barnes, T. R., Davies, L., Dunn, G., Lloyd, H., Hayhurst, K. P., et al. (2006). Randomized controlled trial of the effect on quality of life of second- vs first-generation antipsychotic drugs in schizophrenia: Cost utility of the latest antipsychotic drugs in schizophrenia study (CUtLASS 1). *Archives of General Psychiatry, 63*(10), 1079–1087. https://doi.org/10.1001/archpsyc.63.10.1079.

Juckel, G., Schlagenhauf, F., Koslowski, M., Wustenberg, T., Villringer, A., Knutson, B., et al. (2006). Dysfunction of ventral striatal reward prediction in schizophrenia. *NeuroImage, 29*(2), 409–416. https://doi.org/10.1016/j.neuroimage.2005.07.051.

Kalkman, H. O., & Loetscher, E. (2003). alpha2C-Adrenoceptor blockade by clozapine and other antipsychotic drugs. *European Journal of Pharmacology, 462*(1–3), 33–40.

Kalman, D., Morissette, S. B., & George, T. P. (2005). Co-morbidity of smoking in patients with psychiatric and substance use disorders. *The American Journal on Addictions, 14*(2), 106–123. https://doi.org/10.1080/10550490590924728.

Kamali, M., Kelly, L., Gervin, M., Browne, S., Larkin, C., & O'Callaghan, E. (2000). The prevalence of comorbid substance misuse and its influence on suicidal ideation among in-patients with schizophrenia. *Acta Psychiatrica Scandinavica, 101*(6), 452–456.

Kane, J. M., & Correll, C. U. (2016). The role of clozapine in treatment-resistant schizophrenia. *JAMA Psychiatry, 73*(3), 187–188. https://doi.org/10.1001/jamapsychiatry.2015.2966.

Kane, J., Honigfeld, G., Singer, J., & Meltzer, H. (1988). Clozapine for the treatment-resistant schizophrenic. A double-blind comparison with chlorpromazine. *Archives of General Psychiatry, 45*(9), 789–796.

Kennedy, J. L., Altar, C. A., Taylor, D. L., Degtiar, I., & Hornberger, J. C. (2014). The social and economic burden of treatment-resistant schizophrenia: A systematic literature review. *International Clinical Psychopharmacology, 29*(2), 63–76.

Khantzian, E. J. (1997). The self-medication hypothesis of substance use disorders: A reconsideration and recent applications. *Harvard Review of Psychiatry*, *4*(5), 231–244. https://doi.org/10.3109/10673229709030550.

Khokhar, J. Y., Chau, D. T., Dawson, R., & Green, A. I. (2015). Clozapine reconstructed: Haloperidol's ability to reduce alcohol intake in the Syrian golden hamster can be enhanced through noradrenergic modulation by desipramine and idazoxan. *Drug and Alcohol Dependence*, *152*, 277–281. https://doi.org/10.1016/j.drugalcdep.2015.04.003.

Khokhar, J. Y., Dwiel, L. L., Henricks, A. M., Doucette, W. T., & Green, A. I. (2017). The link between schizophrenia and substance use disorder: A unifying hypothesis. *Schizophrenia Research*. https://doi.org/10.1016/j.schres.2017.04.016.

Khokhar, J. Y., & Green, A. I. (2016). Effects of iloperidone, combined with desipramine, on alcohol drinking in the Syrian golden hamster. *Neuropharmacology*, *105*, 25–34. https://doi.org/10.1016/j.neuropharm.2016.01.017.

Khokhar, J. Y., & Todd, T. P. (2017). Behavioral predictors of alcohol drinking in a neurodevelopmental rat model of schizophrenia and co-occurring alcohol use disorder. *Schizophrenia Research*. https://doi.org/10.1016/j.schres.2017.02.029 (in press).

Kivlahan, D. R., Heiman, J. R., Wright, R. C., Mundt, J. W., & Shupe, J. A. (1991). Treatment cost and rehospitalization rate in schizophrenic outpatients with a history of substance abuse. *Hospital & Community Psychiatry*, *42*(6), 609–614.

Knudsen, P., & Vilmar, T. (1984). Cannabis and neuroleptic agents in schizophrenia. *Acta Psychiatrica Scandinavica*, *69*(2), 162–174.

Kovasznay, B., Fleischer, J., Tanenberg-Karant, M., Jandorf, L., Miller, A. D., & Bromet, E. (1997). Substance use disorder and the early course of illness in schizophrenia and affective psychosis. *Schizophrenia Bulletin*, *23*(2), 195–201.

Lasser, K., Boyd, J. W., Woolhandler, S., Himmelstein, D. U., McCormick, D., & Bor, D. H. (2000). Smoking and mental illness: A population-based prevalence study. *JAMA*, *284*(20), 2606–2610.

Leiberman, J., Johns, C., Pollack, S., Bookstein, P., Cooper, T., Ladorola, M., et al. (1991). Biochemical effects of clozapine in cerebrospinal fluid of patients of schizophrenia. In C. - Tammiga & S. Schultz (Eds.), *Schizophrenia research* (pp. 341–349). New York: Raven Press.

Lewis, S. W., Barnes, T. R., Davies, L., Murray, R. M., Dunn, G., Hayhurst, K. P., et al. (2006). Randomized controlled trial of effect of prescription of clozapine versus other second-generation antipsychotic drugs in resistant schizophrenia. *Schizophrenia Bulletin*, *32*(4), 715–723. https://doi.org/10.1093/schbul/sbj067.

Lieberman, J. A., Stroup, T. S., McEvoy, J. P., Swartz, M. S., Rosenheck, R. A., Perkins, D. O., et al. (2005). Effectiveness of antipsychotic drugs in patients with chronic schizophrenia. *The New England Journal of Medicine*, *353*(12), 1209–1223. https://doi.org/10.1056/NEJMoa051688.

Linszen, D. H., Dingemans, P. M., & Lenior, M. E. (1994). Cannabis abuse and the course of recent-onset schizophrenic disorders. *Archives of General Psychiatry*, *51*(4), 273–279.

Lysaker, P., Bell, M., Beam-Goulet, J., & Milstein, R. (1994). Relationship of positive and negative symptoms to cocaine abuse in schizophrenia. *The Journal of Nervous and Mental Disease*, *182*(2), 109–112.

Machielsen, M. W., Veltman, D. J., van den Brink, W., & de Haan, L. (2014). The effect of clozapine and risperidone on attentional bias in patients with schizophrenia and a cannabis use disorder: An fMRI study. *Journal of Psychopharmacology*, *28*(7), 633–642. https://doi.org/10.1177/0269881114527357.

Machielsen, M. W., Veltman, D. J., van den Brink, W., & de Haan, L. (2017). Comparing the effect of clozapine and risperidone on cue reactivity in male patients with schizophrenia and a cannabis use disorder: A randomized fMRI study. *Schizophrenia Research*. https://doi.org/10.1016/j.schres.2017.03.030 (in press).

Mamo, D., Kapur, S., Shammi, C. M., Papatheodorou, G., Mann, S., Therrien, F., et al. (2004). A PET study of dopamine D2 and serotonin 5-HT2 receptor occupancy in patients with schizophrenia treated with therapeutic doses of ziprasidone. *The American Journal of Psychiatry*, *161*(5), 818–825. https://doi.org/10.1176/appi.ajp.161.5.818.
Marcus, P., & Snyder, R. (1995). Reduction of comorbid substance abuse with clozapine. *The American Journal of Psychiatry*, *152*(6), 959.
Meltzer, H. Y. (1997). Treatment-resistant schizophrenia—The role of clozapine. *Current Medical Research and Opinion*, *14*(1), 1–20. https://doi.org/10.1185/03007999709113338.
Meltzer, H. Y., Alphs, L., Green, A. I., Altamura, A. C., Anand, R., Bertoldi, A., et al. (2003). Clozapine treatment for suicidality in schizophrenia: International Suicide Prevention Trial (InterSePT). *Archives of General Psychiatry*, *60*(1), 82–91.
Meltzer, H. Y., & Baldessarini, R. J. (2003). Reducing the risk for suicide in schizophrenia and affective disorders. *The Journal of Clinical Psychiatry*, *64*(9), 1122–1129.
Meltzer, H. Y., Matsubara, S., & Lee, J. C. (1989). Classification of typical and atypical antipsychotic drugs on the basis of dopamine D-1, D-2 and serotonin2 pKi values. *The Journal of Pharmacology and Experimental Therapeutics*, *251*(1), 238–246.
Mesholam-Gately, R. I., Gibson, L. E., Seidman, L. J., & Green, A. I. (2014). Schizophrenia and co-occurring substance use disorder: Reward, olfaction and clozapine. *Schizophrenia Research*, *155*(1–3), 45–51. https://doi.org/10.1016/j.schres.2014.03.002.
Modestin, J., Dal Pian, D., & Agarwalla, P. (2005). Clozapine diminishes suicidal behavior: A retrospective evaluation of clinical records. *The Journal of Clinical Psychiatry*, *66*(4), 534–538.
Moghaddam, B., & Sesack, S. R. (1996). Cellular interactions in the prefrontal cortex: a major focus of schizophrenia research. In L. Dickstein, M. Riba, & J. Oldham (Eds.), *American psychiatric press review of psychiatry* (pp. 351–372). Washington, D.C.: American Psychiatric Association.
Molina, V., Gispert, J. D., Reig, S., Sanz, J., Pascau, J., Santos, A., et al. (2005). Cerebral metabolic changes induced by clozapine in schizophrenia and related to clinical improvement. *Psychopharmacology*, *178*(1), 17–26. https://doi.org/10.1007/s00213-004-1981-9.
Molina, V., Tamayo, P., Montes, C., De Luxan, A., Martin, C., Rivas, N., et al. (2008). Clozapine may partially compensate for task-related brain perfusion abnormalities in risperidone-resistant schizophrenia patients. *Progress in Neuro-Psychopharmacology & Biological Psychiatry*, *32*(4), 948–954. https://doi.org/10.1016/j.pnpbp.2007.12.028.
Moran, L. V., Sampath, H., Kochunov, P., & Hong, L. E. (2013). Brain circuits that link schizophrenia to high risk of cigarette smoking. *Schizophrenia Bulletin*, *39*(6), 1373–1381. https://doi.org/10.1093/schbul/sbs149.
Moran, L. V., Sampath, H., Stein, E. A., & Hong, L. E. (2012). Insular and anterior cingulate circuits in smokers with schizophrenia. *Schizophrenia Research*, *142*(1–3), 223–229. https://doi.org/10.1016/j.schres.2012.08.033.
Mueser, K. T., Yarnold, P. R., Levinson, D. F., Singh, H., Bellack, A. S., Kee, K., et al. (1990). Prevalence of substance abuse in schizophrenia: Demographic and clinical correlates. *Schizophrenia Bulletin*, *16*(1), 31–56.
Naber, D., & Lambert, M. (2009). The CATIE and CUtLASS studies in schizophrenia: Results and implications for clinicians. *CNS Drugs*, *23*(8), 649–659. https://doi.org/10.2165/00023210-200923080-00002.
Naheed, M., & Green, B. (2001). Focus on clozapine. *Current Medical Research and Opinion*, *17*(3), 223–229. https://doi.org/10.1185/0300799039117069.
Nakajima, S., Takeuchi, H., Fervaha, G., Plitman, E., Chung, J. K., Caravaggio, F., et al. (2015). Comparative efficacy between clozapine and other atypical antipsychotics on depressive symptoms in patients with schizophrenia: Analysis of the CATIE phase 2E

data. *Schizophrenia Research, 161*(2–3), 429–433. https://doi.org/10.1016/j.schres.2014.12.024.
Negrete, J. C., & Knapp, W. P. (1986). The effects of cannabis use on the clinical condition of schizophrenics. *NIDA Research Monograph, 67*, 321–327.
Nielsen, M. O., Rostrup, E., Wulff, S., Bak, N., Broberg, B. V., Lublin, H., et al. (2012a). Improvement of brain reward abnormalities by antipsychotic monotherapy in schizophrenia. *Archives of General Psychiatry, 69*(12), 1195–1204. https://doi.org/10.1001/archgenpsychiatry.2012.847.
Nielsen, M. O., Rostrup, E., Wulff, S., Bak, N., Lublin, H., Kapur, S., et al. (2012b). Alterations of the brain reward system in antipsychotic naive schizophrenia patients. *Biological Psychiatry, 71*(10), 898–905. https://doi.org/10.1016/j.biopsych.2012.02.007.
Nisell, M., Nomikos, G. G., & Svensson, T. H. (1995). Nicotine dependence, midbrain dopamine systems and psychiatric disorders. *Pharmacology & Toxicology, 76*(3), 157–162.
Olfson, M., Gerhard, T., Crystal, S., & Stroup, T. S. (2016). Clozapine for schizophrenia: State variation in evidence-based practice. *Psychiatric Services, 67*(2), 152. https://doi.org/10.1176/appi.ps.201500324.
Olney, J. W., Newcomer, J. W., & Farber, N. B. (1999). NMDA receptor hypofunction model of schizophrenia. *Journal of Psychiatric Research, 33*(6), 523–533.
Patchan, K. M., Richardson, C., Vyas, G., & Kelly, D. L. (2015). The risk of suicide after clozapine discontinuation: Cause for concern. *Annals of Clinical Psychiatry, 27*(4), 253–256.
Peralta, V., & Cuesta, M. J. (1992). Influence of cannabis abuse on schizophrenic psychopathology. *Acta Psychiatrica Scandinavica, 85*(2), 127–130.
Pruessner, M., Cullen, A. E., Aas, M., & Walker, E. F. (2017). The neural diathesis-stress model of schizophrenia revisited: An update on recent findings considering illness stage and neurobiological and methodological complexities. *Neuroscience and Biobehavioral Reviews, 73*, 191–218. https://doi.org/10.1016/j.neubiorev.2016.12.013.
Pycock, C. J., Kerwin, R. W., & Carter, C. J. (1980). Effect of lesion of cortical dopamine terminals on subcortical dopamine receptors in rats. *Nature, 286*(5768), 74–76.
Regier, D. A., Farmer, M. E., Rae, D. S., Locke, B. Z., Keith, S. J., Judd, L. L., et al. (1990). Comorbidity of mental disorders with alcohol and other drug abuse. Results from the Epidemiologic Catchment Area (ECA) Study. *JAMA, 264*(19), 2511–2518.
Rosenheck, R., Cramer, J., Xu, W., Thomas, J., Henderson, W., Frisman, L., et al. (1997). A comparison of clozapine and haloperidol in hospitalized patients with refractory schizophrenia. Department of Veterans Affairs Cooperative Study Group on Clozapine in Refractory Schizophrenia. *The New England Journal of Medicine, 337*(12), 809–815. https://doi.org/10.1056/NEJM199709183371202.
Rosenthal, D. (1970). Genetic theory and abnormal behavior. New York: McGraw Hill.
Sayers, S. L., Campbell, E. C., Kondrich, J., Mann, S. C., Cornish, J., O'Brien, C., et al. (2005). Cocaine abuse in schizophrenic patients treated with olanzapine versus haloperidol. *The Journal of Nervous and Mental Disease, 193*(6), 379–386.
Schulte, P. (2006). Risk of clozapine-associated agranulocytosis and mandatory white blood cell monitoring. *The Annals of Pharmacotherapy, 40*(4), 683–688. https://doi.org/10.1345/aph.1G396.
See, R. E., Fido, A. A., Maurice, M., Ibrahim, M. M., & Salama, G. M. (1999). Risperidone-induced increase of plasma norepinephrine is not correlated with symptom improvement in chronic schizophrenia. *Biological Psychiatry, 45*(12), 1653–1656.
Siris, S. G. (1990). Pharmacological treatment of substance-abusing schizophrenic patients. *Schizophrenia Bulletin, 16*(1), 111–122.
Smith, C. M., Barzman, D., & Pristach, C. A. (1997). Effect of patient and family insight on compliance of schizophrenic patients. *Journal of Clinical Pharmacology, 37*(2), 147–154.

Snyder, S. H. (1976). The dopamine hypothesis of schizophrenia: Focus on the dopamine receptor. *The American Journal of Psychiatry, 133*(2), 197–202. https://doi.org/10.1176/ajp.133.2.197.

Spivak, B., Roitman, S., Vered, Y., Mester, R., Graff, E., Talmon, Y., et al. (1998). Diminished suicidal and aggressive behavior, high plasma norepinephrine levels, and serum triglyceride levels in chronic neuroleptic-resistant schizophrenic patients maintained on clozapine. *Clinical Neuropharmacology, 21*(4), 245–250.

Stille, G., Lauener, H., & Eichenberger, E. (1971). The pharmacology of 8-chloro-11-(4-methyl-1-piperazinyl)-5H-dibenzo(b,e)(1,4)diazepine (clozapine). *Il Farmaco; edizione pratica, 26*(10), 603–625.

Sur, C., Mallorga, P. J., Wittmann, M., Jacobson, M. A., Pascarella, D., Williams, J. B., et al. (2003). *N*-desmethylclozapine, an allosteric agonist at muscarinic 1 receptor, potentiates *N*-methyl-D-aspartate receptor activity. *Proceedings of the National Academy of Sciences of the United States of America, 100*(23), 13674–13679. https://doi.org/10.1073/pnas.1835612100.

Svensson, T. H. (2003). Alpha-adrenoceptor modulation hypothesis of antipsychotic atypicality. *Progress in Neuro-Psychopharmacology & Biological Psychiatry, 27*(7), 1145–1158. doi: S0278-5846(03)00222-7 [pii] https://doi.org/10.1016/j.pnpbp.2003.09.009.

Swendsen, J., Burstein, M., Case, B., Conway, K. P., Dierker, L., He, J., et al. (2012). Use and abuse of alcohol and illicit drugs in US adolescents: Results of the national comorbidity survey-adolescent supplement. *Archives of General Psychiatry, 69*(4), 390–398. https://doi.org/10.1001/archgenpsychiatry.2011.1503.

Thompson, J. L., Urban, N., Slifstein, M., Xu, X., Kegeles, L. S., Girgis, R. R., et al. (2013). Striatal dopamine release in schizophrenia comorbid with substance dependence. *Molecular Psychiatry, 18*(8), 909–915. https://doi.org/10.1038/mp.2012.109.

Tomassi, S., Tosato, S., Mondelli, V., Faravelli, C., Lasalvia, A., Fioravanti, G., et al. (2017). Influence of childhood trauma on diagnosis and substance use in first-episode psychosis. *The British Journal of Psychiatry, 211*, 151–156. https://doi.org/10.1192/bjp.bp.116.194019.

Treffert, D. A. (1978). Marijuana use in schizophrenia: A clear hazard. *The American Journal of Psychiatry, 135*(10), 1213–1215.

van Dijk, D., Koeter, M. W., Hijman, R., Kahn, R. S., & van den Brink, W. (2012). Effect of cannabis use on the course of schizophrenia in male patients: A prospective cohort study. *Schizophrenia Research, 137*(1–3), 50–57.

Warsi, M., Sattar, S. P., Bhatia, S. C., & Petty, F. (2005). Aripiprazole reduces alcohol use. *Canadian Journal of Psychiatry, 50*(4), 244.

Weinberger, D. R. (1987). Implications of normal brain development for the pathogenesis of schizophrenia. *Archives of General Psychiatry, 44*(7), 660–669.

Wenthur, C. J., & Lindsley, C. W. (2013). Classics in chemical neuroscience: Clozapine. *ACS Chemical Neuroscience, 4*(7), 1018–1025. https://doi.org/10.1021/cn400121z.

Wimberley, T., Stovring, H., Sorensen, H. J., Horsdal, H. T., MacCabe, J. H., & Gasse, C. (2016). Predictors of treatment resistance in patients with schizophrenia: A population-based cohort study. *Lancet Psychiatry, 3*(4), 358–366. https://doi.org/10.1016/S2215-0366(15)00575-1.

Wint, D., Dreher, J., Furman, D., Koch, P., Kohn, P., Egan, M., et al. (2005). Altered cerebral processing of reward uncertainty in patients with schizophrenia while medication-free and on atypical neuroleptics. *Neuropsychopharmacology, 30*(Suppl. 1), S262.

Wu, B. J., Chen, H. K., & Lee, S. M. (2013). Do atypical antipsychotics really enhance smoking reduction more than typical ones?: The effects of antipsychotics on smoking reduction in patients with schizophrenia. *Journal of Clinical Psychopharmacology, 33*(3), 319–328. https://doi.org/10.1097/JCP.0b013e31828b2575.

Yoshimura, R., Yanagihara, N., Hara, K., Terao, T., Nakamura, J., Ueno, S., et al. (2000). Inhibitory effects of clozapine and other antipsychotic drugs on noradrenaline transporter in cultured bovine adrenal medullary cells. *Psychopharmacology*, *149*(1), 17–23.

Zimmet, S. V., Strous, R. D., Burgess, E. S., Kohnstamm, S., & Green, A. I. (2000). Effects of clozapine on substance use in patients with schizophrenia and schizoaffective disorder: A retrospective survey. *Journal of Clinical Psychopharmacology*, *20*(1), 94–98.

Zugman, A., Gadelha, A., Assuncao, I., Sato, J., Ota, V. K., Rocha, D. L., et al. (2013). Reduced dorso-lateral prefrontal cortex in treatment resistant schizophrenia. *Schizophrenia Research*, *148*(1–3), 81–86. https://doi.org/10.1016/j.schres.2013.05.002.

CHAPTER EIGHT

Imaging Translocator Protein as a Biomarker of Neuroinflammation in Dementia

William C. Kreisl*[,1], Ioline D. Henter†, Robert B. Innis†
*Taub Institute, Columbia University Medical Center, New York, NY, United States
†Molecular Imaging Branch, National Institute of Mental Health, Bethesda, MD, United States
[1]Corresponding author: e-mail address: wck2107@cumc.columbia.edu

Contents

Abstract

Neuroinflammation has long been considered a potential contributor to neurodegenerative disorders that result in dementia. Accumulation of abnormal protein aggregates in Alzheimer's disease, frontotemporal dementia, and dementia with Lewy bodies is associated with the activation of microglia and astrocytes into proinflammatory states, and chronic low-level activation of glial cells likely contributes to the pathological changes observed in these and other neurodegenerative diseases. The 18kDa translocator protein (TSPO) is a key biomarker for measuring inflammation in the brain via positron emission tomography (PET). Increased TSPO density has been observed in brain tissue from patients with neurodegenerative diseases and colocalizes to activated microglia and reactive astrocytes. Several radioligands have been developed to measure TSPO density in vivo with PET, and these have been used in clinical studies of different dementia syndromes. However, TSPO radioligands have limitations, including low specific-to-nonspecific signal and differential affinity to a polymorphism on the *TSPO* gene, which must be taken into consideration in designing and interpreting human

Advances in Pharmacology, Volume 82
ISSN 1054-3589
https://doi.org/10.1016/bs.apha.2017.08.004

PET studies. Nonetheless, most PET studies have shown that increased TSPO binding is associated with various dementias, suggesting that TSPO has potential as a biomarker to further explore the role of neuroinflammation in dementia pathogenesis and may prove useful in monitoring disease progression.

ABBREVIATIONS

AD Alzheimer's disease
CBD corticobasal degeneration
DLB dementia with Lewy bodies
FDG fluorodeoxyglucose
FTD frontotemporal dementia
MCI mild cognitive impairment
PDD Parkinson's disease dementia
PET positron emission tomography
PSP progressive supranuclear palsy
SNP single nucleotide polymorphism
TSPO translocator protein 18 kDa

1. INTRODUCTION

A number of studies have implicated neuroinflammation, loosely defined here as the activation of microglia and astrocytes into proinflammatory states, as a pathological contributor to various neurodegenerative causes of dementia. Clinically, dementia is defined as a decline in cognitive function severe enough to interfere with daily function. While some forms of dementia—for instance, that caused by cerebrovascular disease—are an exception, most neurodegenerative dementias are associated with a specific proteinopathy: the abnormal accumulation of a misfolded protein. One example is the neurofibrillary tangles associated with Alzheimer's disease (AD), which are composed of the microtubule-associated protein tau in a hyperphosphorylated state, aggregated into paired helical filaments. In vitro studies and animal models suggest that proteinopathies stimulate neuroimmune responses (Gao et al., 2011; Maezawa, Zimm, Wulff, & Jin, 2011; Serrano-Pozo et al., 2011). As a result, several clinical and nonclinical studies have been performed in an attempt to elucidate the relationship between neuroinflammation and neurodegenerative dementias.

Astrocytes and microglia are the primary building blocks of the immune system in brain, but even peripheral immune cells—including monocytes and leukocytes—can enter brain and play important roles (Kanegawa et al., 2016). Glial cells have both pro- and antiinflammatory functions and are key to a number of processes under basal as well as disease conditions; these include cellular repair, free radical reduction, phagocytosis, and steroid release. Proinflammatory functions—for instance, cytokine or reactive oxygen species release—can damage healthy neurons, leading to synaptic dysfunction, synapse loss, and neuronal death. In neuroimmune cells, any imbalance between proinflammatory and reparatory functions can thus result in CNS injury. Although the damaging effects of such potential imbalances are recognized in classic neuroimmunological diseases (e.g., multiple sclerosis), growing evidence nevertheless suggests that chronic low-level activation of glial cells may also contribute to the pathological changes observed in many neurodegenerative diseases. Given the importance of this area of study, one goal of considerable interest is quantifying the current inflammatory state in a living human brain, which would allow investigators to measure disease severity, study pathophysiological mechanisms, and identify novel targets for treatment.

It should be noted here that while frontotemporal dementia (FTD), dementia with Lewy bodies (DLB), and Parkinson's disease dementia (PDD) are all proteinopathies, AD is by far the most studied because it is the most common. Indeed, only a handful of studies have used translocator protein 18 kDa (TSPO) PET imaging (discussed later) to study non-AD dementias. Furthermore, because it is a dual proteinopathy in which both amyloid plaques and tau tangles play a key role, the relationship between AD and inflammation may be more complex, due to different temporal order and topographic location of amyloid and tau pathologies. Thus, this chapter will largely focus on the extant state of research into neuroinflammation in AD.

2. TRANSLOCATOR PROTEIN 18 kDa

A key biomarker for measuring inflammation in the brain via positron emission tomography (PET) has been TSPO (Chauveau, Boutin, Van Camp, Dolle, & Tavitian, 2008). TSPO is a transmembrane protein found mainly in the outer mitochondrial membrane. Previously known as the peripheral benzodiazepine receptor (PBR) because it binds diazepam, TSPO was first discovered as a high-affinity receptor for Ro-4864 in lung, liver, and kidney (Braestrup & Squires, 1977). Studies have shown that TSPO binds to cholesterol and porphyrins and likely plays a role in transporting substrates across membranes (Papadopoulos et al., 2015; Papadopoulos & Miller, 2012). However, recent findings in viable mice genetically depleted of TSPO have called into question its role in some of these functions (Banati et al., 2014; Morohaku et al., 2014; Selvaraj, Stocco, & Tu, 2015; Tu et al., 2014; Tu, Zhao, Stocco, & Selvaraj, 2015). In the periphery, low TSPO levels have been found in immune-competent cells, leukocytes, and macrophages, but TSPO is also found in microglia and astrocytes (Casellas, Galiegue, & Basile, 2002). Glial cells are known to become activated in response to cellular injury, and this morphological and functional change results in increased TSPO expression (Kuhlmann & Guilarte, 2000).

With regard to the scope of this chapter, increased TSPO density has been observed in a number of neurological disorders (see Jacobs, Tavitian, & INMind Consortium, 2012 for a review), including classic neuroimmunological disorders such as multiple sclerosis and HIV encephalopathy (Cosenza-Nashat et al., 2009). Notably, increased TSPO density has also been observed in brain tissue from patients with neurodegenerative diseases and is expected to be increased in proteinopathic dementias (that is, dementias associated with abnormal protein aggregates such as amyloid plaques).

3. RADIOLIGANDS FOR TSPO

Since the racemic version of ^{11}C-PK-11195 was used to image TSPO more than 30 years ago (Le Fur et al., 1983), new radioligands have been developed that have a much greater amount of specific binding in human brain. Nevertheless, a key limitation shared by all ligands, including PK-11195, is that a common single nucleotide polymorphism (SNP) affects the affinity of their binding to TSPO (Kreisl et al., 2010; Owen et al., 2011). This characteristic was first noted with ^{11}C-PBR28, where a 40-fold difference of affinity exists between high- and low-affinity binders (Kreisl et al., 2010). The responsible SNP (rs6971) is codominantly expressed, thereby generating three genotypes: high, mixed, and low-affinity binders (Owen et al., 2011, 2010). This SNP is variably present in different ethnic groups; for instance, it is almost nonexistent among the Japanese but present in roughly 5%–10% of subjects of European and African American descent. This SNP has such a dramatic effect on the binding of ^{11}C-PBR28 that homozygous low-affinity binders provide no quantifiable brain uptake and are typically excluded prior to any scan, based on a genotype test. Excluding low-affinity binders is important to avoid unnecessary exposure to radiation and can be logistically difficult for subjects who live far from the imaging center.

Although still sensitive to genotype, several of the second-generation TSPO radioligands, including ^{11}C-PBR28 and ^{11}C-DPA713, appeared to have greater specific binding than ^{11}C-(*R*)-PK-11195. For example, receptor/transporter blocking studies in monkeys showed that ^{11}C-PBR28 has about 10-fold higher specific binding than ^{11}C-(*R*)-PK-11195, but comparable blocking was only recently reported in humans (Ikawa et al., 2017; Kobayashi et al., 2017; Owen et al., 2014). The blocking drug used in humans was XBD173, which was reported to reduce anxiety symptoms in rodents and to blunt panic attacks in humans (Rupprecht et al., 2009). XBD173 was developed as an anxiolytic specifically because it (and perhaps all TSPO ligands) stimulates production of steroids and neurosteroids, the latter of which may have antianxiety properties. Because XBD173 had been used in humans and found to be relatively well tolerated, research PET Centers at Imanova (London) and at the NIMH (Bethesda) were able to use it to measure the amount of specific binding of four ^{11}C-labeled radioligands for TSPO (Table 1). Baseline and blocking studies were performed in the same healthy subjects. The outcome measure was "binding potential" (BP_{ND}), the ratio at equilibrium of specific to nondisplaceable uptake, which may be roughly viewed as an overall measure of "signal to noise" in PET studies. Indeed, ^{11}C-(*R*)-PK-11195 had a woefully inadequate BP_{ND} value (0.8), followed by ^{11}C-PBR28 (1.2), ^{11}C-ER176 (4.2), and ^{11}C-DPA-713 (7.3). Based on these overall values of "signal to noise," ^{11}C-DPA-713 appeared

Table 1 Comparison of Four ^{11}C-Radiolabeled Ligands for TSPO in Healthy Subjects, Before and After Blockade by XBD173

Ligand	Genotype Sensitivity	BP_{ND} in High-Affinity Binders[a]	Radiometabolite Contamination in Low-Affinity Binders[b]
^{11}C-(*R*)-PK11195	+	0.8	+++
^{11}C-PBR28	+++	1.2	Not reliably measured
^{11}C-DPA-713	++	7.3	+++
^{11}C-ER176	+	4.2	None

[a] BP_{ND} is a unitless measure of the ratio at equilibrium of the concentration of specific to nondisplaceable uptake, which may be roughly interpreted as the overall "signal-to-noise" ratio in PET imaging.
[b] The presence of radiometabolites in brain was indirectly measured as a time-dependent increase of apparent receptor density (i.e., distribution volume (V_T)) during the course of scans in low-affinity binders.

to the best of these four radioligands for measuring TSPO. However, studying these radioligands in homozygous low-affinity binders showed that ^{11}C-ER176 had an unexpected advantage (Table 1); specifically, among the four ^{11}C-radioligands, only ^{11}C-ER176 did not generate radiometabolites that accumulate in brain and confound quantitation of the target. Such accumulation might differ between individuals or between groups and is a common reason for rejecting a radioligand for inadequate quantitation. Although these studies need to be replicated, they suggest that ^{11}C-ER176 may currently be the best radioligand for imaging TSPO. It should be noted here that ^{11}C-ER176 is sensitive to genotype, and the imaging results must thus still be corrected for genotype post hoc, but low-affinity binders need not be excluded a priori.

^{18}F-GE180, a recently developed TSPO radioligand, was reported to have increased binding in amyloid-producing transgenic mice (Brendel et al., 2016; Liu et al., 2015). However, quantitative studies in healthy human subjects have shown that it has such low brain uptake that it is unlikely to be useful in clinical populations. More specifically, ^{18}F-GE180 has very low rate of brain entry, with K_1 estimated to be 0.01 mL cm^{-3} min^{-1} and corresponding first pass extraction of approximately 1% (Feeney et al., 2016). Such a low rate of brain entry may be caused by the radioligand's being a substrate for efflux transporters, such as P-glycoprotein, at the blood–brain barrier. In our opinion, the cause of this low brain uptake should be examined before ^{18}F-GE180 is used in patient populations.

In addition to deficiencies specific to each radioligand, the methods used to quantify TSPO density can also introduce potential confounds in clinical PET studies. The "gold standard" method of quantification for reversible PET radioligands is kinetic modeling using the metabolite-corrected arterial input function. However, this method requires arterial catheterization, which may be a barrier to subject recruitment in populations suffering from dementia and that may introduce errors associated with the relatively high technical demands of precise measurement of parent radioligand concentration in plasma. To avoid these disadvantages, semiquantitative methods have been used in clinical TSPO PET studies. For ^{11}C-(*R*)-PK-11195, the most common method of analysis is a cluster-based approach. With this approach, voxels on the PET image are identified that behave as though there is no specific binding (i.e., reference tissue), and these voxels are used to correct for between-subject differences in radioligand delivery to voxels that have high amounts of specific binding (i.e., target tissue). However, TSPO is expressed throughout the brain, and the identified reference tissue will therefore also contain radioligand that is bound to TSPO to some extent. Thus, this method likely introduces some degree of underestimation bias. Another analytic method that has been used with ^{11}C-(*R*)-PK-11195 and some second-generation radioligands is a tissue-ratio method, where radioligand binding in a target region expected to show disease-related pathology is divided by radioligand binding in a region expected to have little pathology. A previous study from our laboratory validated this approach against the "gold standard" of kinetic modeling, using the cerebellum as a "pseudo-reference" region to compare ^{11}C-PBR28 binding in patients with AD vs healthy controls (Lyoo et al., 2015). However, some studies have used this or similar tissue-ratio approaches with a different radioligand without first validating it against kinetic modeling (Bloomfield et al., 2016; Zurcher et al., 2015).

4. NEUROINFLAMMATION IN ALZHEIMER'S DISEASE

Neuroimmune response is a key pathological contributor to AD (Baik, Kang, Son, & Mook-Jung, 2016; Jin et al., 2015; Lee, McGeer, & McGeer, 2015; McGeer & McGeer, 2013; Raha et al., 2017). β-Amyloid activates microglia at physiologic concentrations (Maezawa et al., 2011), resulting in release of cytokines and activation of complement. The proinflammatory state initiated by activated microglia can cause neuronal loss (Neniskyte, Neher, & Brown, 2011). Inflammation can stimulate hyperphosphorylation of tau, resulting in the aggregation of neurofibrillary tangles (Ghosh et al., 2013). Extracellular tau can also activate microglia, potentially leading to a positive feedback loop of inflammation and tau pathology that propagates without involvement of β-amyloid (Serrano-Pozo et al., 2011). Brain tissue from AD patients revealed activated microglia and reactive astrocytes, which overexpress TSPO when proximal to β-amyloid plaques (Cosenza-Nashat et al., 2009).

Most PET studies conducted to date in AD have shown positive results (Schain & Kreisl, 2017). For instance, studies found that ^{11}C-(*R*)-PK-11195 binding was increased in AD patients and correlated with clinical severity (Cagnin et al., 2001; Edison et al., 2008; Yokokura et al., 2011). Edison and colleagues found that ^{11}C-(*R*)-PK-11195 binding did not correlate with amyloid load (measured with ^{11}C-Pittsburgh compound B (PIB)), despite both ^{11}C-(*R*)-PK-11195 and PIB being elevated in AD patients (Edison et al., 2008). One study using ^{11}C-PBR28 found that binding was greater in amyloid-positive AD patients than in controls or than in amyloid-positive mild cognitive impairment (MCI) patients, especially in temporo-parietal regions; no difference was noted in the cerebellum, which is typically spared of pathology in AD (Kreisl et al., 2013) (Fig. 1). That study further found that ^{11}C-PBR28 binding correlated with volume loss as well as with several cognitive indices, but not with amyloid load. Another study found that ^{11}C-DAA1106 binding was greater in AD patients than controls in several brain regions, including striatum and cerebellum but that binding did not correlate with symptom severity (Yasuno et al., 2008). Autoradiography studies demonstrated greater binding of ^{3}H-DAA1106 to TSPO in both a transgenic AD mouse model (Maeda et al., 2011) and in human tissue from AD brains (Gulyas et al., 2009). In addition, binding with ^{18}F-FEPPA was shown to be greater in AD patients than in controls in hippocampus and white matter regions such as internal capsule and cingulum bundle, as well as in prefrontal, temporal, parietal, and occipital cortices (Suridjan et al., 2015). Greater ^{18}F-FEPPA binding also correlated with worse performance on some cognitive measures (Suridjan et al., 2015). Finally, in studies using ^{11}C-(*R*)-PK-11195 and ^{11}C-PBR28, TSPO binding was found to increase with progression of AD (Fan, Okello, Brooks, & Edison, 2015; Kreisl et al., 2016). Building on this work, Kreisl and colleagues similarly found that patients who showed clinical progression at follow-up had a greater increase in ^{11}C-PBR28 binding than patients who remained clinically stable (Kreisl et al., 2016).

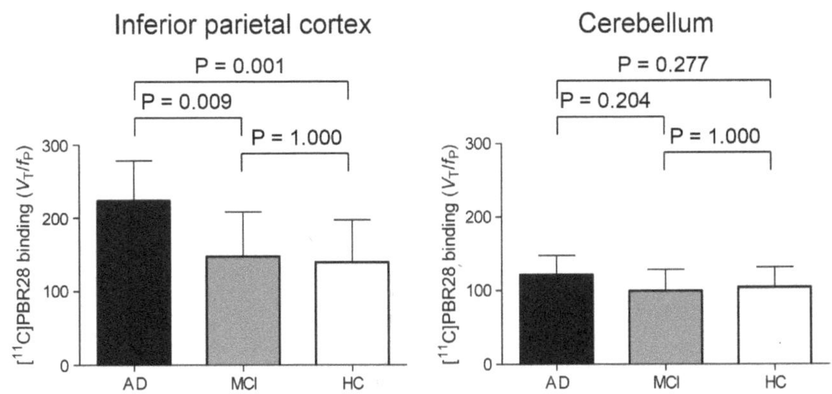

Fig. 1 ^{11}C-PBR28 binding is greater in patients with Alzheimer's disease (AD, $n=19$) than in patients with mild cognitive impairment (MCI, $n=10$) or age-matched healthy controls (HC, $n=13$). Bar graphs show values for ^{11}C-PBR28 binding (V_T/f_P) in inferior parietal lobule (*left*) and cerebellum (*right*), corrected for partial volume effect. ^{11}C-PBR28 binding values were adjusted for *TSPO* genotype, age, and education. Error bars denote SD.

Nevertheless, some negative studies found no difference in TSPO binding between AD patients and controls (Groom, Junck, Foster, Frey, & Kuhl, 1995; Schuitemaker et al., 2013; Varrone et al., 2013; Wiley et al., 2009). Methodological differences may explain some of these mixed results. For instance, one of the negative studies had a control group that included seven patients with unilateral gliomas, and the unaffected hemisphere was used as comparison data (Groom et al., 1995). Also, none of the negative studies using ^{11}C-(*R*)-PK-11195 used absolute quantification of ^{11}C-(*R*)-PK-11195 binding; rather, they used a cluster-based method. In one negative study using ^{18}F-FEDAA1106, *TSPO* genotype was not determined (Varrone et al., 2013). Therefore, it is likely that variance in the PET data caused by the rs6971 SNP contributed to the negative results.

Whether changes in TSPO occur in the preclinical and prodromal stages of AD is less clear. The earliest studies comparing TSPO binding between prodromal AD patients (defined as having MCI) and controls found no difference between the groups (Kreisl et al., 2013; Lyoo et al., 2015; Schuitemaker et al., 2013; Wiley et al., 2009). In contrast, Yasuno and colleagues showed that three MCI patients with ^{11}C-DAA1106 binding >1.5 SD above the mean binding of controls had converted to dementia at follow-up; however, of the seven MCI patients imaged at baseline, two were lost to follow-up and one had ^{11}C-DAA1106 binding similar to that seen in controls but still converted to dementia at follow-up (Yasuno et al., 2012). In another study measuring ^{11}C-(*R*)-PK-11195 binding, Okello and colleagues found that only 5 of 13 MCI patients had elevated ^{11}C-(*R*)-PK-11195 binding and that this was not related to amyloid binding (Okello et al., 2009). Hamelin and colleagues found that amyloid-positive MCI patients had greater ^{18}F-DPA-714 binding than controls (Hamelin et al., 2016). However, in contrast to the findings of Kreisl et al. (2013) and Lyoo et al. (2015)—where AD patients had greater TSPO binding than MCI patients—and those of Yasuno and colleagues, which found that MCI and AD patients both had increased binding compared to controls, Hamelin and colleagues found that binding was greater in MCI than in AD patients (Hamelin et al., 2016); that study further found that ^{18}F-DPA-714 binding was inversely correlated with cognitive measures, with more affected patients having lower TSPO binding. The study by Hamelin and colleagues was the first to present results demonstrating that amyloid-positive control subjects (preclinical AD) had greater TSPO binding than amyloid-negative controls. One interpretation of these data is that TSPO is elevated in the preclinical and prodromal phase of AD and then decreases as the disease progresses. The authors concluded that there was an early and protective microglial activation in AD. This conclusion was predicated on the assumption that decreases in TSPO in the more severely affected patients reflected a loss of protective function of microglia—such as amyloid phagocytosis—and that the loss of this protective microglial function allows AD to progress. While the study by Hamelin and colleagues included an unusually large sample size for a clinical PET study ($n=96$), it was a cross-sectional study, and it has not yet been determined if individual subjects demonstrate increased ^{18}F-DPA-714 binding over time (Hamelin et al., 2016). The study also used a simplified tissue-ratio method to quantify ^{18}F-DPA-714 binding that has not yet been validated against the "gold standard" for reversible radioligands without a true reference region (i.e., kinetic modeling using the metabolite-corrected arterial input function).

A recent study by Fan and colleagues reported decreased ^{11}C-(*R*)-PK-11195 binding in MCI patients after longitudinal follow-up (Fan, Brooks, Okello, & Edison, 2017). The authors concluded that there may be a biphasic pattern of microglial activation, with a peak occurring during MCI that later declines, followed by a second peak during the dementia stage of the disease. In such a scenario, the evidence suggests that the amount of microglial activation in the second peak would continue to rise as the dementia process worsens (Calsolaro & Edison, 2016). These results may resolve the apparent contradictions noted earlier, where TSPO binding was greater in MCI than AD dementia, as well as the evidence from earlier TSPO PET studies that found that TSPO binding increased with disease severity in patients with dementia. However, the paper by Fan and colleagues included only eight MCI patients, half of whom showed no evidence of amyloid plaque deposition on baseline PET imaging. Also, follow-up imaging was not performed on controls in either this or the earlier longitudinal study of ^{11}C-(*R*)-PK-11195 in AD (Fan et al., 2015), and the effects of natural aging or test–retest variability on longitudinal ^{11}C-(*R*)-PK-11195 binding may have influenced these results. Larger, serial-imaging studies with harmonized TSPO-imaging methodology are needed to elucidate the relationship between TSPO and progression along the AD spectrum.

5. NEUROINFLAMMATION IN NON-ALZHEIMER'S DEMENTIAS

5.1 PDD and DLB

Neuroinflammation is a proposed pathogenic contributor to diffuse Lewy body disease (DLBD), which includes the aforementioned PDD and

DLB. DLBD is defined by aggregated α-synuclein inclusions (i.e., Lewy bodies), which activate microglia in vitro and stimulate release of proinflammatory mediators (Zhang et al., 2005). Activated microglia are found proximal to Lewy bodies at autopsy (Mackenzie, 2000; Power & Blumbergs, 2009; Togo et al., 2001). The amount of activated microglia is proportional to both the number of Lewy bodies found at autopsy (Mackenzie, 2000) and, in transgenic mice, to the amount of α-synuclein and measured loss of dopaminergic neurons (Gao et al., 2011). Prior TSPO PET studies in patients with Parkinson's disease without dementia have mostly shown positive results (Bartels et al., 2010; Gerhard et al., 2006; Iannaccone et al., 2013; Ouchi et al., 2005), although there have been a small number of negative studies (Bartels et al., 2010; Ghadery et al., 2017). Two studies also found increased TSPO in PDD or DLB (Edison et al., 2013; Iannaccone et al., 2013). One of these studies found that ^{11}C-(*R*)-PK-11195 binding was greater in basal ganglia and substantia nigra for both PDD and DLB patients than in controls. In addition, the DLB patients had increased binding in the cortex and cerebellum (Iannaccone et al., 2013). Interestingly, all PDD and DLB patients were accrued within 1 year of onset of their clinical symptoms, which suggests that increased TSPO density is detectable in the early stages of disease. The second study performed ^{11}C-(*R*)-PK-11195 PET imaging in patients with Parkinson's disease with and without dementia and found that binding was greater than controls in frontal, temporal, and occipital cortices for both PDD patients and those with Parkinson's disease without dementia; furthermore, ^{11}C-(*R*)-PK-11195 binding was found to be inversely correlated with Mini Mental State Exam score among PDD patients (Edison et al., 2013). In addition, regional increases in ^{11}C-(*R*)-PK-11195 binding overlapped with regional glucose hypometabolism in patients for whom ^{18}F-FDG PET was also performed (Edison et al., 2013).

5.2 Frontotemporal Lobar Degeneration and Related Tauopathies

Frontotemporal lobar degeneration (FTLD) refers to a collection of diseases—including behavioral variant FTD, progressive nonfluent aphasia, and semantic dementia (Ferrari et al., 2014; The Lund and Manchester Groups, 1994)—that are pathologically distinct from AD and the α-synucleinopathies and that can cause synaptic dysfunction and neuronal loss in the frontal and temporal lobes. Both familial and sporadic forms of FTLD often—though not always—result from the aggregation of abnormal tau filaments (Caroppo et al., 2016; Ferrer et al., 2014; He et al., 2016;

Laws et al., 2008; Lee et al., 2013; Lindquist, Schwartz, Batbayli, Waldemar, & Nielsen, 2009). Other disorders considered under the larger umbrella of FTLD include the "Parkinson's plus" disorders such as primary progressive palsy and corticobasal ganglionic degeneration; these are characterized by shared nigrostriatal cell loss and are pathologically defined by tau aggregation (Ioannidis, Konstantinopoulou, Maiovis, & Karacostas, 2012).

One study found that ^{11}C-(*R*)-PK11195 binding was increased in patients with a clinical diagnosis of FTLD ($n=5$), but quantification was performed without either blood sampling or use of a valid reference region (Cagnin, Rossor, Sampson, Mackinnon, & Banati, 2004). Using full quantification with arterial blood sampling, we observed increased ^{11}C-PBR28 binding in patients with behavioral variant FTD (Fig. 2; unpublished data). A study of four patients with corticobasal degeneration (CBD) found increased ^{11}C-(*R*)-PK11195 binding in several cortical regions as well as striatum and brainstem (Gerhard et al., 2004). Another small study found that four patients with progressive supranuclear palsy (PSP) displayed increased ^{11}C-(*R*)-PK11195 binding in striatum, cerebellum, brainstem, thalamus, and the frontal lobe (Gerhard et al., 2006). Both of the latter two studies used the primary visual cortex and occipital white matter as a reference for nonspecific binding. While the authors suggested that these

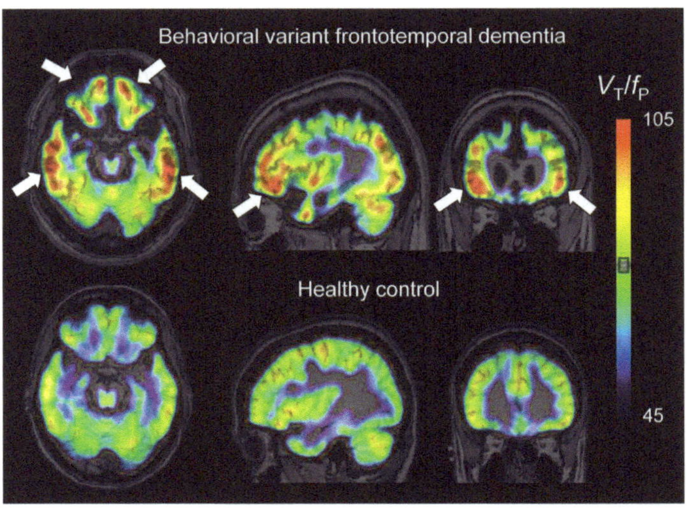

Fig. 2 Representative ^{11}C-PBR28 parametric images (V_T/f_P) for a patient with behavioral variant FTD and a healthy control. Both subjects were high-affinity binders (noncarriers of the rs6971 *TSPO* polymorphism). *Arrows* show increased binding in frontal and temporal cortices.

regions are unaffected in CBD and PSP—though not free from TSPO—the outcome measures may nevertheless be methodologically biased. However, another study found that the distribution of tau pathology commonly seen in CBD overlapped with the location of increased binding (Dickson et al., 2002).

6. ALTERNATIVE TARGETS FOR NEUROINFLAMMATION IN DEMENTIA

Given the limitations associated with TSPO PET imaging, alternative targets for measuring neuroinflammation in vivo have been explored. Monoamine oxidase (MAO)-A and MAO-B are isoenzymes that metabolize neurotransmitters and xenobiotic amines via oxidative deamination (Saura et al., 1994), and hydrolysis of substrates by MAO-B results in reactive oxygen species as a by-product (Corcia et al., 2012). Because MAO-B expression increases with age, the corresponding accumulation of reactive oxygen species may contribute to age-related neurodegeneration (Saura, Richards, & Mahy, 1994a, 1994b). In addition, reactive astrocytes overexpress MAO-B, and the density of this isoenzyme has therefore been used as a marker for neuroinflammatory response (Aquilonius, Jossan, Ekblom, Askmark, & Gillberg, 1992; Jossan, Gillberg, Gottfries, Karlsson, & Oreland, 1991; Nakamura et al., 1990; Oreland, 1980). In studies, the MAO-B radioligand ^{11}*C*-L-deprenyl showed greater binding in AD and MCI patients than in older controls (Carter et al., 2012; Choo, Carter, Scholl, & Nordberg, 2014; Hirvonen et al., 2009; Santillo et al., 2011), suggesting reactive astrocytosis early in AD pathogenesis.

Additional proposed targets for neuroinflammation include arachidonic acid metabolism (Esposito et al., 2008), cyclooxygenase (Shukuri et al., 2016), and the P2X purinoceptor 7, which is expressed by microglia and thought to play a regulatory role in the inflammatory pathway (Han et al., 2017). However, at present, radioligand development for these potential targets is in the early stages.

7. THE CLINICAL SIGNIFICANCE OF INCREASED TSPO IN DEMENTIA

Activated microglia have several functions, including aberrant synaptic pruning and release of reactive oxygen species, driving a more proinflammatory state that can lead to neurodegeneration. Conversely, activated microglia may be involved in phagocytosis and release of trophic factors that promote an overall antiinflammatory state. Broad categories have been used to define two distinct microglial phenotypes: M1 and M2. In neurodegenerative dementias, the potential role of microglia becomes particularly confusing, as evidence exists for both protective and destructive actions. One current theory is that activated microglia play a more protective role early in the AD process that later fails, resulting in increased plaque and tangle deposition, and that later stages of disease are associated with activated microglia that have predominantly cytotoxic functions (Hickman, Allison, & El Khoury, 2008). Under this hypothesis, "switching" microglia from an M1 to an M2 state may be therapeutically useful in treating AD. However, the M1/M2 dichotomy may be overly simplistic, and the concept of polarization of microglial function remains controversial (Ransohoff, 2016).

While the proposed biphasic pattern of microglial activation in AD—an early protective phase followed by a later neurodegenerative phase—conforms to the concept of M1/M2 microglial phenotypes, limitations to this model exist. First, imaging and CSF studies have shown that neurodegenerative changes are frequently detected in the MCI stage of AD (Knopman et al., 2016). Elevations in CSF tau, fluorodeoxyglucose (FDG) hypometabolism, and hippocampal atrophy are all detectable prior to the onset of dementia, and FDG hypometabolism and hippocampal atrophy may accelerate as cerebral amyloid is increasing, prior to obvious clinical symptoms (Insel et al., 2017). These results argue against MCI being a "protected" stage of AD.

Second, amyloid-negative MCI should not be universally equated with early-stage AD, as considerable evidence suggests that in many of these subjects cognitive symptoms may be due to non-AD pathology. For instance, autopsy, CSF, and PET studies have shown significant cerebral amyloidosis in subjects without cognitive symptoms (Jansen et al., 2015; Serrano-Pozo et al., 2013; Toledo et al., 2015), and longitudinal studies suggest that, in most patients, amyloid plaque deposition occurs prior to functional changes in cognition (Bateman et al., 2012; Buchhave et al., 2012; Forster et al., 2012; Landau et al., 2012; Lo et al., 2011). In addition, MCI patients without evidence of amyloidopathy are less likely to have pathologically defined AD at autopsy (Vos et al., 2013), and they show less cognitive decline than amyloid-positive MCI patients (Landau, Horng, Fero, Jagust, & Alzheimer's Disease Neuroimaging Initiative, 2016). The emergence of symptoms that warrant a clinical diagnosis of MCI due to AD without evidence of amyloid plaque pathology is not consistent with the prevailing model of the temporal order of biomarker abnormalities in AD (Jack et al., 2011).

Finally, this biphasic model of microglial activation does not take into account differences in the threshold of detection of different biomarkers (Jack et al., 2013). As noted earlier, all TSPO radioligands are associated with sensitivity limitations that confound accurate quantification. Therefore, it is possible that the amount of TSPO binding seen in prodromal and MCI patients is very close to the threshold of detection achievable with currently available radioligands. The apparent peak and decline of TSPO binding in patients with MCI may represent variation in the noise at a stage where TSPO density is relatively low and therefore difficult to accurately detect.

Most of the agreement in TSPO studies concerns patients in the dementia phase of AD, when the disease phenotype is most severe and TSPO binding is likely at its greatest. Determining the temporal relationship between TSPO binding and AD more precisely will require larger and better-powered studies. Moreover, the detection threshold for TSPO radioligands should be compared to that for other, better-characterized AD biomarkers to avoid erroneous associations between microglial activation, amyloid deposition, tau aggregation, and neurodegeneration. In addition, because human PET studies are associational in nature, the results cannot be used to conclude a cause and effect relationship between microglial function and AD progression. Because the role of microglia in the prevention or progression of AD presently remains unknown, we cannot yet determine whether increased TSPO binding reflects positive, negative, or neutral biological effects. Windows of opportunity may indeed exist for modulating microglial responses with novel therapeutics in order to attenuate the course of AD. However, in order to use TSPO PET to define those windows, we need to better understand the role that TSPO specifically, and microglia generally, plays in the AD process.

8. CONCLUSION

Considerable evidence supports the notion that neuroinflammation is closely related to the neurodegenerative changes seen in dementing disorders and that inflammatory responses can be detected with TSPO PET imaging in patients suffering from these disorders. Therefore, TSPO PET has potential as a biomarker to further study various dementias and may prove useful in monitoring disease progression. However, more information on the role of microglial activation and the causal relationships, if any, between microglial function and dementia pathogenesis is needed if TSPO PET is to be used to monitor response to immunomodulatory treatments.

CONFLICT OF INTEREST STATEMENT

Funding for this work was supported in part by the Intramural Research Program at the National Institute of Mental Health, National Institutes of Health (IRP-NIMH-NIH). Dr. Kreisl has received research funding from AstraZeneca, Merck, and the NIA (K23AG052633). Dr. Innis and Ms. Henter have no conflicts of interest to disclose, financial or otherwise.

REFERENCES

Aquilonius, S. M., Jossan, S. S., Ekblom, J. G., Askmark, H., & Gillberg, P. G. (1992). Increased binding of 3H-L-deprenyl in spinal cords from patients with amyotrophic lateral sclerosis as demonstrated by autoradiography. *Journal of Neural Transmission. General Section*, *89*, 111–122.

Baik, S. H., Kang, S., Son, S. M., & Mook-Jung, I. (2016). Microglia contributes to plaque growth by cell death due to uptake of amyloid beta in the brain of Alzheimer's disease mouse model. *Glia*, *64*, 2274–2290.

Banati, R. B., Middleton, R. J., Chan, R., Hatty, C. R., Kam, W. W., Quin, C., et al. (2014). Positron emission tomography and functional characterization of a complete PBR/TSPO knockout. *Nature Communications*, *5*, 5452.

Bartels, A. L., Willemsen, A. T., Doorduin, J., de Vries, E. F., Dierckx, R. A., & Leenders, K. L. (2010). [11C]-PK11195 PET: Quantification of neuroinflammation and a monitor of anti-inflammatory treatment in Parkinson's disease? *Parkinsonism & Related Disorders*, *16*, 57–59.

Bateman, R. J., Xiong, C., Benzinger, T. L., Fagan, A. M., Goate, A. M., Fox, N. C., et al. (2012). Clinical and biomarker changes in dominantly inherited Alzheimer's disease. *The New England Journal of Medicine*, *367*, 795–804.

Bloomfield, M. A., Bonoldi, I., Kalk, N., Turkheimer, F., McGuire, P., de Vaola, V., et al. (2016). Microglial activity in people at ultra high risk of psychosis and schizophrenia: An [(11)C]PBR28 PET brain imaging study. *The American Journal of Psychiatry*, *173*, 44–52.

Braestrup, C., & Squires, R. F. (1977). Specific benzodiazepine receptors in rat brain characterized by high-affinity (3H)diazepam binding. *Proceedings of the National Academy of Sciences of the United States of America*, *74*(9), 3805–3809.

Brendel, M., Probst, F., Jaworska, A., Overhoff, F., Korzhova, V., Albert, N. L., et al. (2016). Glial activation and glucose metabolism in a transgenic amyloid mouse model: A triple-tracer PET study. *Journal of Nuclear Medicine*, *57*, 954–960.

Buchhave, P., Minthon, L., Zetterberg, H., Wallin, A. K., Blennow, K., & Hansson, O. (2012). Cerebrospinal fluid levels of beta-amyloid 1-42, but not of tau, are fully changed already 5 to 10 years before the onset of Alzheimer dementia. *Archives of General Psychiatry*, *69*, 98–106.

Cagnin, A., Brooks, D. J., Kennedy, A. M., Gunn, R. N., Myers, R., Turkheimer, F. E., et al. (2001). In-vivo measurement of activated microglia in dementia. *Lancet*, *358*(9280), 461–467.

Cagnin, A., Rossor, M., Sampson, E. L., Mackinnon, T., & Banati, R. B. (2004). In vivo detection of microglial activation in frontotemporal dementia. *Annals of Neurology*, *56*(6), 894–897.

Calsolaro, V., & Edison, P. (2016). Neuroinflammation in Alzheimer's disease: Current evidence and future directions. *Alzheimer's and Dementia, 12*, 719–732.

Caroppo, P., Camuzat, A., Guillot-Noel, L., Thomas-Anterion, C., Couratier, P., Wong, T. H., et al. (2016). Defining the spectrum of frontotemporal dementias associated with TARDBP mutations. *Neurology Genetics, 2*(3), e80.

Carter, S. F., Scholl, M., Almkvist, O., Wall, A., Engler, H., Langstrom, B., et al. (2012). Evidence for astrocytosis in prodromal Alzheimer disease provided by 11C-deuterium-L-deprenyl: A multitracer PET paradigm combining 11C-Pittsburgh compound B and 18F-FDG. *Journal of Nuclear Medicine, 53*, 37–46.

Casellas, P., Galiegue, S., & Basile, A. S. (2002). Peripheral benzodiazepine receptors and mitochondrial function. *Neurochemistry International, 40*, 475–486.

Chauveau, F., Boutin, H., Van Camp, N., Dolle, F., & Tavitian, B. (2008). Nuclear imaging of neuroinflammation: A comprehensive review of [11C]PK11195 challengers. *European Journal of Nuclear Medicine and Molecular Imaging, 35*(12), 2304–2319.

Choo, I. L., Carter, S. F., Scholl, M. L., & Nordberg, A. (2014). Astrocytosis measured by (11)C-deprenyl PET correlates with decrease in gray matter density in the parahippocampus of prodromal Alzheimer's patients. *European Journal of Nuclear Medicine and Molecular Imaging, 41*(11), 2120–2126.

Corcia, P., Tauber, C., Vercoullie, J., Arlicot, N., Prunier, C., Praline, J., et al. (2012). Molecular imaging of microglial activation in amyotrophic lateral sclerosis. *PloS One*, 7, e52941.

Cosenza-Nashat, M., Zhao, M. L., Suh, H. S., Morgan, J., Natividad, R., Morgello, S., et al. (2009). Expression of the translocator protein of 18 kDa by microglia, macrophages and astrocytes based on immunohistochemical localization in abnormal human brain. *Neuropathology and Applied Neurobiology, 35*(3), 306–328.

Dickson, D. W., Bergeron, C., Chin, S. S., Duyckaerts, C., Horoupian, D., Ikeda, K., et al. (2002). Office of rare diseases neuropathologic criteria for corticobasal degeneration. *Journal of Neuropathology and Experimental Neurology, 61*(11), 935–946.

Edison, P., Ahmed, I., Fan, Z., Hinz, R., Gelosa, G., Ray Chaudhuri, K., et al. (2013). Microglia, amyloid, and glucose metabolism in Parkinson's disease with and without dementia. *Neuropsychopharmacology, 38*(6), 938–949.

Edison, P., Archer, H. A., Gerhard, A., Hinz, R., Pavese, N., Turkheimer, F. E., et al. (2008). Microglia, amyloid, and cognition in Alzheimer's disease: An [11C](R)PK11195-PET and [11C]PIB-PET study. *Neurobiology of Disease, 32*(3), 412–419.

Esposito, G., Giovacchini, G., Liow, J. S., Bhattacharjee, A. K., Greenstein, D., Schapiro, M., et al. (2008). Imaging neuroinflammation in Alzheimer's disease with radiolabeled arachidonic acid and PET. *Journal of Nuclear Medicine, 49*(9), 1414–1421.

Fan, Z., Brooks, D. J., Okello, A. A., & Edison, P. (2017). An early and late peak in microglial activation in Alzheimer's disease trajectory. *Brain, 140*, 792–803.

Fan, Z., Okello, A. A., Brooks, D. L., & Edison, P. (2015). Longitudinal influence of microglial activation and amyloid on neuronal function in Alzheimer's disease. *Brain, 138*, 3685–3698.

Feeney, C., Scott, G., Raffel, J., Roberts, S., Coello, C., Jolly, A., et al. (2016). Kinetic analysis of the translocator protein positron emission tomography ligand [18F]GE-180 in the human brain. *European Journal of Nuclear Medicine and Molecular Imaging, 43*, 2201–2210.

Ferrari, R., Hernandez, D. G., Nalls, M. A., Rohrer, J. D., Ramasamy, A., Kwok, J. B., et al. (2014). Frontotemporal dementia and its subtypes: A genome-wide association study. *Lancet Neurology, 13*(7), 686–699.

Ferrer, I., Lopez-Gonzalez, I., Carmona, M., Arregui, L., Dalfo, E., Torrejon-Escribano, B., et al. (2014). Glial and neuronal tau pathology in tauopathies: Characterization of

disease-specific phenotypes and tau pathology progression. *Journal of Neuropathology and Experimental Neurology*, *73*, 81–97.
Forster, S., Grimmer, T., Miederer, I., Henriksen, G., Yousefi, B. H., Graner, P., et al. (2012). Regional expansion of hypometabolism in Alzheimer's disease follows amyloid deposition with temporal delay. *Biological Psychiatry*, *71*, 792–797.
Gao, H. M., Zhang, F., Zhou, H., Kam, W., Wilson, B., & Hong, J. S. (2011). Neuroinflammation and α-synuclein dysfunction potentiate each other, driving chronic progression of neurodegeneration in a mouse model of Parkinson's disease. *Environmental Health Perspectives*, *119*, 807–814.
Gerhard, A., Pavese, N., Hotton, G., Turkheimer, F., Es, M., Hammers, A., et al. (2006). In vivo imaging of microglial activation with [11C](R)-PK11195 PET in idiopathic Parkinson's disease. *Neurobiology of Disease*, *21*(2), 404–412.
Gerhard, A., Trender-Gerhard, I., Turkheimer, F., Quinn, N. P., Bhatia, K. P., & Brooks, D. J. (2006). In vivo imaging of microglial activation with [11C](R)-PK11195 PET in progressive supranuclear palsy. *Movement Disorders*, *21*(1), 89–93.
Gerhard, A., Watts, J., Trender-Gerhard, I., Turkheimer, F., Banati, R. B., Bhatia, K., et al. (2004). In vivo imaging of microglial activation with [11C](R)-PK11195 PET in corticobasal degeneration. *Movement Disorders*, *19*(10), 1221–1226.
Ghadery, C., Koshimori, Y., Coakeley, S., Harris, M., Rusjan, P., Kim, J., et al. (2017). Microglial activation in Parkinson's disease using [18F]-FEPPA. *Journal of Neuroinflammation*, *14*, 8.
Ghosh, S., Wu, M. D., Shaftel, S. S., Kyrkanides, S., LaFerla, F. M., Olschowka, J. A., et al. (2013). Sustained interleukin-1β overexpression exacerbates tau pathology despite reduced amyloid burden in an Alzheimer's mouse model. *The Journal of Neuroscience*, *33*, 5053–5064.
Groom, G. N., Junck, L., Foster, N. L., Frey, K. A., & Kuhl, D. E. (1995). PET of peripheral benzodiazepine binding sites in the microgliosis of Alzheimer's disease. *Journal of Nuclear Medicine*, *36*(12), 2207–2210.
Gulyas, B., Makkai, B., Kasa, P., Gulya, K., Bakota, L., Varszegi, S., et al. (2009). A comparative autoradiography study in post mortem whole hemisphere human brain slices taken from Alzheimer patients and age-matched controls using two radiolabelled DAA1106 analogues with high affinity to the peripheral benzodiazepine receptor (PBR) system. *Neurochemistry International*, *54*(1), 28–36.
Hamelin, L., Lagarde, J., Dorothee, G., Leroy, C., Labit, M., Comley, R. A., et al. (2016). Early and protective microglial activation in Alzheimer's disease: A prospective study using 18F-DPA-714 PET imaging. *Brain*, *139*, 1252–1264.
Han, J., Liu, H., Liu, C., Jin, H., Perlmutter, J. S., Egan, T. M., et al. (2017). Pharmacologic characterizations of a P2X7 receptor-specific radioligand, [11C]GSK1482160 for neuroinflammatory response. *Nuclear Medicine Communications*, *38*, 372–382.
He, F., Jones, J. M., Figueroa-Romero, C., Zhang, D., Feldman, E. L., Goutman, S. A., et al. (2016). Screening for novel hexanucleotide repeat expansions at ALS- and FTD-associated loci. *Neurology. Genetics*, *2*(3), e71.
Hickman, S. E., Allison, E. K., & El Khoury, J. (2008). Microglial dysfunction and defective beta-amyloid clearance pathways in aging Alzheimer's disease mice. *The Journal of Neuroscience*, *28*, 8354–8360.
Hirvonen, J., Kailajarvi, M., Haltia, T., Koskimies, S., Nagren, K., Virsu, P., et al. (2009). Assessment of MAO-B occupancy in the brain with PET and [11C]-L-deprenyl-D2: A dose-finding study with a novel MAO-B inhibitor, EVT 301. *Clinical Pharmacology and Therapeutics*, *85*, 506–512.
Iannaccone, S., Cerami, C., Alessio, M., Garibotto, V., Panzacchi, A., Olivieri, S., et al. (2013). In vivo microglia activation in very early dementia with Lewy bodies, comparison with Parkinson's disease. *Parkinsonism & Related Disorders*, *19*(1), 47–52.

Ikawa, M., Lohith, T. G., Shrestha, S., Telu, S., Zoghbi, S. S., Castellano, S., et al. (2017). 11C-ER176, a radioligand for 18-kDa translocator protein, has adequate sensitivity to robustly image all three affinity genotypes in human brain. *Journal of Nuclear Medicine, 58*, 320–325.

Insel, P. S., Ossenkoppele, R., Gessert, D., Jagust, W., Landau, S., Hansson, O., et al. (2017). Time to amyloid positivity and preclinical changes in brain metabolism, atrophy, and cognition: Evidence for emerging amyloid pathology in Alzheimer's disease. *Frontiers in Neuroscience, 11*, 281.

Ioannidis, P., Konstantinopoulou, E., Maiovis, P., & Karacostas, D. (2012). The frontotemporal dementias in a tertiary referral center: Classification and demographic characteristics in a series of 232 cases. *Journal of the Neurological Sciences, 318*, 171–173.

Jack, C. R., Knopman, D. S., Jagust, W., Petersen, R. C., Weiner, M. W., Aisen, P. S., et al. (2013). Tracking pathophysiological processes in Alzheimer's disease: An updated hypothetical model of dynamic biomarkers. *Lancet Neurology, 12*, 207–216.

Jack, C. R., Vemuri, P., Wiste, H. J., Weigand, S. D., Aisen, P. S., Trojanowski, J. Q., et al. (2011). Evidence for ordering of Alzheimer disease biomarkers. *Archives of Neurology, 68*, 1526–1535.

Jacobs, A. H., Tavitian, B., & INMind Consortium. (2012). Noninvasive molecular imaging of neuroinflammation. *Journal of Cerebral Blood Flow and Metabolism, 32*, 1393–1415.

Jansen, W. J., Ossenkoppele, R., Knol, D. L., Tijms, B. M., Scheltens, P., Verhey, F. R., et al. (2015). Prevalence of cerebral amyloid pathology in persons without dementia: A meta-analysis. *JAMA, 313*, 1924–1938.

Jin, S. C., Carrasquillo, M. M., Benitez, B. A., Skorupa, T., Carrell, D., Patel, D., et al. (2015). TREM2 is associated with increased risk for Alzheimer's disease in African Americans. *Molecular Neurodegeneration, 10*, 19.

Jossan, S. S., Gillberg, P. G., Gottfries, C. G., Karlsson, I., & Oreland, L. (1991). Monoamine oxidase B in brains from patients with Alzheimer's disease: A biochemical and autoradiographical study. *Neuroscience, 45*, 1–12.

Kanegawa, N., Collste, K., Forsberg, A., Schain, M., Arakawa, R., Jucaite, A., et al. (2016). In vivo evidence of a functional association between immune cells in blood and brain in healthy human subjects. *Brain, Behavior, and Immunity, 54*, 149–157.

Knopman, D. S., Jack, C. R., Lundt, E. S., Weigand, S. D., Vemuri, P., Lowe, V. J., et al. (2016). Evolution of neurodegeneration-imaging biomarkers from clinically normal to dementia in the Alzheimer disease spectrum. *Neurobiology of Aging, 46*, 32–42.

Kobayashi, M., Jiang, T., Telu, S., Zoghbi, S. S., Gunn, R. N., Rabiner, E. A., … Fujita, M. 2017. 11C-DPA-713 has much greater specific binding to translocator protein 18 kDa (TSPO) in human brain than 11C-(R)-PK11195. *Journal of Cerebral Blood Flow and Metabolism* (in press), [Epub ahead of print].

Kreisl, W. C., Fujita, M., Fujimura, Y., Kimura, N., Jenko, K. J., Kannan, P., et al. (2010). Comparison of [(11)C]-(R)-PK 11195 and [(11)C]PBR28, two radioligands for translocator protein (18 kDa) in human and monkey: Implications for positron emission tomographic imaging of this inflammation biomarker. *NeuroImage, 49*(4), 2924–2932.

Kreisl, W. C., Lyoo, C. H., Liow, J. S., Wei, M., Snow, J., Page, E., et al. (2016). C-PBR28 binding to translocator protein increases with progression of Alzheimer's disease. *Neurobiology of Aging, 44*, 53–61.

Kreisl, W. C., Lyoo, C. H., McGwier, M., Snow, J., Jenko, K. J., Kimura, N., et al. (2013). In vivo radioligand binding to translocator protein correlates with severity of Alzheimer's disease. *Brain, 136*(Pt. 7), 2228–2238.

Kuhlmann, A. C., & Guilarte, T. R. (2000). Cellular and subcellular localization of peripheral benzodiazepine receptors after trimethyltin neurotoxicity. *Journal of Neurochemistry, 74*, 1694–1704.

Landau, S., Horng, A., Fero, A., Jagust, W., & Alzheimer's Disease Neuroimaging Initiative. (2016). Amyloid negativity in patients with clinically diagnosed Alzheimer disease and MCI. *Neurology, 86*, 1377–1385.

Landau, S., Mintun, M. A., Joshi, A. D., Koeppe, R. A., Petersen, R. C., Aisen, P. S., et al. (2012). Amyloid deposition, hypometabolism, and longitudinal cognitive decline. *Annals of Neurology, 72*, 578–586.

Laws, S. M., Friedrich, P., Diehl-Schmid, J., Muller, J., Ibach, B., Baumi, J., et al. (2008). Genetic analysis of MAPT haplotype diversity in frontotemporal dementia. *Neurobiology of Aging, 29*, 1276–1278.

Le Fur, G., Vaucher, N., Perrier, M. L., Flamier, A., Benavides, J., Renault, C., et al. (1983). Differentiation between two ligands for peripheral benzodiazepine binding sites, [3H] RO5-4864 and [3H]PK 11195, by thermodynamic studies. *Life Sciences, 33*(5), 449–457.

Lee, M., McGeer, E., & McGeer, P. L. (2015). Activated human microglia stimulate neuroblastoma cells to upregulate production of beta amyloid protein and tau: Implications for Alzheimer's disease pathogenesis. *Neurobiology of Aging, 36*, 42–52.

Lee, E. B., Russ, J., Jung, H., Elman, L. B., Chahine, L. M., Kremens, D., et al. (2013). Topography of FUS pathology distinguishes late-onset BIBD from aFTLD-U. *Acta Neuropathologica Communications, 1*(9), 1–11.

Lindquist, S. G., Schwartz, M., Batbayli, M., Waldemar, G., & Nielsen, J. E. (2009). Genetic testing in familial AD and FTD: Mutation and phenotype spectrum in a Danish cohort. *Clinical Genetics, 76*, 205–209.

Liu, B., Le, K. X., Park, M. A., Wang, S., Belanger, A. P., Dubey, S., et al. (2015). In vivo detection of age- and disease-related increases in neuroinflammation by 18F-GE180 TSPO microPET imaging in wild-type and Alzheimer's transgenic mice. *The Journal of Neuroscience, 35*, 15716–15730.

Lo, R. Y., Hubbard, A. E., Shaw, L. M., Trojanowski, J. Q., Petersen, R. C., Aisen, P. S., et al. (2011). Longitudinal change of biomarkers in cognitive decline. *Archives of Neurology, 68*, 1257–1266.

Lyoo, C. H., Ikawa, M., Liow, J. S., Zoghbi, S. S., Morse, C., Pike, V. W., et al. (2015). Cerebellum can serve as a pseudo-reference region in Alzheimer's disease to detect neuroinflammation measured with PET radioligand binding to translocator protein (TSPO). *Journal of Nuclear Medicine, 56*, 701–706.

Mackenzie, I. R. (2000). Activated microglia in dementia with Lewy bodies. *Neurology, 55*, 132–134.

Maeda, J., Zhang, M. R., Okauchi, T., Ji, B., Ono, M., Hattori, S., et al. (2011). In vivo positron emission tomographic imaging of glial responses to amyloid-beta and tau pathologies in mouse models of Alzheimer's disease and related disorders. *The Journal of Neuroscience, 31*(12), 4720–4730.

Maezawa, I., Zimm, P. I., Wulff, H., & Jin, L. W. (2011). Amyloid-beta protein oligomer at low nanomolar concentrations activates microglia and induces microglial neurotoxicity. *The Journal of Biological Chemistry, 286*, 3693–3706.

McGeer, P. L., & McGeer, E. G. (2013). The amyloid cascade-inflammatory hypothesis of Alzheimer disease: Implications for therapy. *Acta Neuropathologica, 126*, 479–497.

Morohaku, K., Pelton, S. H., Daugherty, D. J., Butler, W. R., Deng, W., & Selvaraj, V. (2014). Translocator protein/peripheral benzodiazepine receptor is not required for steroid hormone biosynthesis. *Endocrinology, 155*(1), 89–97.

Nakamura, S., Kawamata, T., Akiguchi, I., Kameyama, M., Nakamura, N., & Kimura, H. (1990). Expression of monoamine oxidase B activity in astrocytes of senile plaques. *Acta Neuropathologica, 80*, 419–425.

Neniskyte, U., Neher, J. J., & Brown, G. C. (2011). Neuronal death induced by nanomolar amyloid β is mediated by primary phagocytosis of neurons by microglia. *The Journal of Biological Chemistry, 286*, 39904–39913.

Okello, A., Edison, P., Archer, H. A., Turkheimer, F. E., Kennedy, J., Bullock, R., et al. (2009). Microglial activation and amyloid deposition in mild cognitive impairment: A PET study. *Neurology, 72*(1), 56–62.

Oreland, L. (1980). Monoamine oxidase activity and affective illness. *Acta Psychiatrica Scandinavica Supplementum, 280,* 41–47.

Ouchi, Y., Yoshikawa, E., Sekine, Y., Futatsubashi, M., Kanno, T., Ogusu, T., et al. (2005). Microglial activation and dopamine terminal loss in early Parkinson's disease. *Annals of Neurology, 57,* 168–175.

Owen, D. R., Gunn, R. N., Rabiner, E. A., Bennacef, I., Fujita, M., Kreisl, W. C., et al. (2011). Mixed-affinity binding in humans with 18-kDa translocator protein ligands. *Journal of Nuclear Medicine, 52*(1), 24–32.

Owen, D. R., Guo, Q., Kalk, N. J., Colasanti, A., Kalogiannopoulou, D., Dimber, R., et al. (2014). Determination of [(11)C]PBR28 binding potential in vivo: A first human TSPO blocking study. *Journal of Cerebral Blood Flow and Metabolism, 34*(6), 989–994.

Owen, D. R., Howell, O. W., Tang, S. P., Wells, L. A., Bennacef, I., Bergstrom, M., et al. (2010). Two binding sites for [3H]PBR28 in human brain: Implications for TSPO PET imaging of neuroinflammation. *Journal of Cerebral Blood Flow and Metabolism, 30*(9), 1608–1618.

Papadopoulos, V., Aghazadeh, Y., Fan, J., Campioli, E., Zirkin, B., & Midzak, A. (2015). Translocator protein-mediated pharmacology of cholesterol transport and steroidogenesis. *Molecular and Cellular Endocrinology, 408,* 90–98.

Papadopoulos, V., & Miller, W. L. (2012). Role of mitochondria in steroidogenesis. *Best Practice & Research. Clinical Endocrinology & Metabolism, 26,* 771–790.

Power, J. H., & Blumbergs, P. C. (2009). Cellular glutathione peroxidase in human brain: Cellular distribution, and its potential role in the degradation of Lewy bodies in Parkinson's disease and dementia with Lewy bodies. *Acta Neuropathologica, 117,* 63–73.

Raha, A. A., Henderson, J. W., Stott, S. R., Vuono, R., Foscarin, S., Friedland, R. P., et al. (2017). Neuroprotective effect of TREM-2 in aging and Alzheimer's disease model. *Journal of Alzheimer's Disease, 55,* 199–217.

Ransohoff, R. M. (2016). A polarizing question: Do M1 and M2 microglia exist? *Nature Neuroscience, 19,* 987–991.

Rupprecht, R., Rammes, G., Eser, D., Baghai, T. C., Schule, C., Nothdurfter, C., et al. (2009). Translocator protein (18kD) as target for anxiolytics without benzodiazepine-like side effects. *Science, 325,* 490–493.

Santillo, A. F., Gambini, J. P., Lannfelt, L., Langstrom, B., Ulla-Marja, L., Kilander, L., et al. (2011). In vivo imaging of astrocytosis in Alzheimer's disease: An 11C-L-deuteriodeprenyl and PIB PET study. *European Journal of Nuclear Medicine and Molecular Imaging, 38*(12), 2202–2208.

Saura, J., Luque, J. M., Cesura, A. M., Da Prada, M., Chan-Palay, V., Huber, G., et al. (1994). Increased monoamine oxidase B activity in plaque-associated astrocytes of Alzheimer brains revealed by quantitative enzyme radioautography. *Neuroscience, 62,* 15–30.

Saura, J., Richards, J. G., & Mahy, N. (1994a). Age-related changes on MAO in Bl/C57 mouse tissues: A quantitative radioautographic study. *Journal of Neural Transmission. Supplementum, 41,* 89–94.

Saura, J., Richards, J. G., & Mahy, N. (1994b). Differential age-related changes of MAO-A and MAO-B in mouse brain and peripheral organs. *Neurobiology of Aging, 15,* 399–408.

Schain, M., & Kreisl, W. C. (2017). Neuroinflammation in neurodegenerative disorders—A review. *Current Neurology and Neuroscience Reports, 17,* 25.

Schuitemaker, A., Kropholler, M. A., Boellaard, R., van der Flier, W. M., Kloet, R. W., van der Doef, T. F., et al. (2013). Microglial activation in Alzheimer's disease: An (R)-[(1)(1) C]PK11195 positron emission tomography study. *Neurobiology of Aging, 34*(1), 128–136.

Selvaraj, V., Stocco, D. M., & Tu, L. N. (2015). Translocator protein (Tspo) and steroidogenesis: A reappraisal. *Molecular Endocrinology*, *29*, 490–501.

Serrano-Pozo, A., Mielke, M. L., Gomez-Isla, T., Betensky, R. A., Growdon, J. H., Frosch, M. P., et al. (2011). Reactive glia not only associates with plaques but also parallels tangles in Alzheimer's disease. *The American Journal of Pathology*, *179*, 1373–1384.

Serrano-Pozo, A., Qian, J., Monsell, S. E., Frosch, M. P., Betensky, R. A., & Hyman, B. T. (2013). Examination of the clinicopathologic continuum of Alzheimer disease in the autopsy cohort of the National Alzheimer Coordinating Center. *Journal of Neuropathology and Experimental Neurology*, *72*, 1182–1192.

Shukuri, M., Mawatari, A., Ohno, M., Suzuki, M., Doi, H., Watanabe, Y., et al. (2016). Detection of cyclooxygenase-1 in activated microglia during amyloid plaque progression: PET studies in Alzheimer's disease model mice. *Journal of Nuclear Medicine*, *57*, 291–296.

Suridjan, I., Pollock, B. G., Verhoeff, N. P., Voineskos, A. N., Chow, T., Rusjan, P. M., et al. (2015). In-vivo imaging of grey and white matter neuroinflammation in Alzheimer's disease: A positron emission tomography study with a novel radioligand, [F]-FEPPA. *Molecular Psychiatry*, *20*, 1579–1587.

The Lund and Manchester Groups. (1994). Clinical and neuropathological criteria for frontotemporal dementia. *Journal of Neurology, Neurosurgery, and Psychiatry*, *57*, 416–418.

Togo, T., Iseki, E., Mariu, W., Akiyama, H., Ueda, K., & Kosaka, K. (2001). Glial involvement in the degeneration process of Lewy body-bearing neurons and the degradation process of Lewy bodies in brains of dementia with Lewy bodies. *Journal of the Neurological Sciences*, *184*, 71–75.

Toledo, J. B., Zetterberg, H., van Harten, A. C., Glodzik, L., Martinez-Lage, P., Bocchio-Chiavetto, L., et al. (2015). Alzheimer's disease cerebrospinal fluid biomarker in cognitively normal subjects. *Brain*, *138*, 2701–2715.

Tu, L. N., Morohaku, K., Manna, P. R., Pelton, S. H., Butler, W. R., Stocco, D. M., et al. (2014). Peripheral benzodiazepine receptor/translocator protein global knock-out mice are viable with no effects on steroid hormone biosynthesis. *The Journal of Biological Chemistry*, *289*(40), 27444–27454.

Tu, L. N., Zhao, A. H., Stocco, D. M., & Selvaraj, V. (2015). PK11195 effect on steroidogenesis is not mediated through the translocator protein (TSPO). *Endocrinology*, *156*(3), 1033–1039.

Varrone, A., Mattsson, P., Forsberg, A., Takano, A., Nag, S., Gulyas, B., et al. (2013). In vivo imaging of the 18-kDa translocator protein (TSPO) with [18F]FEDAA1106 and PET does not show increased binding in Alzheimer's disease patients. *European Journal of Nuclear Medicine and Molecular Imaging*, *40*(6), 921–931.

Vos, S. J., Xiong, C., Visser, P. J., Jasielec, M. S., Hassenstab, J., Grant, E. A., et al. (2013). Preclinical Alzheimer's disease and its outcome: A longitudinal cohort study. *Lancet Neurology*, *12*, 957–965.

Wiley, C. A., Lopresti, B. J., Venneti, S., Price, J., Klunk, W. E., DeKosky, S. T., et al. (2009). Carbon 11-labeled Pittsburgh compound B and carbon 11-labeled (R)-PK11195 positron emission tomographic imaging in Alzheimer disease. *Archives of Neurology*, *66*(1), 60–67.

Yasuno, F., Kosaka, J., Ota, M., Higuchi, M., Ito, H., Fujimura, Y., et al. (2012). Increased binding of peripheral benzodiazepine receptor in mild cognitive impairment-dementia converters measured by positron emission tomography with [(1)(1)C]DAA1106. *Psychiatry Research*, *203*(1), 67–74.

Yasuno, F., Ota, M., Kosaka, J., Ito, H., Higuchi, M., Doronbekov, T. K., et al. (2008). Increased binding of peripheral benzodiazepine receptor in Alzheimer's disease measured by positron emission tomography with [11C]DAA1106. *Biological Psychiatry*, *64*(10), 835–841.

Yokokura, M., Mori, N., Yagi, S., Yoshikawa, E., Kikuchi, M., Yoshihara, Y., et al. (2011). In vivo changes in microglial activation and amyloid deposits in brain regions with hypometabolism in Alzheimer's disease. *European Journal of Nuclear Medicine and Molecular Imaging*, *38*(2), 343–351.

Zhang, W., Wang, T., Pei, Z., Miller, D. S., Wu, X., Block, M. L., et al. (2005). Aggregated α-synuclein activates microglia: A process leading to disease progression in Parkinson's disease. *The FASEB Journal*, *19*, 533–542.

Zurcher, N. R., Loggia, M. L., Lawson, R., Chonde, D. B., Izquierdo-Garcia, D., Yasek, J. E., et al. (2015). Increased in vivo glial activation in patients with amyotrophic lateral sclerosis: Assessed with [(11)C]-PBR28. *NeuroImage. Clinical*, 7, 409–414.

FURTHER READING

Fan, Z., Calsolaro, V., Atkinson, R. A., Femminella, G. D., Waldman, A., Buckley, C., et al. (2016). Flutriciclamide (18F-GE180) PET: First-in-human PET study of novel third-generation in vivo marker of human translocator protein. *Journal of Nuclear Medicine*, *57*, 1753–1759.

CHAPTER NINE

RNA-Based Fluorescent Biosensors for Detecting Metabolites in vitro and in Living Cells

Samie R. Jaffrey[1]
Weill Medical College, Cornell University, New York, NY, United States
[1]Corresponding author: e-mail address: srj2003@med.cornell.edu

Contents

Abstract

Genetically encoded sensors are important tools for measuring metabolites and other small molecules in vitro and in live cells. Until recently, genetically encoded sensors exclusively comprised fluorescent proteins that undergo changes in Förster resonance energy transfer upon binding a target analyte. However, recently a new class of fluorescent sensor has been developed composed of RNA. These RNA-based sensors rely on Spinach and other RNA mimics of green fluorescent protein. In each case, the RNA-based sensors contain an analyte-binding aptamer domain which transduces binding of the analyte into a conformational change in Spinach. Two types of sensors have been developed: allosteric Spinach sensors and Spinach riboswitches. Allosteric Spinach sensors exhibit metabolite-induced folding and subsequent fluorescence. Spinach riboswitches are naturally occurring riboswitches that have been modified to contain the Spinach aptamer. The resulting RNA is a fluorogenic riboswitch, and produces fluorescence upon binding its cognate analyte. We describe the development of this new technology, its uses, and future directions to facilitate the use of this assay technology in mammalian cells and in high-throughput applications.

Advances in Pharmacology, Volume 82
ISSN 1054-3589
https://doi.org/10.1016/bs.apha.2017.09.005

ABBREVIATIONS

AMP adenosine monophosphate
ADP adenosine diphosphate
DFHBI 3,5-difluoro-4-hydroxybenzylidene imidazolinone
FRET Förster resonance energy transfer
GMP guanosine monophosphate
GTP guanosine triphosphate
SAM *S*-adenosyl methionine
TPP thiamine pyrophosphate

1. INTRODUCTION

Assays for detecting small molecules and metabolites have been major enabling technologies for the discovery and characterization of cellular signaling pathways and biological processes. Numerous cellular metabolites have been found to have central roles in cell physiology and signaling pathways. Moreover, numerous studies have demonstrated that altered cellular metabolite levels are mediators and indicators of various diseases (Ward et al., 2010). Therefore, the ability to accurately quantify diverse metabolites will likely accelerate our understanding of the role of metabolites in cellular signaling and physiology.

Although most metabolite measurements are performed using traditional methods such as NMR spectroscopy, mass spectrometry, and liquid chromatography, these assays lack the benefit of being high throughput. In order to rapidly screen and characterize multiple samples in a rapid and high-throughput manner, simple, sensitive, and specific assays are needed. Additionally, many established techniques, such as mass spectrometry, do not readily distinguish between isomers of naturally occurring metabolites, including *cis–trans* isomers, structural isomers, and enantiomers. As a result, these assays have difficulty in definitively identifying common metabolites such as D-amino acids vs L-amino acids and anomers of sugars. Therefore, rapid and simple detection methods that are able to differentiate highly related molecules are needed for numerous applications, including drug discovery.

In addition to in vitro assays, there is a long-standing need to detect metabolites in live cells. Metabolite levels can change rapidly in response to signaling pathway, and harvesting the cells for in vitro measurements at predetermined time points can miss metabolite changes that occur at the nonsampled time points. As a result, "discontinuous" assays like mass spectrometry and liquid chromatography cannot reveal the complete time course of metabolite dynamics. Additionally, these methods do not reveal metabolite dynamics in individual cells, potentially masking marked cell-to-cell variability. Therefore, there is considerable interest in developing methods to detect metabolites over time in living cells.

A new approach for detecting metabolites utilizes fluorescent biosensors composed of RNA, rather than proteins. Although most biosensors are composed of protein, we recently described a class of fluorescent biosensors composed of RNA (Paige, Nguyen-Duc, Song, & Jaffrey, 2012; Song, Strack, & Jaffrey, 2013; Song, Strack, Svensen, & Jaffrey, 2014; You, Litke, & Jaffrey, 2015). These RNA-based biosensors can be expressed in cells and exhibit fluorescence in proportion to the cellular concentration of specific intracellular metabolites. These biosensors have been used to detect diverse intracellular metabolites and signaling molecules in bacteria, and have the potential to detect a wide range of intracellular metabolites. Notably, these biosensors are relatively straightforward to develop, although key optimization steps are required to maximize metabolite-induced fluorescence responses and to tune the fluorescent readout so that the biosensor responds to physiologically relevant metabolite levels in cells. Here we describe the development of this new technology, its uses, and future directions to facilitate the use of this assay technology in mammalian cells and in high-throughput applications.

2. ORGANIC DYE AND FLUORESCENT PROTEIN-BASED BIOSENSORS

An important method for detecting small molecules in live cells involves fluorescence imaging. Some of the earliest fluorescent indicators were small molecule organic dyes that bound calcium, resulting in a change in fluorescence emission (Kao & Tsien, 1988). These dyes revealed the dynamic nature of calcium levels inside the cytosol upon the activation of diverse signaling cascades.

More recently developed biosensors are composed of fluorescent proteins, which are capable of undergoing Förster resonance energy transfer (FRET). These sensors typically comprise two fluorescent proteins that are separated by a domain that binds an analyte of interest. Upon binding the analyte, this domain undergoes a conformational change that repositions the fluorescent proteins. By repositioning the fluorescent proteins, the magnitude of FRET between the fluorescent proteins changes. This change in

FRET can be detected in living cells using FRET microscopy (Miyawaki et al., 1997).

A major advantage of this approach over the original fluorescent indicator dyes is that these biosensors can be genetically encoded. Thus, cells can be engineered to express the fluorescent biosensor. This allows the fluorescent biosensor to have access to the cytoplasm of cells with minimal cellular perturbation, and potentially enables the creation of stable cell lines that could be used for screening purposes and other high-throughput applications.

The major challenge with this approach is that these sensors are exceptionally difficult to design. They require a protein that binds the analyte of interest and subsequently undergoes a large conformational change that can reposition fluorescent proteins. However, in many cases, there is no protein that is available that binds the analyte and undergoes a conformational change that would reposition fluorescent proteins. As a result, it is difficult to generate a fluorescent biosensor that detects any arbitrary analyte. This constitutes a major roadblock for understanding the roles and functions of diverse cellular metabolites.

3. SELECTIVE MOLECULAR RECOGNITION BY ENDOGENOUS AND ENGINEERED RNAs

Although receptors are generally thought to be composed of protein, there are numerous examples of receptors that are composed of RNA. The most well-documented examples are the riboswitches (McCown, Corbino, Stav, Sherlock, & Breaker, 2017). Riboswitches are structured RNAs that are highly prevalent in bacterial mRNA transcripts. These structured RNA elements bind to diverse molecules including single atoms, metabolites, and tRNA and undergo conformational changes that ultimately influence the ability of the transcript to be translated or affect mRNA stability. Notably, these RNA sequences fold into highly intricate three-dimensional structures and show all the key features of molecular recognition seen in protein-based receptors. For example, riboswitches exhibit a high degree of selectivity toward their specific targets, while not reacting with other highly similar molecules in cells (Batey, Gilbert, & Montange, 2004; Lu et al., 2008; Luo, Chen, Zhou, Sintim, & Dayie, 2014). Thus, RNA can bind diverse intracellular targets.

In addition to endogenous RNAs that act as receptors, RNAs can be generated by in vitro selection approaches to bind a wide range of metabolites and small molecules. These RNAs are termed aptamers, and are generated using the SELEX technique (Ellington & Szostak, 1990; Tuerk & Gold, 1990). In SELEX, a pool of $\sim 10^{15}$ random RNA sequences are incubated with an immobilized target molecule. The bound RNAs are collected and then amplified by RT-PCR. The amplified DNA is used to generate RNA for the next round of selection. After 8–15 rounds of iterative selection, RNA aptamers with high affinity to the target of interest are enriched and isolated (Ellington & Szostak, 1990; Tuerk & Gold, 1990).

Using SELEX, aptamers that bind a wide range of molecules have been obtained (Stoltenburg, Reinemann, & Strehlitz, 2007). These include amino acids, carbohydrates, antibiotics, and proteins. The selectivity can be enhanced by negative selection protocols such as "counter-SELEX" in which aptamers that bind to a related molecule can be removed from an RNA pool (Jeong, Han, Lee, & Lee, 2010). Indeed, aptamers that bind caffeine were able to discriminate between caffeine and a variety of other related xanthines (Jenison, Gill, Pardi, & Polisky, 1994). Similarly, aptamers that discriminate between phosphorylated peptides and their unphosphorylated forms have been described (Liu et al., 2009). Thus, just like protein-based receptors and naturally occurring riboswitches, RNA aptamers can be highly selective toward their targets.

RNA aptamers can be expressed in cells, much in the same way that protein-based receptors can be expressed. Typically RNA polymerase III promoters, such as the U6 promoter is used to enable high-level expression of RNA in cells (Paul et al., 2003). RNA polymerase III uses a facilitated "recycling" mechanism that allows a polymerase to reenter the promoter after it finishes transcript (Dieci & Sentenac, 1996). Transcription using this promoter is especially valuable for short RNAs, such as aptamers, that lack the U-rich RNA polymerase III termination element.

What are the potential advantages of using RNA as the foundation for constructing a biosensor? Most importantly, RNA-based receptors can be developed very quickly. RNA aptamers that bind with high specificity and selectivity toward a specific metabolite can be generated within a few weeks (Ellington & Szostak, 1990; Tuerk & Gold, 1990). In contrast, developing a protein-based receptor that binds to a target of interest can be exceptionally challenging. Protein engineering is not yet sufficiently developed to enable the simple development of a protein that binds to a target of interest. Thus, the simplicity of generating receptors composed of RNA makes RNA an exceptionally attractive approach for sensor development. Additionally, as will be described below, we have developed straightforward approaches for converting RNA-based receptors into fluorescent biosensors that can be expressed inside cells. This relatively straightforward approach of converting an RNA aptamer into a fluorescent biosensor makes sense using RNA-based receptor components an attractive strategy for biosensor design.

4. THE FIRST ENGINEERED RNA-BASED METABOLITE SENSORS

The concept that RNAs could be engineered into a sensor derived from seminal work involving engineered ribozymes. The initial study describing this novel class of sensors was developed by Breaker and colleagues and utilized the hammerhead ribozyme (Tang & Breaker, 1997). Normally, the hammerhead ribozyme undergoes a self-cleavage reaction. However, the ribozyme was modified so that it only cleaves itself upon exposure to metabolites such as adenosine triphosphate (ATP). The fundamental principle behind this ATP-regulated ribozyme is that the ribozyme was modified to contain an aptamer that binds ATP. The ATP aptamer was inserted into an RNA helical stem that has an essential structural role in the folding of the ribozyme. Importantly, the ATP aptamer is not folded in the absence of ATP. Thus, the aptamer disrupts the folding of the ribozyme and prevents its activity. However, upon binding ATP, the aptamer folds, allowing the stem to form a stable duplex. At this point, the ribozyme can fold and undergo self cleavage. In this way, ATP is detected by the presence of cleaved ribozyme.

This approach was extended to generate ribozyme sensors that detect various molecules, including flavin mononucleotide, theophylline, and cGMP (Koizumi, Soukup, Kerr, & Breaker, 1999; Robertson & Ellington, 1999; Sekella, Rueda, & Walter, 2002; Soukup & Breaker, 1999). The concentration of the metabolite determines the efficiency and rate of cleavage. In this way, the concentration of the analyte can be extrapolated from the rate of cleavage (Soukup & Breaker, 1999).

Although this approach was a major landmark because it introduced the concept of engineering sensing abilities into a ribozyme, and constituted the first RNA-based sensors, these sensors have inherent limitations. First, they are not reversible. Thus, if the concentration of the metabolite drops, there cannot be a reduction in the overall signal—once the cleavage occurs, it is not reversible. Second, this type of sensor is only appropriate for in vitro measurements. The readout is a relatively cumbersome PCR-based assay, or a gel-based measurement to determine whether the ribozyme has undergone cleavage. This is time consuming, and does not lend itself to rapid high-throughput measurements. Additionally, the cleavage would not be readily detectable inside a mammalian cell. Therefore, this concept is largely limited to in vitro diagnostic applications.

5. FLUORESCENT BIOSENSORS COMPOSED OF RNA

Recently we developed a new type of RNA-based sensor that builds upon fluorogenic aptamers (Paige et al., 2012; Song et al., 2013, 2014; You et al., 2015). We developed fluorogenic RNA aptamers by selecting RNAs that could bind to small molecule fluorophores that resemble the fluorophore naturally found in green fluorescent protein. These fluorophores are typically nonfluorescent, but upon binding to their cognate aptamer, become markedly fluorescent. These readily cross cell membranes show minimal nonspecific fluorescence activation in cells and are nontoxic. The first such aptamer, Spinach (Paige, Wu, & Jaffrey, 2011) binds to 3,5-difluoro-4-hydroxybenzylidene imidazolinone (DFHBI), resulting in green fluorescence. Subsequent RNA aptamers include Broccoli (Filonov, Moon, Svensen, & Jaffrey, 2014) and Corn (Song et al., 2017), which exhibit green and yellow fluorescence, respectively, upon binding to their cognate fluorophores. Together, these RNA aptamers are referred to as "RNA mimics of green fluorescent protein" based on their ability to activate GFP-like fluorophores. Their vegetable names reflect a naming system that is parallel to the fruit-based naming system proposed by Tsien for fluorescent proteins (Shaner et al., 2004).

Fluorogenic aptamers can be used to encode fluorescence in mammalian cells (Filonov et al., 2014; Paige et al., 2011; Song et al., 2017; Strack, Disney, & Jaffrey, 2013). Expression of Spinach, Broccoli, and Corn aptamers results in readily detectable cellular fluorescence. These aptamers can be used to tag various types of RNA. Fusion RNAs expressing an RNA of interest and a fluorogenic aptamer tag can be visualized using fluorescence microscopy if the RNA is expressed at a sufficiently high concentration.

We used fluorogenic RNA aptamers to create biosensors that can detect metabolites both in vitro and in cells (Paige et al., 2012; Song et al., 2013, 2014; You et al., 2015). These sensors function in an analogous manner to

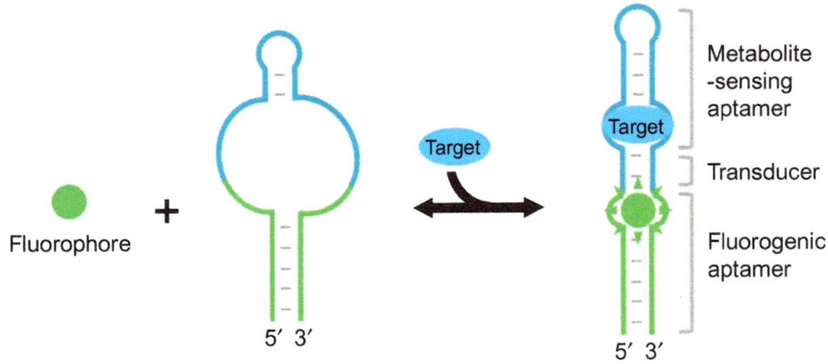

Fig. 1 Metabolite sensors based on fluorogenic aptamers. Metabolite sensors can be generated based on a metabolite-induced allosteric folding mechanism. In these sensors, a metabolite-binding aptamer is fused to Spinach. This aptamer is typically unfolded until the metabolite ("target", *blue*) binds. At this point, the aptamer folds, which facilitates the folding of Spinach. This enables DFHBI, the cognate fluorophore for Spinach, to bind and exhibit fluorescence. In this way, fluorescence is directly correlated to the levels of the metabolite in solution or the cell.

the allosteric ribozymes: a metabolite-binding aptamer is functionally linked to the folding of Spinach, such that metabolite binding leads to fluorescence (Fig. 1). These sensors are genetically encodable since the RNA can be expressed within any cell.

Unlike ribozymes which undergo an irreversible metabolite-induced cleavage, the fluorogenic aptamers are reversibly fluorescent, with changes in metabolite levels causing a relatively rapid change in the fluorescence of the biosensor (Paige et al., 2012).

Two types of sensors have been described: allosteric Spinach sensors (Paige et al., 2012) and Spinach riboswitches (You et al., 2015). A schematic of the structure of allosteric Spinach sensors is shown in Fig. 1. The metabolite-binding aptamer is fused to a critical stem in Spinach via a transducer domain (Paige et al., 2012). When the metabolite is absent, the aptamer is unstructured and destabilizes the transducer domain stem that is essential for Spinach folding. However, when the aptamer binds the metabolite, the aptamer folds, resulting in hybridization of the transducer domain strands and subsequent folding of Spinach. This can be readily detected based on the presence of Spinach fluorescence.

The key feature of an optimized allosteric sensor is low fluorescence in the absence of the metabolite and high fluorescence in the presence of the metabolite. This is fundamentally determined by the transducer sequence, which needs to be optimized to maximize sensor performance.

6. APPLICATIONS OF ALLOSTERIC SPINACH SENSORS

Allosteric Spinach sensors have been used to quantify diverse metabolites in vitro and in cells. The initial Spinach-based biosensors were developed by our lab and included sensors that detected diverse metabolites, including *S*-adenosyl methionine (SAM), adenosine diphosphate (ADP), guanine, adenine, and guanosine triphosphate (GTP) (Paige et al., 2012). The in vivo studies focused on SAM levels and its dynamics in *Escherichia coli*. There are currently no fluorescent biosensors that are composed of proteins that detect endogenous SAM levels. The allosteric Spinach sensor used the aptamer component of an SAM riboswitch (Paige et al., 2012). We fused this aptamer to Spinach in a way that allowed SAM binding to allosterically induce Spinach folding. SAM biosynthesis was measured following application of methionine to methionine-starved cells. One of the notable findings was that different cells showed markedly different rates of SAM biosynthesis, with some cells showing rapid synthesis, while others showing an increase in SAM levels followed by decreases in SAM levels. This suggests that there are cell-to-cell variations in SAM metabolism, which would not have been revealed if entire plates of cells were harvested and analyzed for SAM content using conventional liquid chromatography. Notably, other metabolites, such as ADP, did not show similar cell-to-cell variation when imaged using a Spinach biosensor selective for ADP. This suggests that cell-to-cell variations in metabolite levels are preferentially seen with certain metabolites and not others.

This approach has also been extended to detecting proteins. RNA aptamers can be developed that bind proteins using similar approaches to those used for developing small molecule-binding aptamers (Stoltenburg et al., 2007). We used an endogenous aptamer that binds the coat protein of the MS2 phage to image the expression of the MS2 phage coat protein during phage infection in bacteria (Song et al., 2013). Coat protein was detected in as little as 6 min after infection, demonstrating the ability of Spinach-based sensors to detect rapid changes to intracellular proteins in cells.

Allosteric Spinach sensors have been developed that bind cyclic dinucleotide signaling molecules (Bose, Su, Marcus, Raulet, & Hammond, 2016; Kellenberger, wilson, et al., 2015; Kellenberger, Chen, Whiteley, Portnoy, & Hammond, 2015; Kellenberger, Wilson, Sales-Lee, & Hammond, 2013; Luo et al., 2014; Nakayama, Luo, Zhou, Dayie, & Sintim, 2012), such as cyclic-di-GMP, cyclic-di-AMP, and cyclic AMP-GMP. Thus, in addition to cellular metabolites, Spinach-based sensors can readily detect signaling molecules in cells and in cellular lysates (Bose et al., 2016).

7. RNA-BASED BIOSENSORS MODELED AFTER RIBOSWITCHES

Although allosteric sensors have been utilized successfully for various applications, the development of these sensors requires the identification or generation of a metabolite-binding aptamer that has suitable affinity and selectivity in the complex environment of the cytosol of a cell.

To overcome this, we developed a new type of sensor, termed a Spinach riboswitch. These sensors take advantage of naturally occurring aptamers found in the context of bacterial riboswitches. Riboswitches have evolved to bind their target metabolites at physiologically relevant concentrations with high selectivity and therefore would be highly desirable to adapt into a sensor.

Riboswitches are typically found in the 5′-UTR of certain mRNAs in various prokaryotes, and undergo a conformational switch upon binding metabolites (Mandal & Breaker, 2014; Winkler, Nahvi, & Breaker, 2012). These conformation changes affect mRNA translation or stability. The key mechanism involves the movement of a single strand, i.e., the switching sequence, between the riboswitch's aptamer domain and a semistructured region that can influence mRNA translation or stability, known as the expression platform. The switching sequence can hybridize either to the aptamer or to the expression platform; however, in the absence of the metabolite, hybridization to the aptamer is favored. Metabolite binding liberates the switching strand, which then hybridizes in the expression platform. Hybridization to the expression platform can block ribosome binding or influence mRNA stability. In this way, metabolite binding can alter the fate of the mRNA.

Diverse biochemical and computational approaches have revealed that there are dozens or hundreds of riboswitches that bind different targets (Baker et al., 2012). Therefore, naturally occurring riboswitches constitute a rich pool of naturally occurring and highly optimized metabolite-sensing RNAs that can be exploited for sensor development.

We recently developed a strategy for modifying these riboswitches so that metabolite-induced structural changes lead to folding of Spinach

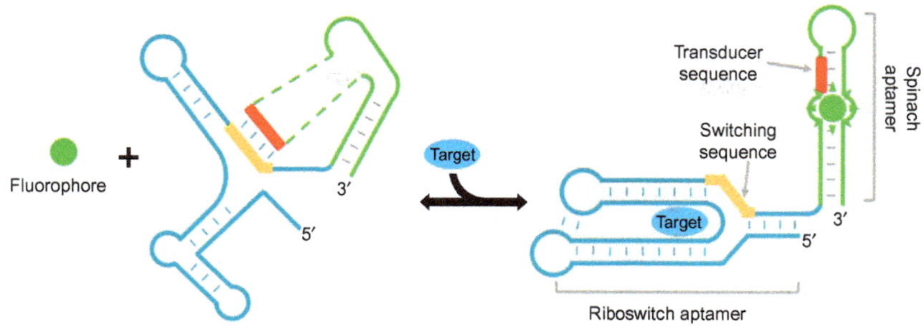

Fig. 2 *Metabolite detection using Spinach riboswitches.* Spinach riboswitches exploit the natural conformational switching in endogenous riboswitches. A riboswitch that binds the target metabolite is identified and the expression platform is replaced with Spinach. The transducer sequence of Spinach and switching sequence of riboswitch hybridize, which allows DFHBI to bind and exhibit fluorescence. During biosensor development, the switching sequence of the riboswitch is modified so that it can interact with Spinach's transducer sequence, which may be slightly modified to maximize sensor performance. To identify the best sensor, variants are synthesized with nucleotide substitutions in the switching strand transducer and linker regions. These are tested in vitro for properties such as signal response, affinity, and kinetics of binding.

(Fig. 2). The initial design of these sensors took advantage of the known structure of Spinach and as well as the structure of riboswitches. We modified four known riboswitches so that the metabolite-released switching sequence triggers the formation of the DFHBI-binding pocket of Spinach.

In Spinach riboswitches, the switching sequence needs to switch Spinach from a conformation that cannot bind its fluorophore to a conformation that binds fluorophore. The Spinach riboswitches rely on the switching sequence creating the binding pocket for the DFHBI fluorophore. The binding pocket of Spinach contains two major structural features: a G-quadruplex structure (Warner et al., 2014), which forms one surface for binding DFHBI, and a U•A•U base triple, which forms the other surface that binds DFHBI. The stem adjacent to the fluorophore-binding pocket includes one of the U residues that form the base triple (Fig. 2). If the switching sequence is designed to form this part of the stem, then the base triple will only form when the switching sequence is liberated from the aptamer by metabolite binding. This approach leads to selective folding of Spinach in response to metabolite binding (You et al., 2015).

Using this approach, four different Spinach riboswitches were developed (You et al., 2015). These riboswitches detected thiamine pyrophosphate (TPP), guanine, adenine, and SAM. The TPP riboswitch was expressed in cells and used to reveal TPP biosynthesis in *E. coli* after application of thiamine (Fig. 3). Notably, the cellular fluorescence was shown to directly correlated with TPP levels measured by liquid chromatography. Thus, the intracellular TPP concentration can be predicted using Spinach-based sensors.

Although we found that Spinach riboswitches can be readily designed even in the absence of structural information of the riboswitch, structural information is very useful for optimizing swapping the expression domain with Spinach in the riboswitch and optimizing the performance of the sensor. The Nucleic Acid Database Project lists over 180 different crystal structures of riboswitches (http://ndbserver.rutgers.edu/). In some cases, the

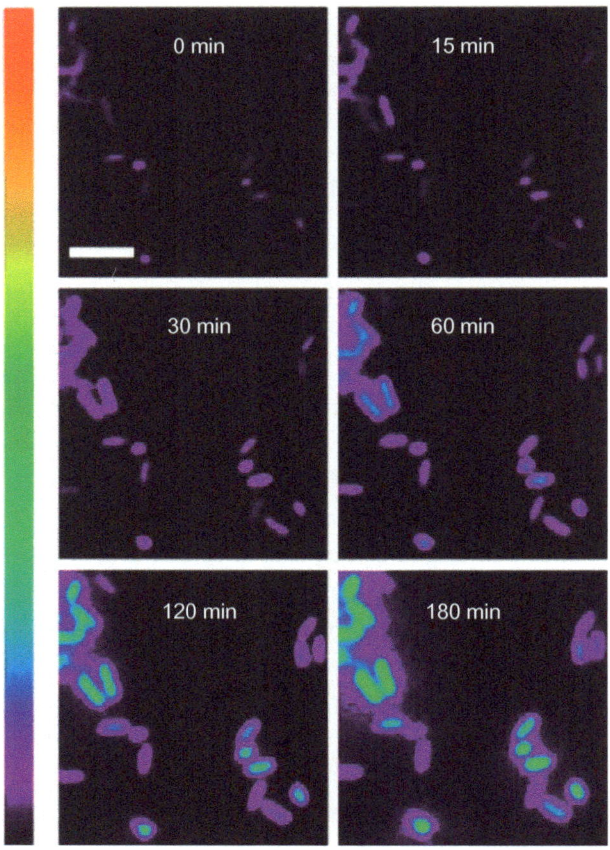

Fig. 3 Representative images of TPP imaging in *E. coli*. *E. coli* are transformed with a plasmid expressing the TPP Spinach riboswitch. A time course of fluorescence imaging after addition of thiamine is shown. Images are presented as a heat map in which the fluorescence at each indicated time is normalized to the fluorescence at $t=0$ min. The color range reflects the increase in fluorescence relative to the 0 min time point.

riboswitches have been crystallized in different switched states (Garst, Heroux, Rambo, & Batey, 2008; Huang, Serganov, & Patel, 2008), which can help indicate identify switching sequences and facilitate the design of Spinach sequences that would become activated once they contain a hybridized switching sequence. Additional information is available based on structure probing methods such as 2′-hydroxyl probing (SHAPE), which reveals nucleotides that have altered conformations upon metabolite binding (Steen, Malhotra, & Weeks, 2010). For several riboswitch classes, bases that are likely to be essential for switching can be predicted based on the identification of conserved nucleotides by genomic alignment of homologous riboswitches (Barrick & Breaker, 2007). Thus, without prior knowledge of the aptamer domain, it may be possible to design Spinach riboswitches.

The relatively straightforward process of developing Spinach riboswitch sensors from endogenous riboswitches demonstrates that this is a generalizable approach that can take advantage of naturally occurring metabolite recognition by riboswitches in nature. In many cases riboswitches were discovered using computational approaches and their endogenous ligands remain unknown (McCown et al., 2017). Because these riboswitches can now be engineered into fluorescent biosensors, discovery of their targets is an important goal.

8. CONCLUSION

The major next step is to develop approaches that allow these sensors to be used in mammalian cells. The current sensor technologies have only been successfully utilized in bacterial cells largely because higher steady-state RNA levels that can be achieved in bacteria compared to mammalian cells. RNA aptamer in bacteria can readily exceed 1 μM (Filonov, Kam, Song, & Jaffrey, 2015; Paige et al., 2011, 2012). The amount of the sensor that is in a fluorescent conformation is directly related to the metabolite concentration, so only a fraction of the sensor will be in a fluorescent conformation. Nevertheless, this level of fluorescence is readily detectable by fluorescence microscopy in *E. coli*. However, expression of the same RNA-based sensors in mammalian cells results in expression that is typically 100-fold lower, with typical expression levels of ~10–40 nM (Filonov et al., 2015). When expressing just the Spinach aptamer at this concentration, fluorescence is relatively low and near the lower limit of detection (Strack et al., 2013).

When a Spinach-based sensor is expressed, and only a fraction of the sensor is in a fluorescent conformation, the fluorescence is not detectable.

A major goal is to express RNAs at high enough expression levels in mammalian cells so that they can be used to measure endogenous metabolite levels. In mammalian cells, fluorescent proteins and protein-based FRET biosensors are routinely expressed at 1–10 μM (Vogel & Marcotte, 2012). A similar concentration of the RNA-based sensor is therefore expected to exhibit readily detectable fluorescence in mammalian cells.

One strategy to achieve high expression in mammalian cells could be to use the mechanisms that confer high-level expression in bacteria. The high bacterial expression reflects both higher RNA expression and lower RNA degradation than mammalian cells. This is most prominent in bacterial strains, such as the BL21 *E. coli* strain, that have been engineered to express T7 RNA polymerase and engineered to lack ribonucleases (Terpe, 2006). Although mammalian cells with heterologous expression of T7 RNA polymerase have been described (Fuerst, Niles, Studier, & Moss, 1986), the requirement for expressing T7 RNA polymerase is cumbersome and could cause unwanted effects on endogenous metabolite expression.

Another approach to achieve high-level expression could be to express the RNA sensors as a circle. RNA circles are RNAs that have the 5′ and 3′ end joined in a phosphodiester bond. This prevents the action of 5′ or 3′ exonucleases. Notably, circular RNAs have half-lives of days to several weeks (Memczak et al., 2013), in contrast to the ~1 h half-life seen for aptamer expression in cells (Filonov et al., 2015; Lu et al., 2015).

New RNA circularization expression constructs may be particularly suited for achieving RNA circle production in cells. For example, a recent expression system takes advantage of the fact that introns that are naturally found in tRNA transcripts are removed and can be circularized by the RtcB, the same RNA ligase that normally reseals the tRNA after intron removal (Lu et al., 2015). When the intron is replaced with an aptamer sequence, such as Broccoli, then Broccoli is expressed as a highly stable circular RNA in mammalian cells (Lu et al., 2015). Notably, although highly stable RNA expression was achieved, the level of expression was not substantially higher than what is achieved for linear RNA. This likely reflects the poor circularization efficiency in this plasmid. Expression systems that result in high-level circular RNA aptamer expression would likely enable the expression of RNA-based sensors at a sufficient concentration for imaging in mammalian cells.

CONFLICT OF INTEREST

S.R.J. is the cofounder of Lucerna Technologies and has equity in this company. Lucerna has licensed commercialization of technology related to Spinach and other RNA–fluorophore complexes.

ACKNOWLEDGMENTS

This work was supported by NIH grants to S.R.J. (R01 NS064516 and R01 EB010249).

REFERENCES

Baker, J. L., Sudarsan, N., Weinberg, Z., Roth, A., Stockbridge, R. B., & Breaker, R. R. (2012). Widespread genetic switches and toxicity resistance proteins for fluoride. *Science, 335*(6065), 233–235.

Barrick, J. E., & Breaker, R. R. (2007). The power of riboswitches. *Scientific American, 296*(1), 50–57.

Batey, R. T., Gilbert, S. D., & Montange, R. K. (2004). Structure of a natural guanine-responsive riboswitch complexed with the metabolite hypoxanthine. *Nature, 432*(7015), 411–415.

Bose, D., Su, Y., Marcus, A., Raulet, D. H., & Hammond, M. C. (2016). An RNA-based fluorescent biosensor for high-throughput analysis of the cGAS-cGAMP-STING pathway. *Cell Chemical Biology, 23*(12), 1539–1549.

Dieci, G., & Sentenac, A. (1996). Facilitated recycling pathway for RNA polymerase III. *Cell, 84*(2), 245–252.

Ellington, A. D., & Szostak, J. W. (1990). In vitro selection of RNA molecules that bind specific ligands. *Nature, 346*(6287), 818–822.

Filonov, G. S., Kam, C. W., Song, W., & Jaffrey, S. R. (2015). In-gel imaging of RNA processing using Broccoli reveals optimal aptamer expression strategies. *Chemistry & Biology, 22*(5), 649–660.

Filonov, G. S., Moon, J. D., Svensen, N., & Jaffrey, S. R. (2014). Broccoli: Rapid selection of an RNA mimic of green fluorescent protein by fluorescence-based selection and directed evolution. *Journal of the American Chemical Society, 136*(46), 16299–16308.

Fuerst, T. R., Niles, E. G., Studier, F. W., & Moss, B. (1986). Eukaryotic transient-expression system based on recombinant vaccinia virus that synthesizes bacteriophage T7 RNA polymerase. *Proceedings of the National Academy of Sciences of the United States of America, 83*(21), 8122–8126.

Garst, A. D., Heroux, A., Rambo, R. P., & Batey, R. T. (2008). Crystal structure of the lysine riboswitch regulatory mRNA element. *The Journal of Biological Chemistry, 283*(33), 22347–22351.

Huang, L., Serganov, A., & Patel, D. J. (2008). Structural insights into ligand recognition by a sensing domain of the cooperative glycine riboswitch. *Molecular Cell, 40*(5), 774–786.

Jenison, R. D., Gill, S. C., Pardi, A., & Polisky, B. (1994). High-resolution molecular discrimination by RNA. *Science, 263*(5152), 1425–1429.

Jeong, S., Han, S. R., Lee, Y. J., & Lee, S. W. (2010). Selection of RNA aptamers specific to active prostate-specific antigen. *Biotechnology Letters, 32*(3), 379–385.

Kao, J. P., & Tsien, R. Y. (1988). Ca2+ binding kinetics of fura-2 and azo-1 from temperature-jump relaxation measurements. *Biophysical Journal, 53*(4), 635–639.

Kellenberger, C. A., Chen, C., Whiteley, A. T., Portnoy, D. A., & Hammond, M. C. (2015). RNA-based fluorescent biosensors for live cell imaging of second messenger cyclic di-AMP. *Journal of the American Chemical Society, 137*(20), 6432–6435.

Kellenberger, C. A., Wilson, S. C., Hickey, S. F., Gonzalez, T. L., Su, Y., Hallberg, Z. F., et al. (2015). GEMM-I riboswitches from Geobacter sense the bacterial second messenger cyclic AMP-GMP. *Proceedings of the National Academy of Sciences of the United States of America*, *112*(17), 5383–5388.

Kellenberger, C. A., Wilson, S. C., Sales-Lee, J., & Hammond, M. C. (2013). RNA-based fluorescent biosensors for live cell imaging of second messengers cyclic di-GMP and cyclic AMP-GMP. *Journal of the American Chemical Society*, *135*, 4906–4909.

Koizumi, M., Soukup, G. A., Kerr, J. N., & Breaker, R. R. (1999). Allosteric selection of ribozymes that respond to the second messengers cGMP and cAMP. *Nature Structural Biology*, *6*(11), 1062–1071.

Liu, Y., Sun, Q. A., Chen, Q., Lee, T. H., Huang, Y., Wetsel, W. C., et al. (2009). Targeting inhibition of GluR1 Ser845 phosphorylation with an RNA aptamer that blocks AMPA receptor trafficking. *Journal of Neurochemistry*, *108*(1), 147–157.

Lu, Z., Filonov, G. S., Noto, J. J., Schmidt, C. A., Hatkevich, T. L., Wen, Y., et al. (2015). Metazoan tRNA introns generate stable circular RNAs in vivo. *RNA*, *21*(9), 1554–1565.

Lu, C., Smith, A. M., Fuchs, R. T., Ding, F., Rajashankar, K., Henkin, T. M., et al. (2008). Crystal structures of the SAM-III/SMK riboswitch reveal the SAM-dependent translation inhibition mechanism. *Nature Structural and Molecular Biology*, *15*(10), 1076–1083.

Luo, Y., Chen, B., Zhou, J., Sintim, H. O., & Dayie, T. K. (2014). E88, a new cyclic-di-GMP class I riboswitch aptamer from Clostridium tetani, has a similar fold to the prototypical class I riboswitch, Vc2, but differentially binds to c-di-GMP analogs. *Molecular BioSystems*, *10*(3), 384–390.

Mandal, M., & Breaker, R. R. (2014). Adenine riboswitches and gene activation by disruption of a transcription terminator. *Nature Structural and Molecular Biology*, *11*(1), 29–35.

McCown, P. J., Corbino, K. A., Stav, S., Sherlock, M. E., & Breaker, R. R. (2017). Riboswitch diversity and distribution. *RNA*, *23*(7), 995–1011.

Memczak, S., Jens, M., Elefsinioti, A., Torti, F., Krueger, J., Rybak, A., et al. (2013). Circular RNAs are a large class of animal RNAs with regulatory potency. *Nature*, *495*(7441), 333–338.

Miyawaki, A., Llopis, J., Heim, R., McCaffery, J. M., Adams, J. A., Ikura, M., et al. (1997). Fluorescent indicators for Ca2+ based on green fluorescent proteins and calmodulin. *Nature*, *388*(6645), 882–887.

Nakayama, S., Luo, Y., Zhou, J., Dayie, T. K., & Sintim, H. O. (2012). Nanomolar fluorescent detection of c-di-GMP using a modular aptamer strategy. *Chemical Communications (Cambridge, England)*, *48*(72), 9059–9061.

Paige, J. S., Nguyen-Duc, T., Song, W., & Jaffrey, S. R. (2012). Fluorescence imaging of cellular metabolites with RNA. *Science*, *335*(6073), 1194.

Paige, J. S., Wu, K. Y., & Jaffrey, S. R. (2011). RNA mimics of green fluorescent protein. *Science*, *333*(6042), 642–646.

Paul, C. P., Good, P. D., Li, S. X., Kleihauer, A., Rossi, J. J., & Engelke, D. R. (2003). Localized expression of small RNA inhibitors in human cells. *Molecular Therapy*, *7*(2), 237–247.

Robertson, M. P., & Ellington, A. D. (1999). In vitro selection of an allosteric ribozyme that transduces analytes to amplicons. *Nature Biotechnology*, *17*(1), 62–66.

Sekella, P. T., Rueda, D., & Walter, N. G. (2002). A biosensor for theophylline based on fluorescence detection of ligand-induced hammerhead ribozyme cleavage. *RNA*, *8*(10), 1242–1252.

Shaner, N. C., Campbell, R. E., Steinbach, P. A., Giepmans, B. N., Palmer, A. E., & Tsien, R. Y. (2004). Improved monomeric red, orange and yellow fluorescent proteins derived from Discosoma sp. red fluorescent protein. *Nature Biotechnology*, *22*(12), 1567–1572.

Song, W., Filonov, G. S., Kim, H., Hirsch, M., Li, X., Moon, J. D., et al. (2017). Imaging RNA polymerase III transcription dynamics using a photostable RNA-fluorophore complex. *Nature Chemical Biology*. https://doi.org/10.1038/nchembio.2477.

Song, W., Strack, R., & Jaffrey, S. R. (2013). Imaging bacterial protein expression using genetically encoded RNA sensors. *Nature Methods, 10*, 873–875.

Song, W., Strack, R. L., Svensen, N., & Jaffrey, S. R. (2014). Plug-and-play fluorophores extend the spectral properties of Spinach. *Journal of the American Chemical Society, 136*(4), 1198–1201.

Soukup, G. A., & Breaker, R. R. (1999). Design of allosteric hammerhead ribozymes activated by ligand-induced structure stabilization. *Structure*, 7(7), 783–791.

Steen, K. A., Malhotra, A., & Weeks, K. M. (2010). Selective 2′-hydroxyl acylation analyzed by protection from exoribonuclease. *Journal of the American Chemical Society, 132*(29), 9940–9943.

Stoltenburg, R., Reinemann, C., & Strehlitz, B. (2007). SELEX—A (r)evolutionary method to generate high-affinity nucleic acid ligands. *Biomolecular Engineering, 24*(4), 381–403.

Strack, R. L., Disney, M. D., & Jaffrey, S. R. (2013). A superfolding Spinach2 reveals the dynamic nature of trinucleotide repeat RNA. *Nature Methods, 10*, 1219–1224.

Tang, J., & Breaker, R. R. (1997). Rational design of allosteric ribozymes. *Chemistry & Biology, 4*, 453–459.

Terpe, K. (2006). Overview of bacterial expression systems for heterologous protein production: From molecular and biochemical fundamentals to commercial systems. *Applied Microbiology and Biotechnology*, 72(2), 211–222.

Tuerk, C., & Gold, L. (1990). Systematic evolution of ligands by exponential enrichment: RNA ligands to bacteriophage T4 DNA polymerase. *Science, 249*(4968), 505–510.

Vogel, C., & Marcotte, E. M. (2012). Insights into the regulation of protein abundance from proteomic and transcriptomic analyses. *Nature Reviews. Genetics, 13*(4), 227–232.

Ward, P. S., Patel, J., Wise, D. R., Abdel-Wahab, O., Bennett, B. D., Coller, H. A., et al. (2010). The common feature of leukemia-associated IDH1 and IDH2 mutations is a neomorphic enzyme activity converting alpha-ketoglutarate to 2-hydroxyglutarate. *Cancer Cell, 17*(3), 225–234.

Warner, K. D., Chen, M. C., Song, W., Strack, R. L., Thorn, A., Jaffrey, S. R., et al. (2014). Structural basis for activity of highly efficient RNA mimics of green fluorescent protein. *Nature Structural and Molecular Biology, 21*(8), 658–663.

Winkler, W., Nahvi, A., & Breaker, R. R. (2012). Thiamine derivatives bind messenger RNAs directly to regulate bacterial gene expression. *Nature, 419*(6910), 952–956.

You, M., Litke, J. L., & Jaffrey, S. R. (2015). Imaging metabolite dynamics in living cells using a Spinach-based riboswitch. *Proceedings of the National Academy of Sciences of the United States of America, 112*(21), E2756–2765.

CHAPTER TEN

Phosphorylation of the Amino Terminus of the Dopamine Transporter: Regulatory Mechanisms and Implications for Amphetamine Action

Caline S. Karam*^,†^, Jonathan A. Javitch*^,†,1^

*College of Physicians & Surgeons, Columbia University, New York, NY, United States
†Division of Molecular Therapeutics, New York State Psychiatric Institute, New York, NY, United States
[1]Corresponding author: e-mail address: javitch@nyspi.columbia.edu

Dedication. Training with Solomon Snyder was extremely inspiring but also profoundly humbling. Sol's interests and knowledge were protean, and his influence has been and continues to be wide ranging and profound, touching on a vast range of scientific topics and discoveries. Sol introduced me to the world of transporters as a graduate student in his lab nearly 40 years ago, and I have studied them ever since. In contrast, after a number of key discoveries, Sol moved on. Nonetheless, a Pubmed search of Sol Snyder and amphetamine leads to 36 hits, whereas a similar search for me, despite my focus in the area reveals just 31! Humbling indeed how great an influence Sol could have on an area in such a short period of time. I just reread Sol's 1972 paper in the *Archives of General Psychiatry* in which he inferred, based on the lack of substantial stereospecificity, that amphetamine induced psychosis through its effects on dopamine and not norepinephrine (Snyder, 1972). This in part led to his discovery of the dopamine receptor as the target for antipsychotic actions (Creese, Burt, & Snyder, 1976), something the field studies to this day. Truly humbling but always inspiring. Sol's influence on all of those he trained is eternal and without measure, and Caline, a scientific granddaughter he has not yet met, and I dedicate this review to him and congratulate him on his profound achievements, both as a scientist, a mentor, a friend, and a true mensch.

Contents

Advances in Pharmacology, Volume 82
ISSN 1054-3589
https://doi.org/10.1016/bs.apha.2017.09.002

Abstract

Amphetamines (AMPHs) are potent psychostimulants that are widely used and abused, with profound medical and societal impact. Their actions at dopaminergic neurons are thought to mediate their therapeutic efficacy as well as their liability for abuse and dependence. AMPHs target the dopamine transporter (DAT), the plasmalemmal membrane protein that mediates the inactivation of released dopamine (DA) through its reuptake. AMPHs act as substrates for DAT and are known to cause mobilization of dopamine (DA) to the cell exterior via DAT-mediated reverse transport (efflux). It has become increasingly evident that the mechanisms that regulate AMPH-induced DA efflux are distinct from those that regulate DA uptake. Central to these mechanisms is the phosphorylation of the DAT amino (N)-terminus, which has been repeatedly demonstrated to facilitate DAT-mediated DA efflux, without impacting other aspects of DAT physiology. This review aims to summarize the current status of knowledge regarding DAT N-terminal phosphorylation and its regulation by protein modulators and the membrane microenvironment. A better understanding of these mechanisms may lead to the identification of novel therapeutic approaches that interfere selectively with the pharmacological effects of AMPHs without altering the physiological function of DAT.

ABBREVIATIONS

AMPH amphetamine
CaMKIIα Ca^{2+}/calmodulin-dependent protein kinase alpha
CaMKIINtide CaMKIIα inhibitor peptide
Cav voltage-gated Ca^{2+} channel
CK2 casein kinase
D_2R dopamine D2 receptor
DA dopamine
DAT dopamine transporter
Flot1 Flotillin-1
MbC methyl-β-cyclodextrin
N-terminus amino terminus
OA okadaic acid

PIP2	phosphatidylinositol 4,5-bisphosphate
PKC	protein kinase C
PMA	phorbol 12-myristate, 13-acetate
PP	protein phosphatase
SERT	serotonin transporter
SLC	solute carrier
STX1	syntaxin
VMAT	vesicular monoamine transporter

1. INTRODUCTION

Prescribed and illicit amphetamines (AMPHs) are widely misused and abused with up to 56 million users worldwide (Vearrier, Greenberg, Miller, Okaneku, & Haggerty, 2012), often leading to aggression and psychosis (Dawe, Davis, Lapworth, & McKetin, 2009), cardiovascular damage, malnutrition, and a host of other medical and psychosocial complications (Heal, Smith, Gosden, & Nutt, 2013). AMPH and its derivatives are also in wide clinical use for the treatment of attention-deficit disorders (Sembower, Ertischek, Buchholtz, Dasgupta, & Schnoll, 2013; Sweeney, Sembower, Ertischek, Shiffman, & Schnoll, 2013). The action of these drugs at dopaminergic neurons is thought to be responsible, in major part, for their therapeutic efficacy as well as their liability for abuse and dependence (Sembower et al., 2013; Sulzer, Sonders, Poulsen, & Galli, 2005; Sweeney et al., 2013). AMPHs target the dopamine transporter (DAT), the plasmalemmal membrane protein that mediates the inactivation of released dopamine (DA) through its reuptake. AMPHs act as substrates for DAT; upon binding to the transporter they are transported into the neuron in a Na^+-dependent manner, eliciting an inward current (Sonders, Zhu, Zahniser, Kavanaugh, & Amara, 1997; Sulzer et al., 2005; Zaczek, Culp, & De Souza, 1991). Once inside neurons, they are transported by the vesicular monoamine transporter (VMAT) into vesicles, causing the release of vesicular DA into the cytoplasm and its mobilization to the cell exterior via DAT through reverse transport (efflux) (Eshleman, Henningsen, Neve, & Janowsky, 1994; Freyberg et al., 2016; Sulzer, 2011; Sulzer et al., 1995). This nonexocytic efflux of DA through DAT results in a dramatic increase of synaptic DA and is believed to play a major role in the psychostimulatory and rewarding properties of AMPHs (Eshleman et al., 1994; Sulzer, 2011; Sulzer et al., 1995).

DAT belongs to the solute carrier 6 (SLC6) family of Na^+/Cl^--dependent neurotransmitter transporters, which also includes the transporters for serotonin (SERT), norepinephrine, GABA, and glycine. DAT comprises 12 transmembrane segments, with cytoplasmic N-terminal and C-terminal domains oriented intracellularly (Amara & Kuhar, 1993; Chen & Reith, 2004; Penmatsa, Wang, & Gouaux, 2013; Torres, Carneiro, et al., 2003). \It primarily functions to regulate the strength and duration of the dopaminergic response by mediating the reuptake of DA from the synaptic cleft, thereby terminating neurotransmission. Accordingly, it plays a critical role in modulating the physiological functions of DA, which include motor control and arousal, as well as higher cognitive functions such as motivation and reward-seeking behavior (Iversen & Iversen, 2007).

Substrate translocation through DAT is driven by the electrochemical gradient generated by the plasma membrane Na^+/K^+ ATPase. It involves the sequential binding of Na^+, Cl^-, and DA, with the movement of Na^+ down its concentration gradient providing the energy necessary to transport DA against its concentration gradient (Krueger, 1990; Torres, Gainetdinov, & Caron, 2003). DAT is thought to function via an alternating access mechanism, whereby binding of substrate and ions triggers a regulated transition of the transporter from an "outward-facing" conformation, in which the substrate binding site is exposed to the extracellular space, to an "inward-facing" conformation, in which the substrate binding site is exposed to the intracellular milieu (Jardetzky, 1966; Loland, Norgaard-Nielsen, & Gether, 2003). It was thus proposed that AMPH-induced DA efflux through DAT occurs via a facilitated exchange mechanism, whereby the transport of AMPH into the cell via DAT increases the number of transporters in the inward-facing conformation, leading to the transport of DA out of the cell by exchange (Fischer & Cho, 1979). However, later studies challenged this model and suggested that AMPH-induced efflux is at least partially uncoupled from uptake function (Pifl & Singer, 1999; Scholze et al., 2002). In fact, it has been proposed that the releasing properties of AMPH may be related to its ability to elicit DAT-mediated inward currents. Consistent with such a model, studies have shown that DAT-mediated DA efflux is voltage sensitive, is influenced by intracellular ionic concentrations, and might involve a channel-like mode of the transporter (Kahlig et al., 2005; Khoshbouei, Wang, Lechleiter, Javitch, & Galli, 2003; Pifl & Singer, 1999; Sitte et al., 1998). AMPH treatment increases intracellular Na^+ and Ca^{2+} (Gnegy et al., 2004; Kantor et al., 2001) which in turn stimulate DA efflux in a concentration-dependent manner. Furthermore, studies over the last two decades have identified various mutations and modulators that differentially affect AMPH-induced DA efflux and DA uptake. Central to these mechanisms is the phosphorylation of the DAT N-terminus, which has been repeatedly demonstrated to promote DAT-mediated DA efflux, without affecting the uptake capacity of DAT, its trafficking, or oligomerization. This review aims to summarize the current status of knowledge regarding DAT N-terminal phosphorylation and its regulation by interacting partners and the membrane environment. A better understanding of these mechanisms may lead to the identification of novel therapeutic approaches that interfere selectively with the pharmacological effects of AMPHs without altering the physiological function of DAT.

2. A ROLE FOR DAT N-TERMINAL PHOSPHORYLATION IN DAT-MEDIATED DA EFFLUX

Analysis of the primary amino acid sequence of DAT (Kilty, Lorang, & Amara, 1991) reveals several putative phosphorylation sites for various kinases in the intracellular domains, and multiple kinases have been shown to regulate DAT function (Foster, Cervinski, Gorentla, & Vaughan, 2006; Foster & Vaughan, 2016; Ramamoorthy, Shippenberg, & Jayanthi, 2011). Early studies demonstrating the ability of DAT to undergo phosphorylation were performed using ^{32}P metabolic labeling in heterologous expression systems (Granas, Ferrer, Loland, Javitch, & Gether, 2003; Huff, Vaughan, Kuhar, & Uhl, 1997) as well as in rat and mouse striatal tissue (Foster, Pananusorn, & Vaughan, 2002; Vaughan, Huff, Uhl, & Kuhar, 1997). More recently, our group developed phosphospecific anti-DAT antibodies to probe the phosphorylation of individual serine resides in DAT in response to various stimuli (Karam, Sen, & Javitch, 2017). These studies showed that DAT phosphorylation is rapidly elevated by activation of protein kinase C (PKC) with phorbol 12-myristate, 13-acetate (PMA) (Huff et al., 1997; Karam et al., 2017; Vaughan et al., 1997), diacylglycerol analogs (Vaughan et al., 1997), or G_q activation by G protein-coupled receptor agonists (Granas et al., 2003). DAT phosphorylation was also shown to be strongly enhanced by treating cells with protein phosphatase inhibitors such as okadaic acid (OA), indicating that the transporter is subject to ongoing kinase activity even in the absence of exogenous kinase activators (Foster, Pananusorn, Cervinski, Holden, & Vaughan, 2003; Foster et al., 2002; Huff et al., 1997; Karam et al., 2017; Vaughan et al., 1997). Critically, treatment with psychostimulants such as AMPH and methamphetamine

(METH) stimulates an increase in DAT phosphorylation in both heterologously expressing cells and in rat brain tissue (Cervinski, Foster, & Vaughan, 2005; Karam et al., 2017). In contrast, the DAT blocker cocaine does not stimulate DAT phosphorylation, but it does prevent the phosphorylation increase induced by METH (Cervinski et al., 2005).

Enzymatic digestion of $^{32}PO_4$-labeled DAT followed by epitope-specific immunoprecipitation showed that most basal, PMA-, and OA-stimulated phosphorylation of DAT occurs at the distal N-terminus in rat striatal tissue (Foster et al., 2002). Consistent with these data, deletion of the first 22 N-terminal residues of DAT (Δ1–22-hDAT) was shown to dramatically decrease incorporation of ^{32}P in response to PKC activation in cultured cells, suggesting that transporter phosphorylation is almost entirely due to phosphorylation of the distal N-terminus, which includes five serine residues at positions 2, 4, 7, 12, and 13 (Granas et al., 2003). Surprisingly, however, truncation of the distal N-terminus (Δ1–22) does not affect surface localization or PKC-mediated internalization of DAT, as shown by surface biotinylation studies (Granas et al., 2003; Khoshbouei et al., 2004), nor does it impair DA reuptake or inhibitor binding in [^3H]tyramine and [^3H]dopamine uptake assays (Khoshbouei et al., 2004). The ability of the transporter to interact with itself and form oligomers in the plasma membrane is also unaffected, as shown by cysteine cross-linking analyses (Hastrup, Karlin, & Javitch, 2001; Hastrup, Sen, & Javitch, 2003). In marked contrast, deletion of the first 22 amino acids or simultaneous mutation of the five N-terminal serines to alanine (hDAT-StoA) dramatically inhibits AMPH-induced DA efflux in heterologous cells, as measured by superfusion of a population of cells or by amperometry combined with the patch-clamp technique in the whole-cell configuration. Mutation of these five serines instead to aspartate (hDAT-StoD), which mimics a constitutive phosphorylation state, preserves efflux (Khoshbouei et al., 2003).

Consistent with these findings, studies of a *Drosophila melanogaster* behavioral model have shown that DAT phosphorylation is also necessary for the stimulatory effects of AMPH in vivo (Pizzo et al., 2013). AMPH stimulates an increase in crawling velocity in *Drosophila* larvae in a DAT-dependent manner; null mutation in the *Drosophila DAT* (*dDAT*) gene inhibits this behavioral response. Expression of human DAT in a *dDAT* null mutant rescues the locomotor response to AMPH, demonstrating the ability of human DAT to substitute functionally for dDAT in the context of this behavioral model (Pizzo et al., 2013). Remarkably, expression of hDAT-StoA fails to rescue the AMPH-induced behavioral response, whereas expression of hDAT-StoD results in robust hyperlocomotion in response to AMPH (Pizzo et al., 2013), consistent with the finding in vitro that phosphorylation is required for AMPH-induced DA efflux (Khoshbouei et al., 2004). In contrast, expression of hDAT-StoA rescues the locomotor response to the psychostimulant methylphenidate (Ritalin®), a DA uptake blocker that does not induce efflux (Pizzo et al., 2013), consistent with the findings that inhibition of DAT phosphorylation does not impair DA reuptake function in vitro. Taken together, these data strongly support an essential and selective role for DAT phosphorylation in AMPH-induced DA efflux and associated behavior.

3. KINASES, PHOSPHATASES, AND SITES OF PHOSPHORYLATION IMPLICATED IN DAT-MEDIATED DA EFFLUX

3.1 Ca^{2+}/Calmodulin-Dependent Protein Kinase Alpha

One critical aspect of AMPH-induced DA efflux through DAT is its dependence on the intracellular Ca^{2+} stores. AMPH treatment increases intracellular Ca^{2+}, which stimulates DA efflux in a concentration-dependent manner (Gnegy et al., 2004; Kantor et al., 2001). Treatment with a Ca^{2+} chelator inhibits AMPH-induced voltage-sensitive currents through DAT, as well as AMPH-induced DA efflux in heterologous cells, and superfusion of rat striatal slices with the Ca^{2+} chelator BAPTA-AM also suppresses AMPH-induced efflux of endogenous DA, without affecting basal DA levels. Interestingly, although it is generally accepted that extracellular Ca^{2+} is not required for reverse transport, it was recently shown that AMPH-induced DAT-mediated currents can robustly activate the voltage-gated L-type Ca^{2+} channels Cav1.3 and Cav1.2 (Cameron, Solis, Ruchala, De Felice, & Eltit, 2015), suggesting that the increase in intracellular Ca^{2+} may be partially mediated by these channels. Consistent with such a model, the increase of intracellular Ca^{2+} in response to low concentrations (but not high concentrations) of AMPH can be inhibited by removal of Ca^{2+} from the extracellular milieu (Gnegy et al., 2004). Taken together, these data establish a fundamental role for Ca^{2+} in AMPH-induced signaling mechanisms, although the precise mechanisms by which AMPH treatment leads to an increase in its intracellular levels will require further investigation.

One cellular target for Ca^{2+} that is highly expressed in neurons is Ca^{2+}/calmodulin-dependent protein kinase alpha (CaMKIIα), which was identified in a yeast two-hybrid screen as a direct interacting partner of DAT via its carboxy (C)-terminus. This interaction was further confirmed by GST-pulldown in vitro and by coimmunoprecipitation in heterologous cells (Fog et al., 2006) and in mouse striatum (Steinkellner et al., 2012). Furthermore, DAT was shown to colocalize with CaMKIIα in midbrain dopaminergic neurons in culture (Fog et al., 2006). Activation of CaMKIIα stimulates DA efflux in heterologous cells and in dopaminergic neurons in culture, most likely through direct interaction with and phosphorylation of DAT, as addition of a synthetic DAT C-terminal peptide that can compete with binding for CaMKIIα inhibits efflux (Fog et al., 2006). In contrast, pharmacological inhibition of CaMKIIα was shown to blunt AMPH-induced DAT phosphorylation and DA efflux in heterologous cells, as well as dopaminergic neurons in culture, striatal slices, and in the striatum of living mice (Fog et al., 2006). Similarly, DAT-mediated efflux is significantly reduced in CaMKIIα knockout (KO) mice, mice that express a permanently self-inhibited CaMKIIα mutant, as well as in a mouse model of Angelman syndrome known to exhibit reduced CaMKIIα activity (Steinkellner et al., 2014, 2012).

Importantly, this observed role for CaMKIIα in AMPH-induced DA efflux also manifests at the level of whole-animal behavior, in several experimental models. CaMKIIα KO mice exhibit a significantly blunted locomotor response to AMPH, as well as a markedly reduced behavioral sensitization to the psychostimulant, suggesting a role for CaMKIIα in both acute and chronic responses to AMPH (Steinkellner et al., 2015, 2014, 2012). Furthermore, expression of a CaMKIIα inhibitory peptide (CaMKIINtide) (Chang, Mukherji, & Soderling, 1998) selectively in DA neurons of *Drosophila* larvae prevents AMPH-induced hyperlocomotion (Pizzo et al., 2014), as does inhibiting DAT phosphorylation by expressing hDAT-StoA (Pizzo et al., 2013), demonstrating that the role of CaMKIIα in AMPH-stimulated behaviors is mediated in DA neurons. Critically, pseudophosphorylation of the hDAT N-terminus by mutation of the five serines to aspartates (hDAT-StoD) leads to robust hyperlocomotion when coexpressed with CaMKNtide, bypassing the need for CaMKIIα activity in AMPH-induced behavior (Pizzo et al., 2014), thereby demonstrating that the role of CaMKIIα in AMPH-induced efflux and behavior is directly related to its role in DAT N-terminal phosphorylation.

Delineating the role of CaMKIIα in DA efflux is especially critical to better understand a possible regulation of efflux by endogenous factors independently of AMPH. Of note, stimulation of the DA D2 receptor (D_2R) has been shown to result in the elevation of intracellular Ca^{2+} concentration and activation of CaMKIIα, most likely through activation of phospholipase C β (PLCβ) and inositol triphosphate (IP_3) production (Morris & Scarlata, 1997; Nishi, Snyder, & Greengard, 1997; Takeuchi, Fukunaga, & Miyamoto, 2002), suggesting that D2 autoreceptors may modulate DA efflux. Consistent with such a model, it was recently shown that treatment with D_2R antagonists inhibits the AMPH-independent, anomalous DA efflux caused by the A559V mutation in hDAT (Bowton et al., 2010), which is associated with autism disorder and attention-deficit hyperactivity disorder (Bowton et al., 2014; Mazei-Robison, Couch, Shelton, Stein, & Blakely, 2005). Cells expressing hDAT-A559V also showed an increase in CaMKIIα activity compared to cells expressing wild-type hDAT, and the increase was reduced by treatment with the D_2R antagonists (Bowton et al., 2010). Given that the anomalous DA efflux was found to be dependent on phosphorylation of N-terminal serines, these findings point to a role for D_2R in regulating DA efflux in a CaMKIIα-dependent manner, although further investigation is needed to determine whether this effect is directly mediated through DAT phosphorylation. It must also be remembered that unlike heterologous cells loaded with DA that can efflux directly from the cytoplasm through DAT, in neurons DA is highly concentrated in synaptic vesicles and must be released from vesicles into the cytoplasm before it can efflux through DAT.

3.2 Protein Kinase C

PKC activators, such as PMA, stimulate N-terminal phosphorylation of DAT in cells in culture (Granas et al., 2003; Huff et al., 1997; Karam et al., 2017) and in rat striatum (Cowell, Kantor, Hewlett, Frey, & Gnegy, 2000; Foster et al., 2002; Granas et al., 2003), and treatment with PKC inhibitors attenuates OA-induced (Foster et al., 2002; Gorentla, Moritz, Foster, & Vaughan, 2009; Huff et al., 1997; Karam et al., 2017; Vaughan et al., 1997) and AMPH-induced DAT phosphorylation (Cervinski et al., 2005; Karam et al., 2017), suggesting a role for PKC in both basal and stimulant-induced DAT phosphorylation. Treatment with a PKC activator was also shown to elicit release of $^{3}[H]$dopamine from striatal synaptosomes that is cocaine-sensitive and independent of extracellular Ca^{2+} (Davis & Patrick, 1990). Furthermore, AMPH increases striatal particulate PKC activity (Giambalvo, 1992) in a manner dependent on intracellular Ca^{2+} (Giambalvo, 2003), implicating PKC as another target of Ca^{2+} signaling in response to AMPH. Furthermore, treatment with PKC inhibitors or down-regulation of PKC attenuates AMPH-induced DAT-mediated DA efflux in cells and in rat striatal tissue (Cowell et al., 2000; Kantor & Gnegy, 1998; Kantor et al., 2001; Zestos, Mikelman, Kennedy, & Gnegy, 2016), as well as AMPH-induced hyperlocomotion (Browman et al., 1998; Carpenter et al., 2017; Zestos et al., 2016) and AMPH-self administration (Carpenter et al., 2017). Investigations using isoform-specific inhibitors have implicated PKCβ as the mediator of DAT-mediated AMPH-induced DA efflux and psychomotor behavior (Johnson, Guptaroy, Lund, Shamban, & Gnegy, 2005; Zestos et al., 2016). Consistent with these observations, PKCβ was also shown to associate in complex with DAT in rat striatal synaptosomal preparations and to colocalize with the transporter in mesencephalic neurons (Johnson et al., 2005; O'Malley, Park, Isom, & Gnegy, 2010).

In summary, there is compelling evidence for a role for both PKC and CaMKIIα in regulating AMPH-induced DA efflux. However, whether these roles are mediated through direct phosphorylation of DAT in vivo remains to be determined. The role of PKC is complicated by its regulation of DAT trafficking (Cervinski et al., 2005; Chen et al., 2009; Foster et al., 2006; Gabriel et al., 2013; Granas et al., 2003), which is in part mediated through DAT interactions with the lipid raft protein Flotillin-1 (Flot1, see below) (Cremona et al., 2011) and the membrane-associated GTPase Rin, which interacts with DAT in membrane microdomains (Navaroli et al., 2011). The two kinases may act in parallel, although the behavioral data from *Drosophila* showing complete inhibition of AMPH-induced hyperlocomotion by CaMKIINtide suggest a more complex interaction (Pizzo et al., 2014). A PKC-mediated mechanism should not be blocked unless CaMKIIα functions downstream of the actions of PKC. Thus, the precise role of PKC activation in DAT phosphorylation and its functional interaction with CaMKIIα will require further study (Fig. 1).

Other kinases, including protein kinase A (PKA), mitogen-activated protein kinase (MAPK) kinases (MEK1/2), and phosphatidylinositol 3-kinase (PI3K), have been shown to regulate the phosphorylation of the DAT N-terminus in vitro and/or in vivo (Batchelor & Schenk, 1998; Gorentla et al., 2009; Lin et al., 2003; Moritz et al., 2013; Page et al., 2004; Ramamoorthy et al., 2011; Vuorenpaa, Ammendrup-Johnsen, Jorgensen, & Gether, 2016). However, there is little evidence thus far to suggest that they play a selective role in AMPH-induced efflux in vivo, but rather have been shown to modulate DA uptake activity and/or DAT surface expression and trafficking.

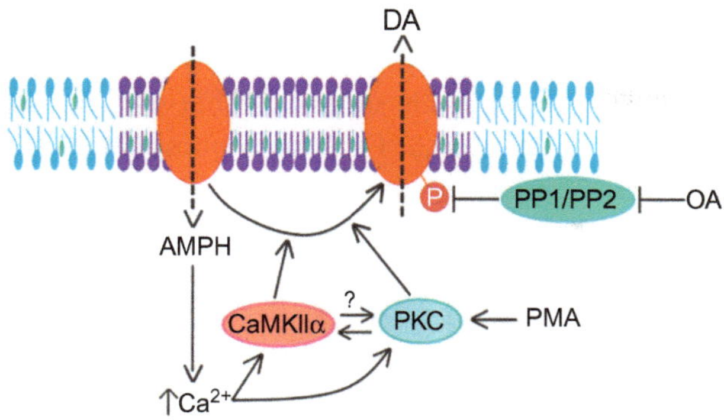

Fig. 1 Regulation of DAT phosphorylation. AMPH acts as a substrate for DAT (orange oval) and is transported into the neuron (dashed arrow pointing intracellularly), which leads to an increase in intracellular Ca^{2+} levels, an increase in CaMKIIα and PKC activity, and an increase in the levels of DAT phosphorylation, all of which have been demonstrated to facilitate AMPH-induced DAT-mediated DA efflux (dashed arrow pointing extracellularly). Activation of PKC by the phorbol ester PMA also increases DAT phosphorylation, as does inhibition of protein phosphatases by okadaic acid (OA). The mechanistic relationship between CaMKII and PKC, with respect to DAT phosphorylation, remains unclear (as indicated by the question mark). Localization of DAT to cholesterol-rich membrane microdomains (purple section of plasma membrane) facilitates its phosphorylation in response to AMPH, and thereby the consequent DA efflux and associated behaviors.

3.3 Phosphatases

As noted earlier, treatment with protein phosphatase inhibitors results in an increase in DAT phosphorylation in the absence of exogenous kinase activation, suggesting that dephosphorylation is another regulatory mechanism of DAT function (Fig. 1). DAT phosphorylation is significantly increased following treatment with OA and other inhibitors of protein phosphatase 1 (PP1) and protein phosphatase 2 (PP2) (Huff et al., 1997; Karam et al., 2017; Vaughan et al., 1997). OA dose–response and peptide inhibitor experiments further suggest a primary role for PP1 in mediating ^{32}P labeling (Foster et al., 2003; Gorentla et al., 2009; Vaughan et al., 1997). On the other hand, biochemical analyses have also identified the catalytic subunit of PP2A in complex with DAT (Bauman et al., 2000), suggesting that the transporter may be regulated by multiple phosphatases.

3.4 Serine Residues

As previously noted, the majority of basal, PMA-induced, and AMPH-induced DAT phosphorylation occurs at a cluster of five serine residues in the proximal N-terminus (S2, S4, S7, S12, and S13). Efforts to identify the specific residues that are phosphorylated have relied on metabolic phosphorylation of DAT with ^{32}P, peptide mapping using specific proteases, and, more recently, immunolabeling of DAT with phosphospecific antibodies. Deletion of the first 22 amino acids of DAT or the simultaneous mutation of the five N-terminal serine residues to alanine eliminates the incorporation of ^{32}P in response to PKC activation (Granas et al., 2003). Mutation of serines at positions 7, 12, and 13 was found to reduce phosphorylation of DAT by PKC, MEK1/2, and PI3K (Lin et al., 2003). In another study, a recombinant rat DAT N-terminal peptide was shown to be phosphorylated in vitro by PKA at S7, CaMKIIα at S13, and at multiple sites (S4, S7, and S13) by PKC (Moritz et al., 2013), while mass spectrometry pointed to S7 as a site for OA-induced phosphorylation of heterologously expressed hDAT (Moritz et al., 2013). Studies with two distinct phosphospecific antibodies that recognize DAT when phosphorylated at either S7 or S12 show that treatment of cells with either AMPH or OA can promote DAT phosphorylation at both these residues, in a PKC- and CaMKIIα-dependent manner (Karam et al., 2017). Consistent with these data, functional analyses of the efflux-deficient hDAT-StoA mutant show that single mutation to aspartate of the alanines at positions 7 and 12, but not at positions 2, 4, and 13, restores a substantial fraction of AMPH-induced DA efflux observed with aspartates at all five positions (hDAT-StoD) (~30% and 45%, respectively) (Fog et al., 2006; Khoshbouei et al., 2004).

4. REGULATION OF DAT-MEDIATED DA EFFLUX BY THE MEMBRANE MICROENVIRONMENT

Evidence has emerged for a critical role of the localization of DAT in the plasma membrane and the surrounding microenvironment in regulating DAT function, and specifically DAT phosphorylation and DAT-mediated DA efflux. Treatment with disruptors of lipid rafts such as nystatin, flipin, or methyl-β-cyclodextrin (MbC) leads to loss of DAT from cholesterol-rich regions in the plasma membrane (Cremona et al., 2011; Foster, Adkins, Lever, & Vaughan, 2008). Treatment with nystatin inhibits AMPH-induced DA efflux, without impairing DAT-mediated DA uptake in heterologous cells (Cremona et al., 2011). In contrast, treatment with MbC has been shown to inhibit transport by DAT and SERT (Adkins et al., 2007; Foster et al., 2008; Magnani, Tate, Wynne, Williams, & Haase, 2004), but this may be reconciled by the different mechanisms by which these drugs disrupt lipid rafts. MbC acts by extracting cholesterol from cell membranes (Ilangumaran & Hoessli, 1998), whereas nystatin and filipin directly insert into the membrane, bind to free cholesterol, and physically disrupt rafts, while maintaining tightly bound cholesterol within the membrane (Coutinho & Prieto, 1995). Given the findings with nystatin (Cremona et al., 2011) and those with filipin (Foster et al., 2008), the effect of MbC likely relates to the removal of cholesterol tightly bound to DAT (Penmatsa et al., 2013), as this could directly impact DAT's ability to undergo the conformational changes associated with transport (Hong & Amara, 2010; Jones, Zhen, & Reith, 2012; North & Fleischer, 1983; Scanlon, Williams, & Schloss, 2001), in addition to the localization of DAT to rafts.

4.1 Flotillin-1

Consistent with a role for raft localization in the regulation of DAT function, we recently showed that the lipid raft-associated protein Flot1 is required to maintain the localization of DAT in cholesterol-rich regions in the plasma membrane and plays a role in regulating PKC-mediated DAT endocytosis, as well as AMPH-induced DA efflux (Cremona et al., 2011). Like nystatin treatment, knockdown of Flot1 also leads to loss of DAT from rafts. This is accompanied by a decrease in PKC-triggered internalization of DAT, although basal levels of DAT at the plasma membrane are unaffected, suggesting that Flot1 is not required for trafficking of DAT to the plasma membrane. Consistent with this, depletion of Flot1 has no effect on the uptake capacity of DAT. In contrast, depletion of Flot1 dramatically inhibits AMPH-induced DA efflux in primary cultures of DA neurons (Cremona et al., 2011). Furthermore, genetic ablation of Flot1, or knockdown of its expression selectively in DA neurons of *Drosophila* larvae, inhibits hyperlocomotion induced by AMPH but not that induced by methylphenidate (Pizzo et al., 2013). Therefore, like DAT phosphorylation, the localization of DAT to lipid rafts is required for its efflux capacity, but not for its ability to transport DA.

The role of raft localization in DA efflux is likely independent of its role in DAT endocytosis, given that inhibition of internalization would leave more DAT at the surface available to efflux DA, resulting in increased AMPH-induced amperometric currents in DA neuronal cultures, as well as enhanced AMPH-induced behavior in flies, whereas we see inhibition of both these measures. Since lipid rafts can scaffold interactions underlying key signaling events that are mediated by kinases, including CaMKIIα

(Jayanthi, Samuvel, & Ramamoorthy, 2004; Suzuki, Du, Tian, Zhang, & Endo, 2008; Tsui, Inagaki, & Schulman, 2005; Weerth, Holtzclaw, & Russell, 2007) and PKC (Evans, Murray, Leslie, & Falke, 2006; Niggli, Meszaros, Oppliger, & Tornay, 2004), it is tempting to speculate that the distribution of DAT within the plasma membrane may regulate its phosphorylation and thereby AMPH-induced DA efflux and behavior. Consistent with such a model, basal and PMA-induced DAT phosphorylation levels are higher in cholesterol-rich fractions of the membrane (Foster et al., 2008), and treatment with nystatin inhibits PMA-induced phosphorylation of DAT at S7 (Karam et al., 2017). Critically, expression of hDAT-StoD in fly DA neurons bypasses the need for Flot1 in AMPH-induced hyperlocomotion (Pizzo et al., 2013), just as it bypasses the requirement for CaMKIIα (Pizzo et al., 2014). This observation that pseudophosphorylation of DAT is able to rescue the AMPH response that is lost despite the mislocalization of DAT away from lipid rafts supports the hypothesis that the role of Flot1 in efflux is to localize DAT to lipid rafts so it can be phosphorylated. These data provide a direct link between the localization of DAT to lipid rafts, its N-terminal phosphorylation, and the consequent behavioral response to AMPH. Furthermore, DAT phosphorylation has been shown to influence palmitoylation of DAT on Cys580, with increased phosphorylation leading to reduced palmitoylation, and vice versa (Moritz et al., 2015; Rastedt, Vaughan, & Foster, 2017). Lipid modification of proteins is thought to drive raft localization (Levental, Lingwood, Grzybek, Coskun, & Simons, 2010; Resh, 2006), suggesting a complex interplay between posttranslational modifications at the termini of DAT, although the mechanisms underlying the concerted regulation of these events remain unclear.

4.2 Phosphatidylinositol 4,5-Bisphosphate

A potential mechanism connecting membrane microdomain localization to DA efflux may relate to DAT N-terminal interactions with charged lipids. Molecular dynamics simulations have revealed the DAT N-terminus to be a highly dynamic domain that engages with lipid membranes through electrostatic interactions between charged residues in the N-terminus and the lipids phosphatidylinositol 4,5-bisphosphate (PIP2) (Khelashvili et al., 2015). PIP2 lipids are strongly anionic and represent a small fraction of the phospholipid composition of the inner leaflets of the plasma membrane (Balla, 2013; McLaughlin, Wang, Gambhir, & Murray, 2002). Yet, they regulate many cellular processes including transmembrane ion fluxes (Gamper & Shapiro, 2007; Hilgemann & Ball, 1996), by affecting the function and organization of various membrane proteins (Balla, 2013; McLaughlin et al., 2002; Suh & Hille, 2008). Ion fluxes have also been observed in neurotransmitter: sodium symporters and are required for AMPH-induced substrate efflux (Khoshbouei et al., 2003; Pifl & Singer, 1999; Sitte et al., 1998).

Association of PIP2 lipids with DAT was established by immunoprecipitation from heterologous cells expressing hDAT and from mouse striatal tissues, as well as by pulldown with a GST-fused hDAT N-terminal construct comprising the first 64 amino acids (Hamilton et al., 2014). Functional analyses further showed that PIP2 depletion or sequestration inhibits AMPH-induced DA efflux without affecting DAT-mediated DA reuptake (Hamilton et al., 2014), similar to its effects on AMPH-induced efflux through SERT (Buchmayer et al., 2013). Consistent with these findings, charge-neutralizing substitutions of lysines at positions 3 and 5 in the hDAT N-terminus to alanine or asparagine (K3A/K5A or K3N/K5N), which significantly inhibit its binding to PIP2 lipids, also blunt AMPH-dependent DA efflux without affecting DA reuptake in heterologous cells. Similarly, expression of hDAT-K3A/K5A in *Drosophila* dopaminergic neurons does not affect DA-dependent basal locomotor activity in adult flies, but rather diminishes AMPH-induced hyperlocomotion (Hamilton et al., 2014). Taken together, these studies support a role for direct electrostatic interactions between specific regions of the DAT N-terminus and PIP2 lipids in AMPH-induced DA efflux. It is possible that these interactions stabilize the N-terminus in a position that facilitates its phosphorylation. Alternatively, they might regulate dynamic intraprotein interactions between the N-terminus and other parts of hDAT to promote a conformation that is favorable for efflux. Curiously, molecular dynamics simulations of the hDAT N-terminus revealed that its phosphorylation disrupts its electrostatic interactions with the negatively charged membrane (Khelashvili et al., 2015), as does, deletion of the first 22 amino acids or the K3A/K5A mutation (Khelashvili et al., 2015). That such distinct manipulations with opposing effects on efflux (Fog et al., 2006; Hamilton et al., 2014) all decrease interactions with the membrane suggest that release of the N-terminus is not sufficient for efflux, and it is more likely that phosphorylation facilitates its interaction either with another part of hDAT, or possibly with another protein, to promote an efflux-competent conformation. Yet another possibility is that phosphorylation of the N-terminus acts as a "latch" that allows for communication between transporters to induce efflux, as proposed in the oligomer-based countertransport model (Seidel et al., 2005; Sitte & Freissmuth, 2010). Oligomerization of DAT has been recognized as an important prerequisite for exit from the endoplasmic reticulum, and DAT has been shown to exist as an oligomer in the plasma membrane (Farhan, Freissmuth, & Sitte, 2006; Hastrup et al., 2001; Kilic & Rudnick, 2000). Furthermore, studies have suggested that oligomerization might play a role in efflux, through a mechanism in which AMPH is taken up by one oligomeric moiety and DA is effluxed via another moiety within the same oligomer (Seidel et al., 2005; Sitte & Freissmuth, 2010). Based on this model, phosphorylation could act as the mechanism by which the two individual subunits communicate, although this remains speculative and has not been tested experimentally.

4.3 Syntaxin

The neuronal soluble N-ethylmaleimide-sensitive factor attachment receptor (SNARE) protein syntaxin 1A (STX1A) plays a central role in vesicular fusion (Han, Pluhackova, & Bockmann, 2017) and is also known to regulate the function of various neurotransmitter transporters, including SERT and NET (Dipace, Sung, Binda, Blakely, & Galli, 2007; Quick, 2002a, 2002b, 2003, 2006). STX1A was identified in a yeast two-hybrid screen as an interacting partner of DAT (Lee, Kim, Kim, & Lee, 2004) and was later shown to coimmunoprecipitate with DAT from heterologous cells and mouse striatal synaptosomes via direct association with the DAT N-terminal tail (Binda et al., 2008; Carvelli, Blakely, & DeFelice, 2008; Cervinski, Foster, & Vaughan, 2010; Lee et al., 2004). This interaction is potentiated by AMPH treatment, both in cultured cells and in mouse striatal synaptosomes, in a manner dependent on CaMKIIα activity, pointing to a possible link between the DAT/STX1 interaction and AMPH-induced DAT phosphorylation. Consistent with this, treatment of rat striatal tissue with the STX1 protease Botulinum Neurotoxin C (BoNT/C) blunts DAT phosphorylation (Cervinski et al., 2010). Furthermore, perfusion of exogenous STX1A into heterologous cells, as well as DA neurons in culture, enhances AMPH-induced DA efflux, and this response is also dependent on CaMKIIα activity. These findings suggest that AMPH activation of CaMKIIα supports DAT/STX1A association, resulting in a mode of DAT that is more efflux competent.

A recent report described the identification and characterization of two independent autism-associated single nucleotide variations in the genes coding for DAT and STX1 (Cartier et al., 2015). Mechanistic examination showed that the functional effects of the two mutations converged to inhibit AMPH-induced DA efflux in heterologous cells, as well as AMPH-mediated hyperlocomotion in *Drosophila*, possibly by inhibiting the DAT/STX1 interaction. Interestingly, the STX1 variant exhibits decreased casein kinase (CK2)-mediated phosphorylation at S14 (Cartier et al., 2015), a modification known to regulate the interaction of STX1 with other proteins (Foletti, Lin, Finley, & Scheller, 2000; Hirling & Scheller, 1996; Khelashvili, Galli, & Weinstein, 2012). Indeed, mutation to alanine of this residue significantly decreases DAT/STX1 interaction, as does inhibition of CK2 activity. Consistent with this, CK2 inhibition also blunts AMPH-induced efflux without affecting DA reuptake in mouse striatal slices, and expression of a dominant-negative CK2 in DA neurons of flies also inhibits AMPH-induced hyperlocomotion (Cartier et al., 2015). Despite these advances, it remains unclear whether STX1 enhances efflux in vivo. The role of STX1 is further complicated by its effect on DAT surface levels; BoNT/C-mediated inhibition of STX1 leads to decreased levels of DAT at the plasma membrane, and thus lower levels of DAT-mediated uptake (Cervinski et al., 2010). Still, this and other recent discoveries of specific mutations in hDAT that affect DA efflux in particular and are linked to various neuropsychiatric disorders underscore the significance of the mechanisms that regulate efflux, and their potential relevance to disease beyond the response to psychostimulants (Hamilton et al., 2013; Hansen et al., 2014; Mazei-Robison et al., 2008; Mergy et al., 2014; Ng et al., 2014).

5. ACUTE ACTION OF AMPH AT THE VMAT

While DAT clearly mediates efflux of cytoplasmic DA across the plasma membrane, how AMPHs release DA from vesicles into the cytoplasm remains controversial. DA is synthesized in the cytosol and concentrated in synaptic vesicles by VMAT, which functions by exporting two H^+ from the vesicle lumen for each cationic monoamine substrate it imports (Knoth, Zallakian, & Njus, 1981). This substrate antiport mechanism is driven by a vesicular pH gradient generated by the vacuolar H^+-ATPase (Edwards, 2007), which also promotes the retention of dopamine in vesicles through its protonation (Maron, Stern, Kanner, & Schuldiner, 1983).

Given VMAT's central role in maintaining DA stores, it follows that its function is essential for the actions of all DA-dependent psychostimulants. However, mechanisms by which AMPH acts directly at VMAT to redistribute DA from vesicles into the cytoplasm are not well defined. Indeed, studies in rodents have shown that the pharmacological inhibition of VMAT prior to treatment with AMPHs blunts the behavioral responses to these drugs (Harrod, Dwoskin, Crooks, Klebaur, & Bardo, 2001; Meyer et al., 2011; Miller et al., 2001; Neugebauer et al., 2007; Wilmouth, Zheng, Crooks, Dwoskin, & Bardo, 2013). These studies, however, were hindered by the fact that early VMAT inhibitors, primarily tetrabenazine, also target DAT (Meyer et al., 2011). This was addressed with the recent development of a novel, more selective VMAT inhibitor, (+)-CYY477, which, when administered $\leq$5 min preceding psychostimulant treatments, completely blocked locomotor and self-administration behaviors stimulated by AMPHs, without affecting those induced by cocaine (Freyberg et al., 2016). These data suggested that, under conditions where DA stores are still available to elicit a behavioral response to a DAT uptake blocker, VMAT function is required for the acute actions of AMPHs to release DA from intraluminal stores prior to its DAT-mediated efflux into the synaptic space.

In an effort to delineate the molecular mechanisms underlying the actions of AMPH at VMAT leading up to the release of DA from the vesicles, we monitored the dynamics of vesicular cargo with a fluorescent false neurotransmitter, as well as real-time changes in synaptic vesicle pH with a genetically encoded pH biosensor in an ex vivo *Drosophila* brain preparation, and showed that AMPH treatment diminishes the vesicular pH gradient and redistributes vesicular contents, in a manner dependent on both DAT and VMAT (Freyberg et al., 2016). Weak bases such as chloroquine can deacidify vesicles by diffusion of the neutral species across the vesicle membrane followed by protonation and trapping within the vesicle lumen (Maron et al., 1983; Sulzer et al., 1995), and it has been proposed that AMPH also acts through a weak base mechanism (Fleckenstein, Volz, Riddle, Gibb, & Hanson, 2007; Sulzer et al., 1995). However, genetic and pharmacological analyses using this optical model provided strong evidence that VMAT-mediated substrate-coupled H^+ antiport itself provides the critical in vivo mechanism for AMPH-induced vesicular deacidification. Notably, the DAT and VMAT substrate 1-methyl-4-phenylpyridinium (MPP^+), which has a fixed positive charge on its quaternary amine (Darchen, Scherman, Desnos, & Henry, 1988; Javitch, D'Amato, Strittmatter, & Snyder, 1985), also leads to vesicle deacidification, even though it is not a weak base. Moreover, chloroquine's actions are not blocked by inhibition of VMAT, whereas vesicle deacidification in response to physiological concentrations of the DAT and VMAT substrates AMPH, DA, and MPP^+ are blocked by selective VMAT inhibitors, consistent with transport by VMAT being the source of proton depletion and not a weak base effect (Freyberg et al., 2016).

Despite these advances, it remains unclear how AMPH transport into vesicles, and their concomitant deacidification, leads to redistribution of DA to the cytoplasm. One hypothesis is that in the presence of a diminished proton gradient, DA simply diffuses out of vesicles as a neutral species and also is less efficiently taken up without the driving force for VMAT transport. However, it has been shown that protonophores dramatically enhance the efflux of MPP^+ from synaptic vesicles (Moriyama, Amakatsu, & Futai, 1993), which suggests that a mechanism other than diffusion may be at play. Computational analyses show a striking similarity between the structure-based properties of the N-terminus of the human VMAT2 and that of hDAT (Khelashvili & Weinstein, 2015), suggesting a potential role of N-terminal phosphorylation of VMAT in modulating DA efflux from synaptic vesicles. Consistent with such a model, it was recently shown that phosphorylation of serines in the N-terminus of VMAT is essential for AMPH-induced DA efflux (Torres & Ruoho, 2014), suggesting the exciting possibility that VMAT might actively mediate the exit of monoamines from vesicles via reverse transport in a phosphorylation-dependent manner, as does DAT at the plasma membrane. However, this hypothesis has not been explored mechanistically nor validated in an in vivo setting.

6. CONCLUSION

The findings reviewed here point to a complex regulatory network that modulates dopamine transporter phosphorylation in a manner that influences the transporter's ability to efflux DA (Table 1). Why multiple transporters in the SLC6 family, including DAT and SERT (Sucic et al., 2010), and possibly VMAT in the SLC18 family, are regulated by N-terminal phosphorylation remains a mystery. Clearly this mode of regulation did not evolve in anticipation of psychostimulants such as AMPH that can coopt the pathway. Whether reverse transport is an alternative means of neurotransmitter release in the absence of psychostimulants but with activation of particular kinases is an intriguing question. One other speculative possibility is that this pathway serves as an "overflow valve" in pathological conditions when cytoplasmic transmitter might be high, particularly in the case of cytoplasmic DA, which can be quite toxic through its reactive species (Kita, Miyazaki, Asanuma, Takeshima, & Wagner, 2009; Segura-Aguilar

Table 1 Modulators of DAT Phosphorylation and AMPH-Induced DAT-Mediated DA Efflux

Modulator	Direct Interaction	Functional Impact
CaMKIIα	With DAT C-terminus based on yeast two-hybrid interaction	Phosphorylates DAT N-terminus in vitro Supports DA efflux in vitro, ex vivo, and in vivo Functions in DA neurons of flies to facilitate AMPH-induced behavior; this can be bypassed by pseudophosphorylation of the DAT N-terminus Supports AMPH-induced behaviors in rodents
PKC	No evidence	Phosphorylates DAT N-terminus in vitro Supports DA efflux in vitro and ex vivo Supports AMPH-induced behavior in rodents
PP1	No evidence	Mediates a major fraction of DAT dephosphorylation
PP2	In complex with DAT, as observed by coimmunoprecipitation	Extent of direct role is unclear
Flotillin-1	In complex with DAT, as observed by coimmunoprecipitation	Necessary for localization of DAT to lipid rafts, which in turn facilitates DAT phosphorylation Supports DA efflux in vitro and ex vivo Functions in DA neurons in flies to support AMPH-induced hyperlocomotion; this can be bypassed by pseudophosphorylation of the DAT N-terminus
PIP2	Electrostatic interaction via DAT N-terminus (K3/K5), as observed by coimmunoprecipitation and GST-pulldown	Interaction with DAT supports DA efflux in vitro and AMPH-induced hyperlocomotion in flies
Syntaxin	With the DAT N-terminus as observed by yeast two-hybrid assay and by coimmunoprecipitation from synaptosomes Interaction is potentiated by AMPH treatment in a CaMKII-dependent manner Interaction is enhanced by CK2-mediated phosphorylation	Interaction with DAT supports efflux in vitro and ex vivo Supports DAT phosphorylation in rat striatal tissue

et al., 2014). While these potential mechanisms are currently purely speculative, further study should reveal clues as to the function of this fascinating means of modulation.

CONFLICT OF INTEREST

The authors have no conflict of interest to declare.

ACKNOWLEDGMENTS

This work was supported by National Institutes of Health Grants R01 DA041510 (J.A.J., C.S.K.) and K05 DA022413 (J.A.J.).

REFERENCES

Adkins, E. M., Samuvel, D. J., Fog, J. U., Eriksen, J., Jayanthi, L. D., Vaegter, C. B., et al. (2007). Membrane mobility and microdomain association of the dopamine transporter studied with fluorescence correlation spectroscopy and fluorescence recovery after photobleaching. *Biochemistry, 46*(37), 10484–10497.

Amara, S. G., & Kuhar, M. J. (1993). Neurotransmitter transporters: Recent progress. *Annual Review of Neuroscience, 16*, 73–93. https://doi.org/10.1146/annurev.ne.16.030193.000445.

Balla, T. (2013). Phosphoinositides: Tiny lipids with giant impact on cell regulation. *Physiological Reviews, 93*(3), 1019–1137. https://doi.org/10.1152/physrev.00028.2012.

Batchelor, M., & Schenk, J. O. (1998). Protein kinase A activity may kinetically upregulate the striatal transporter for dopamine. *The Journal of Neuroscience, 18*(24), 10304–10309.

Bauman, A. L., Apparsundaram, S., Ramamoorthy, S., Wadzinski, B. E., Vaughan, R. A., & Blakely, R. D. (2000). Cocaine and antidepressant-sensitive biogenic amine transporters exist in regulated complexes with protein phosphatase 2A. *The Journal of Neuroscience, 20*(20), 7571–7578.

Binda, F., Dipace, C., Bowton, E., Robertson, S. D., Lute, B. J., Fog, J. U., et al. (2008). Syntaxin 1A interaction with the dopamine transporter promotes amphetamine-induced dopamine efflux. *Molecular Pharmacology, 74*(4), 1101–1108. https://doi.org/10.1124/mol.108.048447.

Bowton, E., Saunders, C., Erreger, K., Sakrikar, D., Matthies, H. J., Sen, N., et al. (2010). Dysregulation of dopamine transporters via dopamine D2 autoreceptors triggers anomalous dopamine efflux associated with attention-deficit hyperactivity disorder. *The Journal of Neuroscience, 30*(17), 6048–6057. https://doi.org/10.1523/JNEUROSCI.5094-09.2010.

Bowton, E., Saunders, C., Reddy, I. A., Campbell, N. G., Hamilton, P. J., Henry, L. K., et al. (2014). SLC6A3 coding variant Ala559Val found in two autism probands alters dopamine transporter function and trafficking. *Translational Psychiatry 4*, e464. https://doi.org/10.1038/tp.2014.90.

Browman, K. E., Kantor, L., Richardson, S., Badiani, A., Robinson, T. E., & Gnegy, M. E. (1998). Injection of the protein kinase C inhibitor Ro31-8220 into the nucleus accumbens attenuates the acute response to amphetamine: Tissue and behavioral studies. *Brain Research, 814*(1–2), 112–119.

Buchmayer, F., Schicker, K., Steinkellner, T., Geier, P., Stubiger, G., Hamilton, P. J., et al. (2013). Amphetamine actions at the serotonin transporter rely on the availability of phosphatidylinositol-4,5-bisphosphate. *Proceedings of the National Academy of Sciences of the United States of America, 110*(28), 11642–11647. https://doi.org/10.1073/pnas.1220552110.

Cameron, K. N., Solis, E., Jr., Ruchala, I., De Felice, L. J., & Eltit, J. M. (2015). Amphetamine activates calcium channels through dopamine transporter-mediated depolarization. *Cell Calcium*, *58*(5), 457–466. https://doi.org/10.1016/j.ceca.2015.06.013.

Carpenter, C., Zestos, A. G., Altshuler, R., Sorenson, R. J., Guptaroy, B., Showalter, H. D., et al. (2017). Direct and systemic administration of a CNS-permeant tamoxifen analog reduces amphetamine-induced dopamine release and reinforcing effects. *Neuropsychopharmacology*, *42*, 1940–1949. https://doi.org/10.1038/npp.2017.95.

Cartier, E., Hamilton, P. J., Belovich, A. N., Shekar, A., Campbell, N. G., Saunders, C., et al. (2015). Rare autism-associated variants implicate syntaxin 1 (STX1 R26Q) phosphorylation and the dopamine transporter (hDAT R51W) in dopamine neurotransmission and behaviors. *eBioMedicine*, *2*(2), 135–146. https://doi.org/10.1016/j.ebiom.2015.01.007.

Carvelli, L., Blakely, R. D., & DeFelice, L. J. (2008). Dopamine transporter/syntaxin 1A interactions regulate transporter channel activity and dopaminergic synaptic transmission. *Proceedings of the National Academy of Sciences of the United States of America*, *105*(37), 14192–14197. https://doi.org/10.1073/pnas.0802214105.

Cervinski, M. A., Foster, J. D., & Vaughan, R. A. (2005). Psychoactive substrates stimulate dopamine transporter phosphorylation and down-regulation by cocaine-sensitive and protein kinase C-dependent mechanisms. *The Journal of Biological Chemistry*, *280*(49), 40442–40449. https://doi.org/10.1074/jbc.M501969200.

Cervinski, M. A., Foster, J. D., & Vaughan, R. A. (2010). Syntaxin 1A regulates dopamine transporter activity, phosphorylation and surface expression. *Neuroscience*, *170*(2), 408–416. https://doi.org/10.1016/j.neuroscience.2010.07.025.

Chang, B. H., Mukherji, S., & Soderling, T. R. (1998). Characterization of a calmodulin kinase II inhibitor protein in brain. *Proceedings of the National Academy of Sciences of the United States of America*, *95*(18), 10890–10895.

Chen, R., Furman, C. A., Zhang, M., Kim, M. N., Gereau, R. W. T., Leitges, M., et al. (2009). Protein kinase Cbeta is a critical regulator of dopamine transporter trafficking and regulates the behavioral response to amphetamine in mice. *The Journal of Pharmacology and Experimental Therapeutics*, *328*(3), 912–920. https://doi.org/10.1124/jpet.108.147959.

Chen, N., & Reith, M. E. (2004). Interaction between dopamine and its transporter: Role of intracellular sodium ions and membrane potential. *Journal of Neurochemistry*, *89*(3), 750–765. https://doi.org/10.1111/j.1471-4159.2004.02409.x.

Coutinho, A., & Prieto, M. (1995). Self-association of the polyene antibiotic nystatin in dipalmitoylphosphatidylcholine vesicles: A time-resolved fluorescence study. *Biophysical Journal*, *69*(6), 2541–2557.

Cowell, R. M., Kantor, L., Hewlett, G. H., Frey, K. A., & Gnegy, M. E. (2000). Dopamine transporter antagonists block phorbol ester-induced dopamine release and dopamine transporter phosphorylation in striatal synaptosomes. *European Journal of Pharmacology*, *389*(1), 59–65.

Creese, I., Burt, D. R., & Snyder, S. H. (1976). Dopamine receptors and average clinical doses. *Science*, *194*(4264), 546. https://doi.org/10.1126/science.194.4264.546.

Cremona, M. L., Matthies, H. J., Pau, K., Bowton, E., Speed, N., Lute, B. J., et al. (2011). Flotillin-1 is essential for PKC-triggered endocytosis and membrane microdomain localization of DAT. *Nature Neuroscience*, *14*(4), 469–477. https://doi.org/10.1038/nn.2781.

Darchen, F., Scherman, D., Desnos, C., & Henry, J. P. (1988). Characteristics of the transport of the quaternary ammonium 1-methyl-4-phenylpyridinium by chromaffin granules. *Biochemical Pharmacology*, *37*(22), 4381–4387.

Davis, M. E., & Patrick, R. L. (1990). Diacylglycerol-induced stimulation of neurotransmitter release from rat brain striatal synaptosomes. *Journal of Neurochemistry*, *54*(2), 662–668.

Dawe, S., Davis, P., Lapworth, K., & McKetin, R. (2009). Mechanisms underlying aggressive and hostile behavior in amphetamine users. *Current Opinion in Psychiatry*, *22*(3), 269–273. https://doi.org/10.1097/YCO.0b013e32832a1dd4.

Dipace, C., Sung, U., Binda, F., Blakely, R. D., & Galli, A. (2007). Amphetamine induces a calcium/calmodulin-dependent protein kinase II-dependent reduction in norepinephrine transporter surface expression linked to changes in syntaxin 1A/transporter complexes. *Molecular Pharmacology*, *71*(1), 230–239. https://doi.org/10.1124/mol.106.026690.

Edwards, R. H. (2007). The neurotransmitter cycle and quantal size. *Neuron*, *55*(6), 835–858. https://doi.org/10.1016/j.neuron.2007.09.001.

Eshleman, A. J., Henningsen, R. A., Neve, K. A., & Janowsky, A. (1994). Release of dopamine via the human transporter. *Molecular Pharmacology*, *45*(2), 312–316.

Evans, J. H., Murray, D., Leslie, C. C., & Falke, J. J. (2006). Specific translocation of protein kinase C alpha to the plasma membrane requires both Ca2+ and PIP2 recognition by its C2 domain. *Molecular Biology of the Cell*, *17*(1), 56–66.

Farhan, H., Freissmuth, M., & Sitte, H. H. (2006). Oligomerization of neurotransmitter transporters: A ticket from the endoplasmic reticulum to the plasma membrane. *Handbook of Experimental Pharmacology*, *175*, 233–249.

Fischer, J. F., & Cho, A. K. (1979). Chemical release of dopamine from striatal homogenates: Evidence for an exchange diffusion model. *The Journal of Pharmacology and Experimental Therapeutics*, *208*(2), 203–209.

Fleckenstein, A. E., Volz, T. J., Riddle, E. L., Gibb, J. W., & Hanson, G. R. (2007). New insights into the mechanism of action of amphetamines. *Annual Review of Pharmacology and Toxicology*, *47*, 681–698. https://doi.org/10.1146/annurev.pharmtox.47.120505.105140.

Fog, J. U., Khoshbouei, H., Holy, M., Owens, W. A., Vaegter, C. B., Sen, N., et al. (2006). Calmodulin kinase II interacts with the dopamine transporter C terminus to regulate amphetamine-induced reverse transport. *Neuron*, *51*(4), 417–429. https://doi.org/10.1016/j.neuron.2006.06.028.

Foletti, D. L., Lin, R., Finley, M. A., & Scheller, R. H. (2000). Phosphorylated syntaxin 1 is localized to discrete domains along a subset of axons. *The Journal of Neuroscience*, *20*(12), 4535–4544.

Foster, J. D., Adkins, S. D., Lever, J. R., & Vaughan, R. A. (2008). Phorbol ester induced trafficking-independent regulation and enhanced phosphorylation of the dopamine transporter associated with membrane rafts and cholesterol. *Journal of Neurochemistry*, *105*(5), 1683–1699. https://doi.org/10.1111/j.1471-4159.2008.05262.x.

Foster, J. D., Cervinski, M. A., Gorentla, B. K., & Vaughan, R. A. (2006). Regulation of the dopamine transporter by phosphorylation. *Handbook of Experimental Pharmacology*, *175*, 197–214.

Foster, J. D., Pananusorn, B., Cervinski, M. A., Holden, H. E., & Vaughan, R. A. (2003). Dopamine transporters are dephosphorylated in striatal homogenates and in vitro by protein phosphatase 1. *Brain Research. Molecular Brain Research*, *110*(1), 100–108.

Foster, J. D., Pananusorn, B., & Vaughan, R. A. (2002). Dopamine transporters are phosphorylated on N-terminal serines in rat striatum. *The Journal of Biological Chemistry*, *277*(28), 25178–25186. https://doi.org/10.1074/jbc.M200294200.

Foster, J. D., & Vaughan, R. A. (2016). Phosphorylation mechanisms in dopamine transporter regulation. *Journal of Chemical Neuroanatomy*, *83–84*, 10–18. https://doi.org/10.1016/j.jchemneu.2016.10.004.

Freyberg, Z., Sonders, M. S., Aguilar, J. I., Hiranita, T., Karam, C. S., Flores, J., et al. (2016). Mechanisms of amphetamine action illuminated through optical monitoring of dopamine synaptic vesicles in Drosophila brain. *Nature Communications*, 7, 10652. https://doi.org/10.1038/ncomms10652.

Gabriel, L. R., Wu, S., Kearney, P., Bellve, K. D., Standley, C., Fogarty, K. E., et al. (2013). Dopamine transporter endocytic trafficking in striatal dopaminergic neurons: Differential dependence on dynamin and the actin cytoskeleton. *The Journal of Neuroscience*, *33*(45), 17836–17846. https://doi.org/10.1523/JNEUROSCI.3284-13.2013.

Gamper, N., & Shapiro, M. S. (2007). Regulation of ion transport proteins by membrane phosphoinositides. *Nature Reviews. Neuroscience*, *8*(12), 921–934. https://doi.org/10.1038/nrn2257.

Giambalvo, C. T. (1992). Protein kinase C and dopamine transport—1. Effects of amphetamine in vivo. *Neuropharmacology*, *31*(12), 1201–1210.

Giambalvo, C. T. (2003). Differential effects of amphetamine transport vs. dopamine reverse transport on particulate PKC activity in striatal synaptoneurosomes. *Synapse*, *49*(2), 125–133. https://doi.org/10.1002/syn.10223.

Gnegy, M. E., Khoshbouei, H., Berg, K. A., Javitch, J. A., Clarke, W. P., Zhang, M., et al. (2004). Intracellular Ca2+ regulates amphetamine-induced dopamine efflux and currents mediated by the human dopamine transporter. *Molecular Pharmacology*, *66*(1), 137–143. https://doi.org/10.1124/mol.66.1.137.

Gorentla, B. K., Moritz, A. E., Foster, J. D., & Vaughan, R. A. (2009). Proline-directed phosphorylation of the dopamine transporter N-terminal domain. *Biochemistry*, *48*(5), 1067–1076. https://doi.org/10.1021/bi801696n.

Granas, C., Ferrer, J., Loland, C. J., Javitch, J. A., & Gether, U. (2003). N-terminal truncation of the dopamine transporter abolishes phorbol ester- and substance P receptor-stimulated phosphorylation without impairing transporter internalization. *The Journal of Biological Chemistry*, *278*(7), 4990–5000. https://doi.org/10.1074/jbc.M205058200.

Hamilton, P. J., Belovich, A. N., Khelashvili, G., Saunders, C., Erreger, K., Javitch, J. A., et al. (2014). PIP2 regulates psychostimulant behaviors through its interaction with a membrane protein. *Nature Chemical Biology*, *10*(7), 582–589. https://doi.org/10.1038/nchembio.1545.

Hamilton, P. J., Campbell, N. G., Sharma, S., Erreger, K., Herborg Hansen, F., Saunders, C., et al. (2013). De novo mutation in the dopamine transporter gene associates dopamine dysfunction with autism spectrum disorder. *Molecular Psychiatry*, *18*(12), 1315–1323. https://doi.org/10.1038/mp.2013.102.

Han, J., Pluhackova, K., & Bockmann, R. A. (2017). The multifaceted role of SNARE proteins in membrane fusion. *Frontiers in Physiology*, *8*, 5. https://doi.org/10.3389/fphys.2017.00005.

Hansen, F. H., Skjorringe, T., Yasmeen, S., Arends, N. V., Sahai, M. A., Erreger, K., et al. (2014). Missense dopamine transporter mutations associate with adult parkinsonism and ADHD. *The Journal of Clinical Investigation*, *124*(7), 3107–3120. https://doi.org/10.1172/JCI73778.

Harrod, S. B., Dwoskin, L. P., Crooks, P. A., Klebaur, J. E., & Bardo, M. T. (2001). Lobeline attenuates d-methamphetamine self-administration in rats. *The Journal of Pharmacology and Experimental Therapeutics*, *298*(1), 172–179.

Hastrup, H., Karlin, A., & Javitch, J. A. (2001). Symmetrical dimer of the human dopamine transporter revealed by cross-linking Cys-306 at the extracellular end of the sixth transmembrane segment. *Proceedings of the National Academy of Sciences of the United States of America*, *98*(18), 10055–10060. https://doi.org/10.1073/pnas.181344298.

Hastrup, H., Sen, N., & Javitch, J. A. (2003). The human dopamine transporter forms a tetramer in the plasma membrane: Cross-linking of a cysteine in the fourth transmembrane segment is sensitive to cocaine analogs. *The Journal of Biological Chemistry*, *278*(46), 45045–45048. https://doi.org/10.1074/jbc.C300349200.

Heal, D. J., Smith, S. L., Gosden, J., & Nutt, D. J. (2013). Amphetamine, past and present—A pharmacological and clinical perspective. *Journal of Psychopharmacology*, *27*(6), 479–496. https://doi.org/10.1177/0269881113482532.

Hilgemann, D. W., & Ball, R. (1996). Regulation of cardiac Na+, Ca2+ exchange and KATP potassium channels by PIP2. *Science, 273*(5277), 956–959.

Hirling, H., & Scheller, R. H. (1996). Phosphorylation of synaptic vesicle proteins: Modulation of the alpha SNAP interaction with the core complex. *Proceedings of the National Academy of Sciences of the United States of America, 93*(21), 11945–11949.

Hong, W. C., & Amara, S. G. (2010). Membrane cholesterol modulates the outward facing conformation of the dopamine transporter and alters cocaine binding. *The Journal of Biological Chemistry, 285*(42), 32616–32626. https://doi.org/10.1074/jbc.M110.150565.

Huff, R. A., Vaughan, R. A., Kuhar, M. J., & Uhl, G. R. (1997). Phorbol esters increase dopamine transporter phosphorylation and decrease transport Vmax. *Journal of Neurochemistry, 68*(1), 225–232.

Ilangumaran, S., & Hoessli, D. C. (1998). Effects of cholesterol depletion by cyclodextrin on the sphingolipid microdomains of the plasma membrane. *The Biochemical Journal, 335*(Pt. 2), 433–440.

Iversen, S. D., & Iversen, L. L. (2007). Dopamine: 50 Years in perspective. *Trends in Neurosciences, 30*(5), 188–193. https://doi.org/10.1016/j.tins.2007.03.002.

Jardetzky, O. (1966). Simple allosteric model for membrane pumps. *Nature, 211*(5052), 969–970.

Javitch, J. A., D'Amato, R. J., Strittmatter, S. M., & Snyder, S. H. (1985). Parkinsonism-inducing neurotoxin, N-methyl-4-phenyl-1,2,3,6-tetrahydropyridine: Uptake of the metabolite N-methyl-4-phenylpyridine by dopamine neurons explains selective toxicity. *Proceedings of the National Academy of Sciences of the United States of America, 82*(7), 2173–2177.

Jayanthi, L. D., Samuvel, D. J., & Ramamoorthy, S. (2004). Regulated internalization and phosphorylation of the native norepinephrine transporter in response to phorbol esters. Evidence for localization in lipid rafts and lipid raft-mediated internalization. *The Journal of Biological Chemistry, 279*(18), 19315–19326. https://doi.org/10.1074/jbc.M311172200.

Johnson, L. A., Guptaroy, B., Lund, D., Shamban, S., & Gnegy, M. E. (2005). Regulation of amphetamine-stimulated dopamine efflux by protein kinase C beta. *The Journal of Biological Chemistry, 280*(12), 10914–10919. https://doi.org/10.1074/jbc.M413887200.

Jones, K. T., Zhen, J., & Reith, M. E. (2012). Importance of cholesterol in dopamine transporter function. *Journal of Neurochemistry, 123*(5), 700–715. https://doi.org/10.1111/jnc.12007.

Kahlig, K. M., Binda, F., Khoshbouei, H., Blakely, R. D., McMahon, D. G., Javitch, J. A., et al. (2005). Amphetamine induces dopamine efflux through a dopamine transporter channel. *Proceedings of the National Academy of Sciences of the United States of America, 102*(9), 3495–3500. https://doi.org/10.1073/pnas.0407737102.

Kantor, L., & Gnegy, M. E. (1998). Protein kinase C inhibitors block amphetamine-mediated dopamine release in rat striatal slices. *The Journal of Pharmacology and Experimental Therapeutics, 284*(2), 592–598.

Kantor, L., Hewlett, G. H., Park, Y. H., Richardson-Burns, S. M., Mellon, M. J., & Gnegy, M. E. (2001). Protein kinase C and intracellular calcium are required for amphetamine-mediated dopamine release via the norepinephrine transporter in undifferentiated PC12 cells. *The Journal of Pharmacology and Experimental Therapeutics, 297*(3), 1016–1024.

Karam, C. S., Sen, N., & Javitch, J. A. (2017). Phospho-specific antibodies targeting the amino terminus of the human dopamine transporter. *Journal of Chemical Neuroanatomy, 83-84*, 91–98. https://doi.org/10.1016/j.jchemneu.2017.05.003.

Khelashvili, G., Doktorova, M., Sahai, M. A., Johner, N., Shi, L., & Weinstein, H. (2015). Computational modeling of the N-terminus of the human dopamine transporter and its interaction with PIP2-containing membranes. *Proteins, 83*(5), 952–969. https://doi.org/10.1002/prot.24792.

Khelashvili, G., Galli, A., & Weinstein, H. (2012). Phosphatidylinositol 4,5-biphosphate (PIP(2)) lipids regulate the phosphorylation of syntaxin N-terminus by modulating both its position and local structure. *Biochemistry*, *51*(39), 7685–7698. https://doi.org/10.1021/bi300833z.

Khelashvili, G., & Weinstein, H. (2015). Functional mechanisms of neurotransmitter transporters regulated by lipid-protein interactions of their terminal loops. *Biochimica et Biophysica Acta*, *1848*(9), 1765–1774. https://doi.org/10.1016/j.bbamem.2015.03.025.

Khoshbouei, H., Sen, N., Guptaroy, B., Johnson, L., Lund, D., Gnegy, M. E., et al. (2004). N-terminal phosphorylation of the dopamine transporter is required for amphetamine-induced efflux. *PLoS Biology*, *2*(3), E78. https://doi.org/10.1371/journal.pbio.0020078.

Khoshbouei, H., Wang, H., Lechleiter, J. D., Javitch, J. A., & Galli, A. (2003). Amphetamine-induced dopamine efflux. A voltage-sensitive and intracellular Na+-dependent mechanism. *The Journal of Biological Chemistry*, *278*(14), 12070–12077. https://doi.org/10.1074/jbc.M212815200.

Kilic, F., & Rudnick, G. (2000). Oligomerization of serotonin transporter and its functional consequences. *Proceedings of the National Academy of Sciences of the United States of America*, *97*(7), 3106–3111. https://doi.org/10.1073/pnas.060408997.

Kilty, J. E., Lorang, D., & Amara, S. G. (1991). Cloning and expression of a cocaine-sensitive rat dopamine transporter. *Science*, *254*(5031), 578–579.

Kita, T., Miyazaki, I., Asanuma, M., Takeshima, M., & Wagner, G. C. (2009). Dopamine-induced behavioral changes and oxidative stress in methamphetamine-induced neurotoxicity. *International Review of Neurobiology*, *88*, 43–64. https://doi.org/10.1016/S0074-7742(09)88003-3.

Knoth, J., Zallakian, M., & Njus, D. (1981). Stoichiometry of H+-linked dopamine transport in chromaffin granule ghosts. *Biochemistry*, *20*(23), 6625–6629.

Krueger, B. K. (1990). Kinetics and block of dopamine uptake in synaptosomes from rat caudate nucleus. *Journal of Neurochemistry*, *55*(1), 260–267.

Lee, K. H., Kim, M. Y., Kim, D. H., & Lee, Y. S. (2004). Syntaxin 1A and receptor for activated C kinase interact with the N-terminal region of human dopamine transporter. *Neurochemical Research*, *29*(7), 1405–1409.

Levental, I., Lingwood, D., Grzybek, M., Coskun, U., & Simons, K. (2010). Palmitoylation regulates raft affinity for the majority of integral raft proteins. *Proceedings of the National Academy of Sciences of the United States of America*, *107*(51), 22050–22054. https://doi.org/10.1073/pnas.1016184107.

Lin, Z., Zhang, P. W., Zhu, X., Melgari, J. M., Huff, R., Spieldoch, R. L., et al. (2003). Phosphatidylinositol 3-kinase, protein kinase C, and MEK1/2 kinase regulation of dopamine transporters (DAT) require N-terminal DAT phosphoacceptor sites. *The Journal of Biological Chemistry*, *278*(22), 20162–20170. https://doi.org/10.1074/jbc.M209584200.

Loland, C. J., Norgaard-Nielsen, K., & Gether, U. (2003). Probing dopamine transporter structure and function by Zn2+-site engineering. *European Journal of Pharmacology*, *479*(1–3), 187–197.

Magnani, F., Tate, C. G., Wynne, S., Williams, C., & Haase, J. (2004). Partitioning of the serotonin transporter into lipid microdomains modulates transport of serotonin. *The Journal of Biological Chemistry*, *279*(37), 38770–38778. https://doi.org/10.1074/jbc.M400831200.

Maron, R., Stern, Y., Kanner, B. I., & Schuldiner, S. (1983). Functional asymmetry of the amine transporter from chromaffin granules. *The Journal of Biological Chemistry*, *258*(19), 11476–11481.

Mazei-Robison, M. S., Bowton, E., Holy, M., Schmudermaier, M., Freissmuth, M., Sitte, H. H., et al. (2008). Anomalous dopamine release associated with a human dopamine transporter coding variant. *The Journal of Neuroscience*, *28*(28), 7040–7046. https://doi.org/10.1523/JNEUROSCI.0473-08.2008.

Mazei-Robison, M. S., Couch, R. S., Shelton, R. C., Stein, M. A., & Blakely, R. D. (2005). Sequence variation in the human dopamine transporter gene in children with attention deficit hyperactivity disorder. *Neuropharmacology, 49*(6), 724–736. https://doi.org/10.1016/j.neuropharm.2005.08.003.

McLaughlin, S., Wang, J., Gambhir, A., & Murray, D. (2002). PIP(2) and proteins: Interactions, organization, and information flow. *Annual Review of Biophysics and Biomolecular Structure, 31*, 151–175. https://doi.org/10.1146/annurev.biophys.31.082901.134259.

Mergy, M. A., Gowrishankar, R., Gresch, P. J., Gantz, S. C., Williams, J., Davis, G. L., et al. (2014). The rare DAT coding variant Val559 perturbs DA neuron function, changes behavior, and alters in vivo responses to psychostimulants. *Proceedings of the National Academy of Sciences of the United States of America, 111*(44), E4779–4788. https://doi.org/10.1073/pnas.1417294111.

Meyer, A. C., Horton, D. B., Neugebauer, N. M., Wooters, T. E., Nickell, J. R., Dwoskin, L. P., et al. (2011). Tetrabenazine inhibition of monoamine uptake and methamphetamine behavioral effects: Locomotor activity, drug discrimination and self-administration. *Neuropharmacology, 61*(4), 849–856. https://doi.org/10.1016/j.neuropharm.2011.05.033.

Miller, D. K., Crooks, P. A., Teng, L., Witkin, J. M., Munzar, P., Goldberg, S. R., et al. (2001). Lobeline inhibits the neurochemical and behavioral effects of amphetamine. *The Journal of Pharmacology and Experimental Therapeutics, 296*(3), 1023–1034.

Moritz, A. E., Foster, J. D., Gorentla, B. K., Mazei-Robison, M. S., Yang, J. W., Sitte, H. H., et al. (2013). Phosphorylation of dopamine transporter serine 7 modulates cocaine analog binding. *The Journal of Biological Chemistry, 288*(1), 20–32. https://doi.org/10.1074/jbc.M112.407874.

Moritz, A. E., Rastedt, D. E., Stanislowski, D. J., Shetty, M., Smith, M. A., Vaughan, R. A., et al. (2015). Reciprocal phosphorylation and palmitoylation control dopamine transporter kinetics. *The Journal of Biological Chemistry, 290*(48), 29095–29105. https://doi.org/10.1074/jbc.M115.667055.

Moriyama, Y., Amakatsu, K., & Futai, M. (1993). Uptake of the neurotoxin, 4-methylphenylpyridinium, into chromaffin granules and synaptic vesicles: A proton gradient drives its uptake through monoamine transporter. *Archives of Biochemistry and Biophysics, 305*(2), 271–277. https://doi.org/10.1006/abbi.1993.1422.

Morris, A. J., & Scarlata, S. (1997). Regulation of effectors by G-protein alpha- and beta gamma-subunits. Recent insights from studies of the phospholipase c-beta isoenzymes. *Biochemical Pharmacology, 54*(4), 429–435.

Navaroli, D. M., Stevens, Z. H., Uzelac, Z., Gabriel, L., King, M. J., Lifshitz, L. M., et al. (2011). The plasma membrane-associated GTPase Rin interacts with the dopamine transporter and is required for protein kinase C-regulated dopamine transporter trafficking. *The Journal of Neuroscience, 31*(39), 13758–13770. https://doi.org/10.1523/JNEUROSCI.2649-11.2011.

Neugebauer, N. M., Harrod, S. B., Stairs, D. J., Crooks, P. A., Dwoskin, L. P., & Bardo, M. T. (2007). Lobelane decreases methamphetamine self-administration in rats. *European Journal of Pharmacology, 571*(1), 33–38. https://doi.org/10.1016/j.ejphar.2007.06.003.

Ng, J., Zhen, J., Meyer, E., Erreger, K., Li, Y., Kakar, N., et al. (2014). Dopamine transporter deficiency syndrome: Phenotypic spectrum from infancy to adulthood. *Brain, 137*(Pt. 4), 1107–1119. https://doi.org/10.1093/brain/awu022.

Niggli, V., Meszaros, A. V., Oppliger, C., & Tornay, S. (2004). Impact of cholesterol depletion on shape changes, actin reorganization, and signal transduction in neutrophil-like HL-60 cells. *Experimental Cell Research, 296*(2), 358–368.

Nishi, A., Snyder, G. L., & Greengard, P. (1997). Bidirectional regulation of DARPP-32 phosphorylation by dopamine. *The Journal of Neuroscience, 17*(21), 8147–8155.

North, P., & Fleischer, S. (1983). Alteration of synaptic membrane cholesterol/phospholipid ratio using a lipid transfer protein. Effect on gamma-aminobutyric acid uptake. *The Journal of Biological Chemistry, 258*(2), 1242–1253.

O'Malley, H. A., Park, Y., Isom, L. L., & Gnegy, M. E. (2010). PKCbeta co-localizes with the dopamine transporter in mesencephalic neurons. *Neuroscience Letters, 480*(1), 40–43. https://doi.org/10.1016/j.neulet.2010.05.091.

Page, G., Barc-Pain, S., Pontcharraud, R., Cante, A., Piriou, A., & Barrier, L. (2004). The up-regulation of the striatal dopamine transporter's activity by cAMP is PKA-, CaMK II- and phosphatase-dependent. *Neurochemistry International, 45*(5), 627–632. https://doi.org/10.1016/j.neuint.2004.04.002.

Penmatsa, A., Wang, K. H., & Gouaux, E. (2013). X-ray structure of dopamine transporter elucidates antidepressant mechanism. *Nature, 503*(7474), 85–90. https://doi.org/10.1038/nature12533.

Pifl, C., & Singer, E. A. (1999). Ion dependence of carrier-mediated release in dopamine or norepinephrine transporter-transfected cells questions the hypothesis of facilitated exchange diffusion. *Molecular Pharmacology, 56*(5), 1047–1054.

Pizzo, A. B., Karam, C. S., Zhang, Y., Ma, C. L., McCabe, B. D., & Javitch, J. A. (2014). Amphetamine-induced behavior requires CaMKII-dependent dopamine transporter phosphorylation. *Molecular Psychiatry, 19*(3), 279–281. https://doi.org/10.1038/mp.2013.29.

Pizzo, A. B., Karam, C. S., Zhang, Y., Yano, H., Freyberg, R. J., Karam, D. S., et al. (2013). The membrane raft protein Flotillin-1 is essential in dopamine neurons for amphetamine-induced behavior in Drosophila. *Molecular Psychiatry, 18*(7), 824–833. https://doi.org/10.1038/mp.2012.82.

Quick, M. W. (2002a). Role of syntaxin 1A on serotonin transporter expression in developing thalamocortical neurons. *International Journal of Developmental Neuroscience, 20*(3–5), 219–224.

Quick, M. W. (2002b). Substrates regulate gamma-aminobutyric acid transporters in a syntaxin 1A-dependent manner. *Proceedings of the National Academy of Sciences of the United States of America, 99*(8), 5686–5691. https://doi.org/10.1073/pnas.082712899.

Quick, M. W. (2003). Regulating the conducting states of a mammalian serotonin transporter. *Neuron, 40*(3), 537–549.

Quick, M. W. (2006). The role of SNARE proteins in trafficking and function of neurotransmitter transporters. *Handbook of Experimental Pharmacology, 175*, 181–196.

Ramamoorthy, S., Shippenberg, T. S., & Jayanthi, L. D. (2011). Regulation of monoamine transporters: Role of transporter phosphorylation. *Pharmacology & Therapeutics, 129*(2), 220–238. https://doi.org/10.1016/j.pharmthera.2010.09.009.

Rastedt, D. E., Vaughan, R. A., & Foster, J. D. (2017). Palmitoylation mechanisms in dopamine transporter regulation. *Journal of Chemical Neuroanatomy, 83-84*, 3–9. https://doi.org/10.1016/j.jchemneu.2017.01.002.

Resh, M. D. (2006). Palmitoylation of ligands, receptors, and intracellular signaling molecules. *Science's STKE, 2006*(359), re14. https://doi.org/10.1126/stke.3592006re14.

Scanlon, S. M., Williams, D. C., & Schloss, P. (2001). Membrane cholesterol modulates serotonin transporter activity. *Biochemistry, 40*(35), 10507–10513.

Scholze, P., Norregaard, L., Singer, E. A., Freissmuth, M., Gether, U., & Sitte, H. H. (2002). The role of zinc ions in reverse transport mediated by monoamine transporters. *The Journal of Biological Chemistry, 277*(24), 21505–21513. https://doi.org/10.1074/jbc.M112265200.

Segura-Aguilar, J., Paris, I., Munoz, P., Ferrari, E., Zecca, L., & Zucca, F. A. (2014). Protective and toxic roles of dopamine in Parkinson's disease. *Journal of Neurochemistry, 129*(6), 898–915. https://doi.org/10.1111/jnc.12686.

Seidel, S., Singer, E. A., Just, H., Farhan, H., Scholze, P., Kudlacek, O., et al. (2005). Amphetamines take two to tango: An oligomer-based counter-transport model of neurotransmitter transport explores the amphetamine action. *Molecular Pharmacology*, *67*(1), 140–151. https://doi.org/10.1124/mol.67.1.

Sembower, M. A., Ertischek, M. D., Buchholtz, C., Dasgupta, N., & Schnoll, S. H. (2013). Surveillance of diversion and nonmedical use of extended-release prescription amphetamine and oral methylphenidate in the United States. *Journal of Addictive Diseases*, *32*(1), 26–38. https://doi.org/10.1080/10550887.2012.759880.

Sitte, H. H., & Freissmuth, M. (2010). The reverse operation of Na(+)/cl(−)-coupled neurotransmitter transporters—Why amphetamines take two to tango. *Journal of Neurochemistry*, *112*(2), 340–355. https://doi.org/10.1111/j.1471-4159.2009.06474.x.

Sitte, H. H., Huck, S., Reither, H., Boehm, S., Singer, E. A., & Pifl, C. (1998). Carrier-mediated release, transport rates, and charge transfer induced by amphetamine, tyramine, and dopamine in mammalian cells transfected with the human dopamine transporter. *Journal of Neurochemistry*, *71*(3), 1289–1297.

Snyder, S. H. (1972). Catecholamines in the brain as mediators of amphetamine psychosis. *Archives of General Psychiatry*, *27*(2), 169–179.

Sonders, M. S., Zhu, S. J., Zahniser, N. R., Kavanaugh, M. P., & Amara, S. G. (1997). Multiple ionic conductances of the human dopamine transporter: The actions of dopamine and psychostimulants. *The Journal of Neuroscience*, *17*(3), 960–974.

Steinkellner, T., Montgomery, T. R., Hofmaier, T., Kudlacek, O., Yang, J. W., Rickhag, M., et al. (2015). Amphetamine action at the cocaine- and antidepressant-sensitive serotonin transporter is modulated by alphaCaMKII. *The Journal of Neuroscience*, *35*(21), 8258–8271. https://doi.org/10.1523/JNEUROSCI.4034-14.2015.

Steinkellner, T., Mus, L., Eisenrauch, B., Constantinescu, A., Leo, D., Konrad, L., et al. (2014). In vivo amphetamine action is contingent on alphaCaMKII. *Neuropsychopharmacology*, *39*(11), 2681–2693. https://doi.org/10.1038/npp.2014.124.

Steinkellner, T., Yang, J. W., Montgomery, T. R., Chen, W. Q., Winkler, M. T., Sucic, S., et al. (2012). Ca(2+)/calmodulin-dependent protein kinase IIalpha (alphaCaMKII) controls the activity of the dopamine transporter: Implications for Angelman syndrome. *The Journal of Biological Chemistry*, *287*(35), 29627–29635. https://doi.org/10.1074/jbc.M112.367219.

Sucic, S., Dallinger, S., Zdrazil, B., Weissensteiner, R., Jorgensen, T. N., Holy, M., et al. (2010). The N terminus of monoamine transporters is a lever required for the action of amphetamines. *The Journal of Biological Chemistry*, *285*(14), 10924–10938. https://doi.org/10.1074/jbc.M109.083154.

Suh, B. C., & Hille, B. (2008). PIP2 is a necessary cofactor for ion channel function: How and why? *Annual Review of Biophysics*, *37*, 175–195. https://doi.org/10.1146/annurev.biophys.37.032807.125859.

Sulzer, D. (2011). How addictive drugs disrupt presynaptic dopamine neurotransmission. *Neuron*, *69*(4), 628–649. https://doi.org/10.1016/j.neuron.2011.02.010.

Sulzer, D., Chen, T. K., Lau, Y. Y., Kristensen, H., Rayport, S., & Ewing, A. (1995). Amphetamine redistributes dopamine from synaptic vesicles to the cytosol and promotes reverse transport. *The Journal of Neuroscience*, *15*(5 Pt. 2), 4102–4108.

Sulzer, D., Sonders, M. S., Poulsen, N. W., & Galli, A. (2005). Mechanisms of neurotransmitter release by amphetamines: A review. *Progress in Neurobiology*, *75*(6), 406–433. https://doi.org/10.1016/j.pneurobio.2005.04.003.

Suzuki, T., Du, F., Tian, Q. B., Zhang, J., & Endo, S. (2008). Ca2+/calmodulin-dependent protein kinase IIalpha clusters are associated with stable lipid rafts and their formation traps PSD-95. *Journal of Neurochemistry*, *104*(3), 596–610. https://doi.org/10.1111/j.1471-4159.2007.05035.x.

Sweeney, C. T., Sembower, M. A., Ertischek, M. D., Shiffman, S., & Schnoll, S. H. (2013). Nonmedical use of prescription ADHD stimulants and preexisting patterns of drug abuse. *Journal of Addictive Diseases*, *32*(1), 1–10. https://doi.org/10.1080/10550887.2012.759858.

Takeuchi, Y., Fukunaga, K., & Miyamoto, E. (2002). Activation of nuclear Ca(2+)/calmodulin-dependent protein kinase II and brain-derived neurotrophic factor gene expression by stimulation of dopamine D2 receptor in transfected NG108-15 cells. *Journal of Neurochemistry*, *82*(2), 316–328.

Torres, G. E., Carneiro, A., Seamans, K., Fiorentini, C., Sweeney, A., Yao, W. D., et al. (2003). Oligomerization and trafficking of the human dopamine transporter. Mutational analysis identifies critical domains important for the functional expression of the transporter. *The Journal of Biological Chemistry*, *278*(4), 2731–2739. https://doi.org/10.1074/jbc.M201926200.

Torres, G. E., Gainetdinov, R. R., & Caron, M. G. (2003). Plasma membrane monoamine transporters: Structure, regulation and function. *Nature Reviews. Neuroscience*, *4*(1), 13–25. https://doi.org/10.1038/nrn1008.

Torres, B., & Ruoho, A. E. (2014). N-terminus regulation of VMAT2 mediates methamphetamine-stimulated efflux. *Neuroscience*, *259*, 194–202. https://doi.org/10.1016/j.neuroscience.2013.11.059.

Tsui, J., Inagaki, M., & Schulman, H. (2005). Calcium/calmodulin-dependent protein kinase II (CaMKII) localization acts in concert with substrate targeting to create spatial restriction for phosphorylation. *The Journal of Biological Chemistry*, *280*(10), 9210–9216. https://doi.org/10.1074/jbc.M407653200.

Vaughan, R. A., Huff, R. A., Uhl, G. R., & Kuhar, M. J. (1997). Protein kinase C-mediated phosphorylation and functional regulation of dopamine transporters in striatal synaptosomes. *The Journal of Biological Chemistry*, *272*(24), 15541–15546.

Vearrier, D., Greenberg, M. I., Miller, S. N., Okaneku, J. T., & Haggerty, D. A. (2012). Methamphetamine: History, pathophysiology, adverse health effects, current trends, and hazards associated with the clandestine manufacture of methamphetamine. *Disease-a-Month*, *58*(2), 38–89. https://doi.org/10.1016/j.disamonth.2011.09.004.

Vuorenpaa, A., Ammendrup-Johnsen, I., Jorgensen, T. N., & Gether, U. (2016). A kinome wide screen identifies novel kinases involved in regulation of monoamine transporter function. *Neurochemistry International*, *98*, 103–114. https://doi.org/10.1016/j.neuint.2016.03.013.

Weerth, S. H., Holtzclaw, L. A., & Russell, J. T. (2007). Signaling proteins in raft-like microdomains are essential for Ca2+ wave propagation in glial cells. *Cell Calcium*, *41*(2), 155–167. https://doi.org/10.1016/j.ceca.2006.06.006.

Wilmouth, C. E., Zheng, G., Crooks, P. A., Dwoskin, L. P., & Bardo, M. T. (2013). Oral administration of GZ-793A, a VMAT2 inhibitor, decreases methamphetamine self-administration in rats. *Pharmacology, Biochemistry, and Behavior*, *112*, 29–33. https://doi.org/10.1016/j.pbb.2013.09.006.

Zaczek, R., Culp, S., & De Souza, E. B. (1991). Interactions of [3H]amphetamine with rat brain synaptosomes. II. Active transport. *The Journal of Pharmacology and Experimental Therapeutics*, *257*(2), 830–835.

Zestos, A. G., Mikelman, S. R., Kennedy, R. T., & Gnegy, M. E. (2016). PKCbeta inhibitors attenuate amphetamine-stimulated dopamine efflux. *ACS Chemical Neuroscience*, 7(6), 757–766. https://doi.org/10.1021/acschemneuro.6b00028.

CHAPTER ELEVEN

Anti-NMDA Receptor Encephalitis: Clinical Features and Basic Mechanisms

David R. Lynch[*,†,1], Amy Rattelle[*], Yi Na Dong[*], Kylie Roslin[*], Amy J. Gleichman[†,2], Jessica A. Panzer[*,†]

[*]Children's Hospital of Philadelphia, Philadelphia, PA, United States
[†]Perelman School of Medicine, University of Pennsylvania, Philadelphia, PA, United States
[1]Corresponding author: e-mail address: lynchd@mail.med.upenn.edu

Contents

Abstract

In slightly more than 10 years, anti-NMDA receptor (NMDAR) encephalitis has changed from a rare paraneoplastic syndrome to the most common cause of nonviral encephalitis. It presents fulminantly with progressive psychosis, seizures, and autonomic dysfunction, leading to death if untreated. However, rapid recognition and treatment can lead to survival and a return to baseline levels of functioning in many patients. While initially associated with ovarian teratomas, it is now associated with other tumors and can reflect a postviral event. The antibodies to the NMDAR made in this syndrome are

[2] Current address: Department of Neurology, David Geffen School of Medicine, University of California—Los Angeles, Los Angeles, CA, United States.

Advances in Pharmacology, Volume 82
ISSN 1054-3589
https://doi.org/10.1016/bs.apha.2017.08.005

pathogenic and are directed at the extracellular domain of the GluN1 subunit. Such antibodies lead to internalization of NMDARs in model systems, leading to a physiological state characterized by NMDAR hypofunction. Analogous disorders, characterized by antibodies to other synaptic receptors, present with neurological and psychiatric dysfunction and also appear to reflect antibody-induced internalization of receptors. However, this simple pathophysiology may be too simplistic to reflect the complexity of events in anti-NMDAR encephalitis. Future scientific investigations may allow a more complete understanding of this disorder and improve treatment of anti-NMDAR encephalitis.

ABBREVIATIONS

AMPA α-amino-3-hydroxy-5-methyl-4-isoxazolepropionic acid
anti-NMDARE anti-NMDA receptor encephalitis
NMDA *N*-methyl D-aspartate
PtAbs anti-NMDARE patients' antibodies

1. INTRODUCTION

In the context of this commemorative volume, it seems appropriate to remember what Sol Snyder, Chair of Neuroscience at Johns Hopkins for decades, taught one of us (D.R.L.) 35 years ago in graduate school. First, the core of many discoveries, particularly Sol's, begins with a clinical observation that demands scientific explanation (e.g., the biological basis of opiate action). In addition, Sol's work always stressed that crucial neuroscientific findings have implications outside the nervous system, and vice versa. Thus, during the time there of Dr. Lynch, work in the lab included not only collaborations with neurologists and psychiatrists but also endocrinologists, hypertension specialists, pathologists, and physiologists. Understanding all these fields prepares one for the breadth of modern investigation. Finally, through working with Sol, one comes to realize a collaborative spirit that must unite investigators and science advances. Crucial in this is that one can learn from one's close collaborators and friends, but also from essentially all others in the field. These principles have exemplified the work of Sol over the past 50+ years.

The ongoing elucidation of the disorder now known as anti-NMDA receptor (NMDAR) encephalitis demonstrates all of these principles. First described as a clinical syndrome of acute onset psychosis followed by progressive, but treatable, encephalopathy in 2005, then linked to the NMDAR in 2007, anti-NMDAR encephalitis (anti-NMDARE) is now one of the most common nonviral encephalitides worldwide (Dalmau et al., 2007). With the discovery of an increased incidence of anti-NMDARE also has come the realization of the seriousness of the disorder. Thus, there is an urgent need for increased clinical and scientific understanding that could lead to improved treatment. In this chapter, we will review the basic pharmacology and neurobiology of the NMDAR, the present understanding of the clinical phenomenology and pathophysiology of anti-NMDARE, and possible concepts and future directions for ameliorating the effect of this disorder.

2. NMDA RECEPTORS

Glutamate, the most important excitatory transmitter in the mammalian brain, acts synaptically at a series of receptors named for their prototypical agonist (Lynch & Guttmann, 2002). The major fast excitatory receptor in the mammalian brain is the AMPA receptor, a glutamate-gated sodium channel. In contrast, the other main postsynaptic ionotropic glutamate receptor, the NMDAR, is a ligand-gated cation channel that is highly permeable to calcium. Consequently, calcium entering through the NMDAR readily modifies the long-term biochemical proprieties of the cell and mediates the effects of intracellular calcium changes on both normal physiological events and pathophysiological processes. NMDARs are formed from four subunits: each receptor contains two GluN1 subunits in combination with two GluN2 or GluN3 subunits. GluN1, the so-called obligatory subunit, is found as eight different splice variants (GluN1–1a to GluN1–4a and GluN1–1b to GluN1–4b), while GluN2 and GluN3 are made from four (2A–2D) and two (A–B) genes, respectively (Monyer et al., 1992; Regan, Romero-Hernandez, & Furukawa, 2015; Traynelis et al., 2010; Zhu & Paoletti, 2015). GlunN3 subunits are less well understood. GluN2 subunits bind glutamate or its competitive analogs (NMDA for example), while GluN1 and GluN3 bind the obligatory coagonist glycine. D-Serine substitutes for glycine in certain physiological situations or anatomic locations and may be the endogenous agonist at synaptic NMDARs (Papouin et al., 2012). Different subunit combinations create receptors with distinct physiological and pharmacological properties and are differentially expressed regionally and developmentally in vivo (Lynch & Guttmann, 2001).

Specific properties make NMDARs conceptually distinct from other ligand-gated ion channels. First, NMDARs require two agonists (glutamate and glycine) to open. NMDARs are also blocked by magnesium in a voltage-dependent manner; membrane depolarization from adjacent AMPA receptors is needed to open NMDARs (Kupper, Ascher, & Neyton,1996;

Traynelis et al., 2010). A variety of regulated posttranslational modifications also influence receptor opening and localization. These unusual features of the NMDAR allow it to be a coincidence detector in the nervous system in that it opens only when a series of events occur; this makes it a crucial modulator of long-term change. Thus interference with NMDAR function represents a likely site for pathophysiological events to occur in human disease.

In addition, NMDARs are heterogeneous in the manner in which they signal downstream of the receptor. Calcium entering through the NMDAR can activate many pathways and be either neuroprotective or neurotoxic. At present, most paradigms suggest that synaptic NMDARs are protective against neuronal toxicity, while extrasynaptic NMDAR activation leads to cell death. This paradigm is based on results from excitotoxicity, in which NMDAR overactivation leads to neurotoxicity. Although there are combinations of different GluN receptor subunits that are more likely to be synaptic vs extrasynaptic, this varies between brain regions so that the properties of synaptic and extrasynaptic receptors do not always correlate with subunit combinations. Consequently, the differentiation between synaptic and extrasynaptic receptors is defined anatomically rather than pharmacologically.

Until the discovery of anti-NMDARE, the toxicology of NMDARs involved two types of diseases. The first are those of excitotoxicity, in which excess glutamatergic stimulation through the NMDAR leads to acute or chronic neuronal death. Excitotoxicity has been implicated in numerous disorders, including acute insults such as stroke and epilepsy and chronic diseases like Huntington's, Parkinson's, and Alzheimer's diseases. In addition, although less explored, NMDAR hypofunction can lead to human diseases or clinical syndromes. Schizophrenia has features of NMDAR hypofunction, as do forms of developmental disability such as autism (Balu & Coyle, 2015; Coyle, 2012; Schade & Paulus, 2016). The well-established roles of NMDARs in synaptic plasticity and learning lend credence to the idea that NMDAR hypofunction may play a role in these developmental disorders. Given the many varied and crucial roles of every component of the receptor, it is therefore to be expected that interfering with the NMDAR via antibody binding would have dramatic neurological consequences.

3. ANTI-NMDAR ENCEPHALITIS

3.1 Essential Clinical Features

Anti-NMDARE was initially described as a paraneoplastic process, in which the immune reaction to a tumor leads to cross-reacting sequelae in the brain

(Dalmau et al., 2007). In the initial description, a cohort of young women presented with mental status changes of acute psychosis including severe short-term memory loss. This cohort overall contained 12 young women with teratomas (benign tumors containing all three germ cell layers): 11 teratomas were ovarian and 1 mediastinal. Over the course of weeks, neurological function worsened until individuals developed ongoing psychosis, dyskinesias, autonomic dysfunction, decreased consciousness, hypoventilation, and death (if untreated). There was also a high frequency of response to plasmapheresis or other forms of immunotherapy, leading to patients recovering with no memory of the events or the illness. This is suggestive of antibodies to a specific protein mediating the events, as T cell-mediated immunity seen in classical paraneoplastic processes is far less responsive. In individuals with antibody-mediated paraneoplastic processes, when patient sera or cerebrospinal fluid (CSF) is applied to tissue sections, antibodies from the sera react with the particular antigen involved in the process in the brain. The immunological properties of the antibodies in patients' serum and CSF in this new syndrome were distinct from those found in individuals with other forms of limbic encephalitis, as when sera from the individuals with teratomas were applied to brain sections, they recognized an antigen found in high levels in the cortex and particularly hippocampus, with lower levels in brainstem and cerebellum.

In a search for the novel antigen, the distribution closely resembled that of the NMDAR. The role of the NMDAR as the autoantigen was shown by the introduction of GluN1/GluN2 heteromeric receptors into heterologous cells; the NMDAR-transfected cells were recognized by patients' serum and CSF, while untransfected cells or cells transfected with other antigens were not. As all subjects in this initial cohort contained antibodies to GluN1/GluN2 heteromers, this led to a definition of anti-NMDARE as an appropriate clinical syndrome in the context of serum or CSF antibodies staining specific items:

1. Reactivity to brain involving the hippocampus.
2. Cell-surface staining of cultured cortical or hippocampal neurons.
3. Staining of heterologous cells transfected with GluN1 and GluN2 (forming GluN1–GluN2 heteromers of the NMDAR) in a pattern matching that of other antibodies to GluN1 (Fig. 1).

These three features characterize the antibody response of anti-NMDARE.

Using the criteria defined in the initial report, the number of identified patients with anti-NMDARE has expanded rapidly and has revised much of the concept of anti-NMDARE (Dalmau et al., 2008). Although the

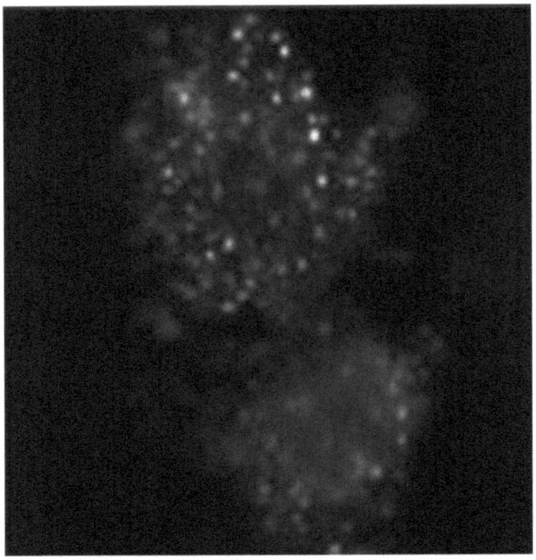

Fig. 1 Staining of NMDAR in transfected cells by anti-NMDAR antibodies. HEK cells transfected with GluN1 and GluN2A were stained with PtAbs. Puncta representing staining of NMDA receptors are noted on the cell surface. No such staining is found with control antibodies.

recognition of anti-NMDARE occurred in young adults with paraneoplastic processes, not all individuals have identified tumors and anti-NMDARE is found in all age groups (Armangue et al., 2013; Florance et al., 2009; Rainey, Gholkar, & Cheesman, 2014; Titulaer et al., 2013). Anti-NMDAR encephalitis also occurs in children and in older adults. If anti-NMDARE is viewed as a nonviral encephalitis, then its frequency surpasses that of any identified virus, and it becomes the most common single form of nonviral encephalitis identified (Gable, Sheriff, Dalmau, Tilley, & Glaser, 2012; Kamei et al., 2009; Prüss et al., 2010). Thus anti-NMDARE is not a rare disease limited to neurooncology, but instead a far more common disorder affecting thousands of people every year.

With time, the identification of large cohorts demonstrates a continuum of findings across patients with anti-NMDARE (Dalmau et al., 2008; Zekeridou et al., 2015). In general, patients with anti-NMDARE are young (mean age 23 in an early large series) and predominantly women, matching the sex difference in many immune disorders. The presentation is dominantly psychiatric (particularly in adults), in association with memory difficulties, autonomic instability, seizures, and hypoventilation in greater than half of adult patients. More than 30%–60% of patients have neoplasms, mainly ovarian teratomas. However, in contrast to the earliest series, only

75% of subjects recover to their baseline level of functioning; 25% have residual functional deficits (Thomas et al., 2013; Titulaer et al., 2013). In addition, neuropsychological testing reveals persistent cognitive dysfunction in many patients, and people still die on occasion from anti-NMDARE (Chi et al., 2017; McKeon et al., 2017). In broadening the features of the disease, a variety of new presentations have appeared. These include unilateral dyskinesia movements in children, status epilepticus, isolated epilepsy, fever of unknown origin, irritable insomnia, exercise-induced foot weakness, late-onset autism, anorexia nervosa, and, rarely, opsoclonus myoclonus (Baizabal-Carvallo, Stocco, Muscal, & Jankovic, 2013; Creten et al., 2011; Hur, 2015; Johnson, Henry, Fessler, & Dalmau, 2010; Kurian, Lalive, Dalmau, & Horvath, 2010; Labate, Quattrone, Dalmau, & Gambardella, 2013; Mechelhoff et al., 2015; Player et al., 2015). Interestingly, isolated seizures as a presentation are more frequent in men than women for reasons that are unclear. Similarly, a large number of novel tumors are associated with anti-NMDAR, including hepatic neuroendocrine tumors, uterine neuroendocrine tumors, small cell lung cancer, and carcinoma of unknown origin (Afanasiev et al., 2016; Hara et al., 2011; Jeraiby, Depincé-Berger, Bossy, Antoine, & Paul, 2016; Wu, He, Zhang, Shi, & Zhang, 2016).

The pathology of anti-NMDARE is consistent with a paraneoplastic limbic encephalitis. Inflammatory infiltrates are found in the hippocampus, and there is a specific decrease in the number of NMDARs in the hippocampus. Complement-mediated mechanisms are not prominent in anti-NMDARE, showing that it is likely a direct effect of antibodies on NMDARs that mediate the disease process (Martinez-Hernandez et al., 2011). Plasma cell infiltration of the CNS though does occur and may be crucial to the disease process (Dale, Pillai, & Brilot, 2013).

Relapses can occur in anti-NMDARE (Gabilondo et al., 2011; Kayser, Titulaer, Gresa-Arribas, & Dalmau, 2013; Ramanathan, Wong, & Fung, 2013). However, while antibody titer correlates with severity, improvement may not be fully correlated with falling titer as intrathecal synthesis can remain for years after functional recovery (Alexopoulos, Kosmidis, Dalmau, & Dalakas, 2011; Dalmau, Lancaster, Martinez-Hernandez, Rosenfeld, & Balice-Gordon, 2011; Gresa-Arribas et al., 2014; Hansen et al., 2013; Wali, Cai, Rossor, & Clough, 2011). This suggests that mechanisms unrelated to NMDAR biology may play some role in recovery, particularly in individuals with spontaneous recovery and those with persistent intrathecal synthesis.

3.2 Relationship With Viral Infection

While the trigger for anti-NMDARE is neoplastic in greater than half of individuals, viral illness appears to precede this disorder in another large set of individuals. Paraneoplastic anti-NMDARE is less common in children, a group in which viral exposure is more common. Although direct links to viral illness are most commonly found with herpes virus infection, it has also been noted with varicella zoster, measles virus, and other viruses (Grillo & da Silva, 2013; Ioannidis, Papadopoulos, Koufou, Parissis, & Karacostas, 2015, Phan et al., 2016; Solís, Salazar, & Hasbun, 2016). In many cases of anti-NMDARE, a link to viral illness is missed, but might account for the seasonal variability in anti-NMDARE in children (Adang, Lynch, & Panzer, 2014). In addition, in some situations viral infection is remote, and anti-NMDARE represents a late sequelae.

However, the most well- defined postviral association of anti-NMDARE occurs in herpes encephalitis, in which an initial viral encephalitis leads to a secondary anti-NMDARE (Nosadini et al., 2017). Such individuals are recognized as persons in which the initial presentation is consistent with herpes encephalitis (with PCR confirmation), but is followed by persistent and advancing neurological sequelae (Geoghegan et al., 2016; Hacohen et al., 2014; Höftberger, Armangue, Leypoldt, Graus, & Dalmau, 2013; Leypoldt et al., 2013). These events include both cognitive events and movement disorder (chorea). Treatment thus must be aimed not only at the original viral encephalitis but also at the secondary immune phenomenon of anti-NMDARE.

With the growing frequency of anti-NMDARE, it is possible that other disorders could be linked to anti-NMDARE. The first is schizophrenia, based on the hypothesis that a subset of this disorder could represent chronic anti-NMDARE. While some studies have detected anti-NMDAR antibodies in schizophrenic patients, the type of antibodies seems to differ and the number of patients is low (Pollak, McCormack, Peakman, Nicholson, & David, 2014; Tsutsui et al., 2012). Thus, it seems unlikely that chronic anti-NMDARE represents a major subgroup of schizophrenic patients (de Witte et al., 2015). Similarly, studies show no large association between anti-NMDAR antibodies and epilepsy of unknown origin. In addition, there have been some links between anti-NMDARE and other immune disorders such as progressive systemic sclerosis (Suzuki et al., 2011). Isolated patients have been identified with multiple sclerosis and neuromyelits optica following anti-NMDARE, and a true association appears to be present based on some series (Baheerathan et al., 2017; Ran et al., 2017; Titulaer et al., 2014; Uzawa et al., 2012; Zoccarato et al., 2013). As immune disorders frequently coassociate, an association of anti-NMDARE with other immune-mediated disorders would not be surprising.

3.3 Treatment

One of the most exciting aspects of anti-NMDARE is its response to therapy. Even in the early studies the majority of patients return to relatively normal function with basic immunotherapies such as plasmapheresis or IV IgG (DeSena et al., 2015). In addition, a number of reports also demonstrate spontaneous recovery, usually after extended periods of time (Evoli et al., 2012; Iizuka et al., 2008). Still the quality of recovery on average reflects the speed with which definitive treatment occurs (Breese, Dalmau, Lennon, Apiwattanakul, & Sokol, 2010; Byrne, McCoy, Lynch, Webb, & King, 2014; Kurian, Fluss, & Korff, 2012).

In those individuals with anti-NMDARE as a paraneoplastic process, the first consideration in treatment is tumor removal (Iizuka et al., 2008). Ovarian teratomas do not typically metastasize and are usually benign, so tumor removal can be accomplished expeditiously in most situations. As these tumors contain neural tissue leading to production of NMDAR antibodies, then this step should lead to falling antibody levels and ideal clinical response.

However, anti-NMDARE is an immune disease at the time it presents in all patients. Thus, immunomodulation must begin in parallel with tumor removal, including plasmapheresis, IV IgG, and potentially corticosteroids as first-line therapies. In some individuals, improvement does not occur and bolder therapies including rituximab and cyclophosphamide may be used; these of course carry greater risk (Hachiya et al., 2013; Ikeguchi et al., 2012; Ishiuraet et al., 2008; Kashyape et al., 2012). A novel approach is the use of a proteosomal inhibitor for therapy, though the mechanisms for such protection is not fully known (Scheibe et al., 2017). Perhaps the most difficult aspect of anti-NMDAR treatment is ascertaining who requires more aggressive therapy. Early series emphasize the surprisingly large number of individuals who return to baseline in anti-NMDAR, while more recent perspectives have addressed the substantial portion who remain disabled. Treating such refractory individuals earlier might improve outcome. However, identifying such individuals early in their course (when they might be most responsive) is challenging and to this point no specific identifiers of whom are most likely to be refractory to therapy have been defined.

4. BASIC MECHANISMS OF ANTI-NMDARE

In the initial characterizations of anti-NMDAR encephalitis, the crucial step was identification of the antigen. While this step happened mainly by chance, the physiological properties of the NMDAR suggest it as a potential antibody target based on the clinical phenomena. NMDAR blockade using agents like phencyclidine leads to acute psychosis, a phenotype matching that of typical anti-NMDARE (Javitt & Zukin, 1991). In addition, NMDA knockdown in mice leads to hypoventilation, the cause of death in many patients with anti-NMDARE (Forrest et al., 1994). Finally, NMDAR modulation is linked to control of dyskinesias, an aspect that could be associated with the prominent dyskinesia in anti-NMDARE (Blanchet, Papa, Metman, Mouradian, & Chase, 1997). Thus, studies identifying NMDARs as the autoantigen in this disorder are consistent with the expected features of dysfunctional NMDARs.

Biochemically, the site of epitope recognition for the antibodies of anti-NMDARE is on GluN1, the glycine-binding subunit. Expression of GluN1 in heterologous systems, such as HEK cells, is necessary and sufficient for binding of patients' antibodies (PtAbs). There is no difference among any naturally occurring GluN1 splice variants in their ability to be recognized by PtAbs. Expression of GluN2 subunits (as performed in the initial studies) may alter the recognition of the epitope on GluN1, perhaps by altering the conformation of the GluN1 subunit, but is not required for epitope formation. A variety of manipulations to the GluN1 subunit alter epitope recognition (Gleichman, Spruce, Dalmau, Seeholzer, & Lynch, 2012). Development of immunoreactivity to PtAbs is blocked by tunicamycin, an agent altering glycosylation of proteins, and removal of a single glycosylation site (N368) removes the epitope of GluN1. However, alternative mutations that remove glycosylation but not N368 still retain the ability to be recognized by PtAbs. Thus, multiple mutations in the region around N368 remove epitope recognition, but they do not correlate perfectly with glycosylation, suggesting that this region creates a conformation of GluN1 that is necessary for generating epitope recognition. It also does not prove that this region is sufficient for immunoreactivity; the smallest portion of GluN1 that still generates immunoreactivity includes the full N-terminal domain linked to a transmembrane region, a much larger region that that which is necessary. These data are most easily interpreted as showing that GluN1 contains a conformational epitope in the first 381 amino acids of

GluN1 that requires the region near amino acid 368 to develop proper conformation.

Anti-NMDARE antibodies also alter the physiology of the receptor and of glutamatergic transmission. In patch-clamp experiments, receptors with mutant GluN1s having shorter open times bind lower levels of PtAbs, and PtAbs appear to bind to an open form of the receptor. This could lead receptors to remain in an open conformation when the receptor is bound. This would explain the observation that intracellular calcium levels in neurons increase with low-level exposure to PtAbs, suggesting an initial effect of PtAbs in activating NMDARs before decreasing by 24 h in culture (Fig. 2). Such an observation also might explain some of the discrepancies in the distribution of immunoreactivity to PtAbs in the brain. While the initial studies suggested lower levels of binding to cerebellar NMDARs, this result has not always been replicated. However, cerebellar receptors open less frequently than forebrain NMDAR under similar activation paradigms. As different studies have not closely matched protocols for incubation with antibody, the level of activation across different studies might explain this variability. The effects of PtAbs are also apparent in larger physiological contexts, as they

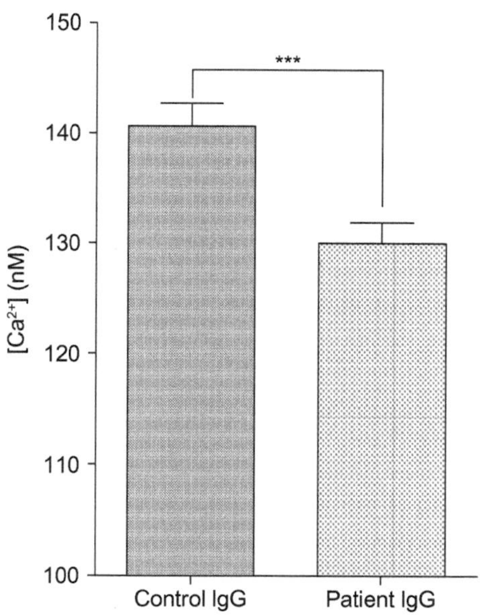

Fig. 2 Effect of PtAbs on neuronal calcium levels. Cultured cortical neurons were exposed to PtAbs (IgG) for 24 h. Levels of intracellular calcium were lower in PtAbs treated cells, consistent with NMDAR hypofunction. ***The basal Ca^{2+} levels are $P < 0.0001$ (T-test).

facilitate afferent cortical motor response when injected into rodent brain, consistent with glutamatergic dysfunction in cortical neurons (Manto, Dalmau, Didelot, Rogemond, & Honnorat, 2010). They also produce cognitive loss in rodents, similar to the features of anti-NMDARE (Planagumà et al., 2016). Finally, such antibodies suppress synaptic plasticity in vitro, consistent with blocking the role of the NMDAR in many paradigms of synaptic modification.

While PtAbs alter the physiology of the receptor, their direct pathogenicity more likely reflects antibody-induced changes in synaptic NMDAR levels. PtAbs induce internalization of NMDARs from synapses, without loss of associated synaptic proteins. This internalization correlates with antibody titer and requires receptor cross-linking, as Fab fragments of antibody do not lead to receptor internalization, while exogenously cross-linked Fab' fragments do (Hughes et al., 2010). After internalization, receptors are destroyed in a proteasome-dependent manner, suggesting that proteosomal inhibition may be one avenue for treatment (Fig. 3). Synaptic NMDAR currents decrease, but other synaptic receptors are spared. In addition, a key aspect of the pathophysiology is the movement of NMDAR to extrasynaptic sites by PtAbs; this along with the internalization is blocked by the activation/presence of EphB receptors (Mikasova et al., 2012). Thus, the selective internalization of NMDAR receptors can be controlled by synaptic messenger systems in addition to PtAbs. Cellular mechanisms also block the full effect of internalization by mobilizing a compensatory increase in inhibitory mechanisms (Moscato et al., 2014). Thus, the events involved in creation of the NMDAR hypofunction state of anti-NMDARE require both PtAbs-based events and neuronal reactions.

Are these PtAbs truly the cause of the disease or merely an epiphenomenon? Ongoing experiments demonstrate the pathogenicity of the antibodies, as they meet the basic principles of Koch's postulates for demonstrating causal relationships as applied to this form of limbic encephalitis. First, antibodies with specific anti-NMDAR reactivity have been found in all individuals with anti-NMDARE, though this is somewhat circular as such antibodies define the specific type of limbic encephalitis. The antibodies have been partially purified from patients to antibody types (IgG vs IgA) and retain their basic biochemical properties; they continue to react with NMDAR in transfected cells and on the surface of cultured neurons (Desestret et al., 2015). In addition, such antibodies lead to internalization of receptors and to behavioral changes in mice, consistent with PtAbs reproducing the phenotype of the disease. Finally, cloning of B cells from patients' CSF produces antibodies that recapitulate the features of

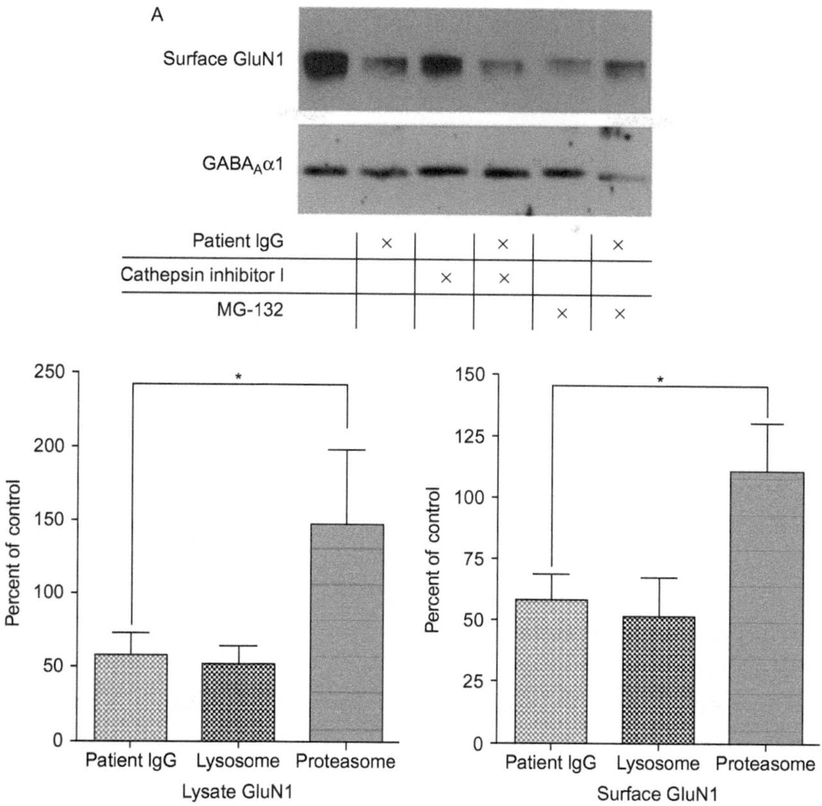

Fig. 3 Effect of proteosomal and lysosomal inhibition on the effect of PtAbs. Application of PtAbs to cortical neurons in culture leads to lower levels of GluN1 compared to untreated neurons. The effect is blocked by proteosomal inhibition but not by cathepsin (lysosomal) inhibition (Western blot in A). This increase is found in both the overall lysate and surface receptors, suggesting proteosomal control of the effect of PtAbs. $*P < 0.05$ (one way ANOVA with Dunnett's Multiple Comparison Test).

disease when injected into animals (Kreye et al., 2016). Further preliminary reports suggest that antibodies derived from peripheral B cells from patients also recognize NMDAR and have some of the features of pathogenic antibodies. Consequently, substantial data show that the PtAbs are pathogenic as they essentially satisfy all of Koch's postulates for disease reproduction.

4.1 NMDAR Antibodies From Other Human Disorders

While the PtAbs associated with anti-NMDARE have a defined target specificity, other antibodies to NMDAR have been characterized from other disorders and occasionally from normal people. Recent reports suggest that some individuals produce IgA antibodies to the NMDAR in association with a clinical syndrome of dementia (Doss et al., 2014). Though their exact epitope specificity is unknown, they lead to cell death in culture and do not have the selectivity of anti-NMDARE antibodies for synaptic structures. They are also found in individuals with a broad variety of dementias, thus lacking the clinical specificity associated with typical anti-NMDARE. Thus, in contrast to PtAbs of NMDARE that are selective for a specific clinical phenotype, synaptic pattern, and epitope specificity, the meaning of the IgA antibodies in these dementias is unclear.

A second type of anti-NMDAR antibody is associated with systemic lupus erythematosus (SLE). Such antibodies recognize GluN2A/2B subunits and parallel the presence of clinical neuropsychiatric syndromes in SLE (Fragoso-Loyo et al., 2008; Harrison, Ravdin, & Lockshin, 2006; Lapteva et al., 2006). However, there is little evidence of a causal nature of the antibodies, and the basic science data on their epitopes, and how they alter synaptic function and animal models is limited. Thus these most likely represent markers of CNS SLE rather than direct causes of CNS dysfunction.

Still, while clinical phenotyping and substantial data dissociate the effects of PtAbs from anti-NMDARE from other forms of NMDAR antibodies found in humans, it remains possible that other NMDAR antibodies could be pathogenic in specific situations. In model systems such as heterologous systems, all human NMDAR antibodies to extracellular epitopes appear to be capable of internalizing NMDAR (Castillo-Gómez et al., 2016). While this seems to conflict with the clinical data and the remainder of the basic science data on PtAbs in anti-NMDARE, there are several possible ways to reconcile these results. First, in anti-NMDAR and other immune disorders, the blood–brain barrier allows increased penetration of antibodies into the CNS allowing plasma cells to reside there. While blood–brain barrier opening is clearly a feature of anti-NMDARE, what leads to this is unclear. Creation of anti-NMDAR antibodies outside of anti-NMDARE may not be associated with blood–brain barrier dysfunction. In addition, there may be concentration differences in antibody accumulation in vivo between PtAbs of anti-NMDARE and other antibodies. Finally, while internalization is part of the pathogenesis of anti-NMDARE, it is possible that other events are also required. The immune response of anti-NMDARE is not monoclonal. Other anti-NMDARE antibodies besides those that lead to internalization may facilitate or even be necessary for complete disease pathogenesis. The diversity of the immune response in anti-NMDARE remains incompletely explored, but might provide a perspective on this concept.

4.2 Other Synaptic Encephalitides

Anti-NMDARE serves as a model for other antibody-generated disorders of the synapse, collectedly called "synaptic encephalitides," in which the pathophysiology reflects antibody binding to synaptic neurotransmitter receptors rather than more destructive traditional immune responses (Panzer, Gleichman, & Lynch, 2014; Rosenfeld & Dalmau, 2011). The most well-known of these (besides anti-NMDARE) is anti-AMPA receptor encephalitis. Like NMDAR, AMPA receptors are tetrameric complexes made from four receptor subunits (GluA1–4) that are assembled into homomeric (identical subunits) or heteromeric (differing subunits) receptors. Most AMPA receptors in vivo are GluA1/GluA2 or GluA2/GluA3 heterotetramers (Geiger et al., 1995; Sans et al., 2003; Wenthold, Petralia, Blahos, & Niedzielski, 1996). Distinct genes encode GluA1–4, all of which have multiple splice variants (Traynelis et al., 2010). AMPA receptors activate and deactivate faster than NMDAR (ms timescale) and thus control fast glutamatergic neurotransmission in most synapses. AMPA receptor activation removes the magnesium block on NMDARs, thus allowing AMPA receptors to modulate NMDAR-mediated events.

Anti-AMPA receptor encephalitis presents distinctly from anti-NMDARE, being primarily a disorder of memory (De Bruijn & Titulaer, 2016). Subjects present with memory issues and seizures, but lack much of the psychotic behavior (Höftberger et al., 2015). As in anti-NMDARE, about 50% of AMPAR encephalitis is paraneoplastic, and the antibodies give rise to internalization of AMPA receptors with sparing of other glutamatergic receptors, analogous to the events of anti-NMDARE (Lai et al., 2009; Peng et al., 2015). However, anti-AMPAR encephalitis is much less common, with less than 30 identified patients. In addition, the receptor regions controlling epitope recognition are less specific as antibodies can be to GluA2 subunits, GluA1 subunits, or sometimes both. This contrasts with anti-NMDARE, in which receptor recognition of PtAbs can be modulated selectively by the small region around N368. In antibodies from a large group of AMPAR encephalitis patients, the epitope resides in the N-terminus of the subunit based on epitope mapping using both deletion mutants and fusion proteins, but cannot be further localized (Gleichman, Panzer, Baumann, Dalmau, &

Lynch, 2014). In addition, the exact receptor conformation appears less critical for epitope recognition in AMPA receptor encephalitis, as PtAbs recognize not only heterologous receptors but also denatured portions of receptor found in fusion proteins. Unfortunately, while AMPA receptor encephalitis contributes to the concept of the importance of synaptic encephalitides, the small number of patients prohibits further mechanistic characterization at this time.

Other synaptic encephalitides have been identified to nonglutamatergic receptors. These include anti-GABAB receptor encephalitis, anti-mGluR1 receptor encephalitis, and anti-mGluR5 encephalitis (Boronat, Sabater, Saiz, Dalmau, & Graus, 2011; Höftberger, Titulaer, et al., 2013; Jarius & Wildemann, 2015; Lancaster et al., 2011; Petit-Pedrol et al., 2014; Spatola et al., 2017). In general, these are less well characterized than anti-NMDAR encephalitis but appear to have similar mechanisms, and internalization of receptors is a crucial component of the pathophysiology. They can have very specific clinical syndromes attached to them such as the "Ophelia syndrome" associated with mGluR5 antibodies. In addition, a variety of clinical syndromes such as Rasmussen's encephalitis (GluA3) and opsoclonus myoclonus (unknown antigens) exist in which subgroups of patients exist with antibodies to synaptic components (Gurcharran & Karkare, 2017). Such disorders likely represent overlapping syndromes rather than a specific disease, and the mechanisms of these disorders may or may not match the antibody-dependent internalization of receptors found in anti-NMDARE.

5. NMDARE: A NEW CONCEPTUALIZATION

Given that many patients with anti-NMDARE have poor recovery despite aggressive treatment with potentially risky immunotherapies, innovative treatments are needed. Such treatments must be based on a better understanding of the neurobiology of the disorder. The published dogma is that anti-NMDAR encephalitis is a disease of global NMDAR hypofunction, in many ways analogous to schizophrenia. However, published data conflict with this hypothesis including the findings that PtAbs can prolong NMDAR channel open time and appear to activate the receptor initially before leading to a later NMDAR hypofunction state. In addition, antibodies have decreased affinity for GluN1 mutants with shorter channel open time. These data support the possibility that PtAbs act as NMDAR agonists in some situations and that antibody impact may vary depending on NMDAR open conformation and subtype. At active excitatory synapses, PtAbs may preferentially bind to open synaptic (often GluN2A-containing) NMDARs. In contrast, on tonically active inhibitory neurons, extrasynaptic NMDARs are more likely to be open from glutamate spillover and may be preferentially bound by PtAbs. This concept suggests that PtAbs cause a shift from synaptic to extrasynaptic NMDAR signaling *specifically at the sites of greatest NMDAR activity* (Fig. 4). This hypothesis can account for unexplained clinical features of anti-NMDAR encephalitis: (1) it is known that treatment with NMDAR agonists, excess extrasynaptic NMDAR signaling, and inhibitory neuron dysfunction all can trigger seizures, a surprising clinical feature of a purely NMDAR hypofunction state; and (2) both dyskinesias and catatonia are associated with excessive extrasynaptic GluN2B signaling. Thus, this hypothesis has the potential to explain the core symptoms of anti-NMDAR encephalitis in a way that simple NMDAR hypofunction does not (Table 1). Thus as Dr. Snyder has demonstrated throughout his career, scientific and clinical hypotheses are intimately interrelated in a way that drives both forward.

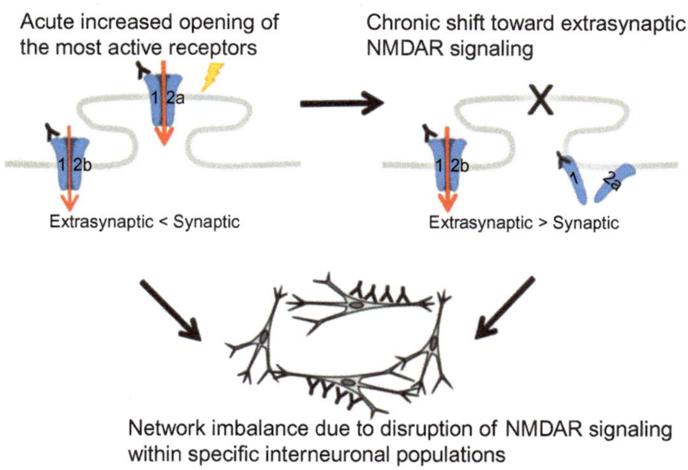

Fig. 4 Proposed pathophysiology of anti-NMDARE. Application of PtAbs leads to increased opening of synaptic receptors (lightning bolt) (GluN1/2A receptors more commonly) followed by their movement to extrasynaptic sites and/or internalization. Extrasynaptic (more commonly GluN1/2B) receptors open less frequently and are unaffected by PtAbs. This leads to an imbalance between extrasynaptic and synaptic receptors that could account for the complex neurological features of anti-NMDARE.

Table 1 Proposed relationship between synaptic effects and symptoms in anti-NMDARE

NMDAR Dysregulation	Proposed Symptoms
Agonist effect on NMDARs	Seizures
Synaptic NMDAR hypofunction	Amnesia, psychosis, hypoventilation
Extrasynaptic NMDAR hyperfunction	Catatonia, dyskinesias, seizures
Neuronal network imbalance with impaired intraneuronal activity	Seizures

6. CONCLUSION

For a disorder as common as anti-NMDARE, there is surprisingly little basic science information available. As the outcome is not always benign, such information is crucial to advancing therapy and preventing adverse outcomes. Early intervention based on the properties of antibody–NMDAR interactions could provide a logical methodology for improving long-term outcome.

There are many questions to be addressed including the following:

1. Is there any selectivity to the in vivo recognition process of NMDAR by PtAbs? In vitro systems suggest that all receptors containing a GluN1 subunit should be recognized by PtAbs, but the stereotypic presentation of the disease suggests that it is not that simple. If subtypes of NMDAR are the key targets, does it reflect differing subunits, differing synaptic locations, differing activation states, or other properties?
2. How diverse is the immune response in anti-NMDARE and which antibodies mediate disease? While single monoclonal antibodies appear capable of generating the crucial phenomena of anti-NMDARE, antibody production is almost certainly polyclonal. There could be multiple types of antibody involved in disease pathogenesis, or perhaps the diagnostic antibodies do not necessarily match the true disease generating antibodies. This might explain instances of recovery without disappearance of immunoreactivity to NMDAR.
3. Is internalization the only event mediating pathogenesis? While the role of internalization in vitro is well defined, the observation that NMDAR antibodies other than those found in anti-NMDARE can also cause internalization suggests that other factors may be involved. Such factors could include opening the blood–brain barrier, or other actions at the

NMDAR such as direct receptor antagonism. Answering this question almost certainly requires better knowledge of the diversity of the immune response in anti-NMDARE.

4. Are there downstream mechanisms for interaction? One of the crucial events of excitotoxicity is a differential effect on downstream pathways, which provides a novel methodology for facilitating neuronal repair in excitotoxic disorders. Does a similar diversity in messenger systems exist after internalization that might be modulated? The modest success of proteosomal inhibition could represent a way to modulate such pathways.

Through further scientific investigations, many of these questions may be answered. This should lead to new understanding of anti-NMDARE and related disorders and facilitate development of definitive therapies.

ACKNOWLEDGMENTS

Dr. Lynch is supported by R21 NS088148, Dr. Panzer by K08-099506 and the Pablove and Rally foundations. Dr. Gleichman is supported by NIH F32 NS087783. This chapter is dedicated to the Memory of Dr. Panzer, who provided many of the conceptualizations behind the ongoing work on anti-NMDAR encephalitis.

CONFLICT OF INTEREST

No conflicts of interest exist in this chapter for all authors. Dr. Lynch receives grants from the Friedreich Ataxia Research Alliance and the National Institutes of Health.

REFERENCES

Adang, L. A., Lynch, D. R., & Panzer, J. A. (2014). Pediatric anti-NMDA receptor encephalitis is seasonal. *Annals of Clinical Translational Neurology*, *1*, 921–925.

Afanasiev, V., Brechemier, M. L., Boisseau, W., Ducoudray, R., Mayeur, M. E., Meyronet, D., et al. (2016). Anti-NMDA receptor antibody encephalitis and neuroendocrine pancreatic tumor: Causal link? *Neurology*, *87*, 112–113.

Alexopoulos, H., Kosmidis, M. L., Dalmau, J., & Dalakas, M. C. (2011). Paraneoplastic anti-NMDAR encephalitis: Long term follow-up reveals persistent serum antibodies. *Journal of Neurology*, *258*, 1568–1570.

Armangue, T., Titulaer, M. J., Málaga, I., Bataller, L., Gabilondo, I., Graus, F., et al. (2013). Spanish anti-N-methyl-D-aspartate receptor (NMDAR) encephalitis work group. Pediatric anti-N-methyl-D-aspartate receptor encephalitis-clinical analysis and novel findings in a series of 20 patients. *The Journal of Pediatrics*, *162*, 850–856.

Baheerathan, A., Brownlee, W. J., Chard, D. T., Shields, K., Gregory, R., & Trip, S. A. (2017). Antecedent anti-NMDA receptor encephalitis in two patients with multiple sclerosis. *Multiple Sclerosis and Related Disorders*, *12*, 20–22.

Baizabal-Carvallo, J. F., Stocco, A., Muscal, E., & Jankovic, J. (2013). The spectrum of movement disorders in children with anti-NMDA receptor encephalitis. *Movement Disorders*, *28*, 543–547.

Balu, D. T., & Coyle, J. T. (2015). The NMDA receptor 'glycine modulatory site' in schizophrenia: D-serine, glycine, and beyond. *Current Opinion in Pharmacology*, *20*, 109–115.
Blanchet, P. J., Papa, S. M., Metman, L. V., Mouradian, M. M., & Chase, T. N. (1997). Modulation of levodopa-induced motor response complications by NMDA antagonists in Parkinson's disease. *Neuroscience and Biobehavioral Reviews*, *21*, 447–453.
Boronat, A., Sabater, L., Saiz, A., Dalmau, J., & Graus, F. (2011). GABA(B) receptor antibodies in limbic encephalitis and anti-GAD-associated neurologic disorders. *Neurology*, *76*, 795–800.
Breese, E. H., Dalmau, J., Lennon, V. A., Apiwattanakul, M., & Sokol, D. K. (2010). Anti-N-methyl-D-aspartate receptor encephalitis: Early treatment is beneficial. *Pediatric Neurology*, *42*, 213–214.
Byrne, S., McCoy, B., Lynch, B., Webb, D., & King, M. D. (2014). Does early treatment improve outcomes in N-methyl-D-aspartate receptor encephalitis? *Developmental Medicine and Child Neurology*, *56*, 794–796.
Castillo-Gómez, E., Oliveira, B., Tapken, D., Bertrand, S., Klein-Schmidt, C., Pan, H., et al. (2016). All naturally occurring autoantibodies against the NMDA receptor subunit NR1 have pathogenic potential irrespective of epitope and immunoglobulin class. *Molecular Psychiatry*, [in press].
Chi, X., Wang, W., Huang, C., Wu, M., Zhang, L., Li, J., et al. (2017). Risk factors for mortality in patients with anti-NMDA receptor encephalitis. *Acta Neurologica Scandinavica*, *136*, 298–304.
Coyle, J. T. (2012). NMDA receptor and schizophrenia: A brief history. *Schizophrenia Bulletin*, *38*, 920–926.
Creten, C., van der Zwaan, S., Blankespoor, R. J., Maatkamp, A., Nicolai, J., van Os, J., et al. (2011). Late onset autism and anti-NMDA-receptor encephalitis. *The Lancet*, *378*, 98.
Dale, R. C., Pillai, S., & Brilot, F. (2013). Cerebrospinal fluid CD19(+) B-cell expansion in N-methyl-D-aspartate receptor encephalitis. *Developmental Medicine and Child Neurology*, *55*, 191–193.
Dalmau, J., Gleichman, A. J., Hughes, E. G., Rossi, J. E., Peng, X., Lai, M., et al. (2008). Anti-NMDA-receptor encephalitis: Case series and analysis of the effects of antibodies. *Lancet Neurology*, *7*, 1091–1098.
Dalmau, J., Lancaster, E., Martinez-Hernandez, E., Rosenfeld, M. R., & Balice-Gordon, R. (2011). Clinical experience and laboratory investigations in patients with anti-NMDAR encephalitis. *Lancet Neurology*, *10*, 63–74.
Dalmau, J., Tüzün, E., Wu, H. Y., Masjuan, J., Rossi, J. E., Voloschin, A., et al. (2007). Paraneoplastic anti-N-methyl-D-aspartate receptor encephalitis associated with ovarian teratoma. *Annals of Neurology*, *61*, 25–36.
De Bruijn, M. A., & Titulaer, M. J. (2016). Anti-NMDAR encephalitis and other glutamate and GABA receptor antibody encephalopathies. *Handbook of Clinical Neurology*, *133*, 199–217.
DeSena, A. D., Noland, D. K., Matevosyan, K., King, K., Phillips, L., Qureshi, S. S., et al. (2015). Intravenous methylprednisolone versus therapeutic plasma exchange for treatment of anti-N-methyl-D-aspartate receptor antibody encephalitis: A retrospective review. *Journal of Clinical Apheresis*, *30*, 212–216.
de Witte, L. D., Hoffmann, C., van Mierlo, H. C., Titulaer, M. J., Kahn, R. S., & Martinez-Martinez, P. (2015). European consortium of autoimmune mental disorders (CAIMED). Absence of N-methyl-D-aspartate receptor IgG autoantibodies in schizophrenia: The importance of cross-validation studies. *JAMA Psychiatry*, *72*, 731–733.
Desestret, V., Chefdeville, A., Viaccoz, A., Bost, C., Ducray, F., Picard, G., et al. (2015). CSF IgA NMDAR antibodies are potential biomarkers for teratomas in anti-NMDAR encephalitis. *Neurology: Neuroimmunology & Neuroinflammation*, *2*, e166.

Doss, S., Wandinger, K. P., Hyman, B. T., Panzer, J. A., Synofzik, M., Dickerson, B. M., et al. (2014). High prevalence of NMDA receptor IgA/IgM antibodies in different dementia types. *Annals of Clinical Translational Neurology, 1*, 822–832.

Evoli, A., Spinelli, P., Frisullo, G., Alboini, P. E., Servidei, S., & Marra, C. (2012). Spontaneous recovery from anti-NMDAR encephalitis. *Journal of Neurology, 259*, 1964–1966.

Florance, N. R., Davis, R. L., Lam, C., Szperka, C., Zhou, L., Ahmad, S., et al. (2009). Anti-N-methyl-D-aspartate receptor (NMDAR) encephalitis in children and adolescents. *Annals of Neurology, 66*, 11–18.

Forrest, D., Yuzaki, M., Soares, H. D., Ng, L., Luk, D. C., Sheng, M., et al. (1994). Targeted disruption of NMDA receptor 1 gene abolishes NMDA response and results in neonatal death. *Neuron, 13*, 325–338.

Fragoso-Loyo, H., Cabiedes, J., Orozco-Narváez, A., Dávila-Maldonado, L., Atisha-Fregoso, Y., et al. (2008). Serum and cerebrospinal fluid autoantibodies in patients with neuropsychiatric lupus erythematosus. Implications for diagnosis and pathogenesis. *PLoS One, 3*, e3347.

Gabilondo, I., Saiz, A., Galán, L., González, V., Jadraque, R., Sabater, L., et al. (2011). Analysis of relapses in anti-NMDAR encephalitis. *Neurology, 77*, 996–999.

Gable, M. S., Sheriff, H., Dalmau, J., Tilley, D. H., & Glaser, C. A. (2012). The frequency of autoimmune N-methyl-D-aspartate receptor encephalitis surpasses that of individual viral etiologies in young individuals enrolled in the California Encephalitis Project. *Clinical Infectious Diseases, 54*, 899–904.

Geiger, J. R., Melcher, T., Koh, D. S., Sakmann, B., Seeburg, P. H., Jonas, P., et al. (1995). Relative abundance of subunit mRNAs determines gating and Ca2+ permeability of AMPA receptors in principal neurons and interneurons in rat CNS. *Neuron, 15*, 193–204.

Geoghegan, S., Walsh, A., King, M. D., Lynch, B., Webb, D., & Twomey, E. (2016). Anti-N-methyl-D-aspartate receptor antibody mediated neurologic relapse post herpes simplex encephalitis: A case series. *The Pediatric Infectious Disease Journal, 35*, e258–61.

Gleichman, A. J., Panzer, J. A., Baumann, B. H., Dalmau, J., & Lynch, D. R. (2014). Antigenic and mechanistic characterization of anti-AMPA receptor encephalitis. *Annals of Clinical Translational Neurology, 1*, 180–189.

Gleichman, A. J., Spruce, L. A., Dalmau, J., Seeholzer, S. H., & Lynch, D. R. (2012). Anti-NMDA receptor encephalitis antibody binding is dependent on amino acid identity of a small region within the GluN1 amino terminal domain. *The Journal of Neuroscience, 32*, 11082–11094.

Gresa-Arribas, N., Titulaer, M. J., Torrents, A., Aguilar, E., McCracken, L., Leypoldt, F., et al. (2014). Antibody titres at diagnosis and during follow-up of anti-NMDA receptor encephalitis: A retrospective study. *The Lancet. Neurology, 13*, 167–177.

Grillo, E., & da Silva, R. J. (2013). Anti-N-methyl-D-aspartate receptor encephalitis and parvovirus B19: A possible link? *The Journal of Pediatrics, 163*(4), 1233.

Gurcharran, K., & Karkare, S. (2017). Anti-N-methyl-D-aspartate receptor encephalitis and Rasmussen-like syndrome: An association? *Pediatric Neurology, 66*, 104–107.

Hachiya, Y., Uruha, A., Kasai-Yoshida, E., Shimoda, K., & Satoh-Shirai, I. (2013). Rituximab ameliorates anti-N-methyl-D-aspartate receptor encephalitis by removal of short-lived plasmablasts. *Journal of Neuroimmunology, 265*, 128–130.

Hacohen, Y., Deiva, K., Pettingill, P., Waters, P., Siddiqui, A., & Chretien, P. (2014). N-Methyl-D-aspartate receptor antibodies in post-herpes simplex virus encephalitis neurological relapse. *Movement Disorders, 29*, 90–96.

Hansen, H. C., Klingbeil, C., Dalmau, J., Li, W., Weissbrich, B., & Wandinger, K. P. (2013). Persistent intrathecal antibody synthesis 15 years after recovering from anti-N-methyl-D-aspartate receptor encephalitis. *JAMA Neurology, 70*, 117–119.

Hara, M., Morita, A., Kamei, S., Yamaguchi, M., Homma, T., Nemoto, N., et al. (2011). Anti-N-methyl-D-aspartate receptor encephalitis associated with carcinosarcoma with neuroendocrine differentiation of the uterus. *Journal of Neurology, 258*, 1351–1353.
Harrison, M. J., Ravdin, L. D., & Lockshin, M. D. (2006). Relationship between serum NR2a antibodies and cognitive dysfunction in systemic lupus erythematosus. *Arthritis and Rheumatism, 54*, 2515–2522.
Höftberger, R., Armangue, T., Leypoldt, F., Graus, F., & Dalmau, J. (2013). Clinical neuropathology practice guide 4-2013: Post-herpes simplex encephalitis: N-methyl-D-aspartate receptor antibodies are part of the problem. *Clinical Neuropathology, 32*, 251–254.
Höftberger, R., Titulaer, M. J., Sabater, L., Dome, B., Rózsás, A., Hegedus, B., et al. (2013). Encephalitis and GABAB receptor antibodies: Novel findings in a new case series of 20 patients. *Neurology, 81*, 1500–1506.
Höftberger, R., van Sonderen, A., Leypoldt, F., Houghton, D., Geschwind, M., Gelfand, J., et al. (2015). Encephalitis and AMPA receptor antibodies: Novel findings in a case series of 22 patients. *Neurology, 84*, 2403–2412.
Hughes, E. G., Peng, X., Gleichman, A. J., Lai, M., Zhou, L., Tsou, R., et al. (2010). Cellular and synaptic mechanisms of anti-NMDA receptor encephalitis. *The Journal of Neuroscience, 30*, 5866–5875.
Hur, J. (2015). Fever of unknown origin: An unusual presentation of anti-N-methyl-D-aspartate receptor encephalitis. *Infection & Chemotherapy, 47*, 129–132.
Iizuka, T., Sakai, F., Ide, T., Monzen, T., Yoshii, S., Iigaya, M., et al. (2008). Anti-NMDA receptor encephalitis in Japan: Long-term outcome without tumor removal. *Neurology, 70*, 504–511.
Ikeguchi, R., Shibuya, K., Akiyama, S., Hino, S., Kubom, H., & Takeda, T. (2012). Rituximab used successfully in the treatment of anti-NMDA receptor encephalitis. *Internal Medicine, 51*, 1585–1589.
Ioannidis, P., Papadopoulos, G., Koufou, E., Parissis, D., & Karacostas, D. (2015). Anti-NMDA receptor encephalitis possibly triggered by measles virus. *Acta Neurologica Belgica, 115*, 801–802.
Ishiura, H., Matsuda, S., Higashihara, M., Hasegawa, M., Hida, A., Hanajima, R., et al. (2008). Response of anti-NMDA receptor encephalitis without tumor to immunotherapy including rituximab. *Neurology, 71*, 1921–1923.
Jarius, S., & Wildemann, B. (2015). 'Medusa-head ataxia': The expanding spectrum of Purkinje cell antibodies in autoimmune cerebellar ataxia. Part 1: Anti-mGluR1, anti-Homer-3, anti-Sj/ITPR1 and anti-CARP VIII. *Journal of Neuroinflammation, 12*, 166.
Javitt, D. C., & Zukin, S. R. (1991). Recent advances in the phencyclidine model of schizophrenia. *The American Journal of Psychiatry, 148*, 1301–1308.
Jeraiby, M., Depincé-Berger, A., Bossy, V., Antoine, J. C., & Paul, S. (2016). A case of anti-NMDA receptor encephalitis in a woman with a NMDA-R(+) small cell lung carcinoma (SCLC). *Clinical Immunology, 166–167*, 96–99.
Johnson, N., Henry, C., Fessler, A. J., & Dalmau, J. (2010). Anti-NMDA receptor encephalitis causing prolonged nonconvulsive status epilepticus. *Neurology, 75*, 1480–1482.
Kamei, S., Kuzuhara, S., Ishihara, M., Morita, A., Taira, N., Togo, M., et al. (2009). Nationwide survey of acute juvenile female non-herpetic encephalitis in Japan: Relationship to anti-N-methyl-D-aspartate receptor encephalitis. *Internal Medicine, 48*(9), 673.
Kashyape, P., Taylor, E., Ng, J., Krishnakumar, D., Kirkham, F., & Whitney, A. (2012). Successful treatment of two paediatric cases of anti-NMDA receptor encephalitis with cyclophosphamide: The need for early aggressive immunotherapy in tumour negative paediatric patients. *European Journal of Paediatric Neurology, 16*, 74–78.
Kayser, M. S., Titulaer, M. J., Gresa-Arribas, N., & Dalmau, J. (2013). Frequency and characteristics of isolated psychiatric episodes in anti-N-methyl-D-aspartate receptor encephalitis. *JAMA Neurology, 70*(9), 1133.

Kreye, J., Wenke, N. K., Chayka, M., Leubner, J., Murugan, R., Maier, N., et al. (2016). Human cerebrospinal fluid monoclonal N-methyl-D-aspartate receptor autoantibodies are sufficient for encephalitis pathogenesis. *Brain, 139*, 2641–2652.

Kupper, J., Ascher, P., & Neyton, J. (1996). Probing the pore region of recombinant N-methyl-D-aspartate channels using external and internal magnesium block. *Proceedings of the National Academy of Sciences of the United States of America, 93*, 8648–8653.

Kurian, M., Fluss, J., & Korff, C. (2012). Anti-NMDA receptor encephalitis: The importance of early diagnosis and aggressive immunotherapy in tumor negative pediatric patients. *European Journal of Paediatric Neurology, 16*, 764–765.

Kurian, M., Lalive, P. H., Dalmau, J. O., & Horvath, J. (2010). Opsoclonus-myoclonus syndrome in anti-N-methyl-D-aspartate receptor encephalitis. *Archives of Neurology, 67*, 118–121.

Labate, A., Quattrone, A., Dalmau, J., & Gambardella, A. (2013). Anti-N-methyl-D-aspartate-glutamic-receptor encephalitis presenting as paroxysmal exercise-induced foot weakness. *Movement Disorders, 28*, 820–822.

Lai, M., Hughes, E. G., Peng, X., Zhou, L., Gleichman, A. J., Shu, H., et al. (2009). AMPA receptor antibodies in limbic encephalitis alter synaptic receptor location. *Annals of Neurology, 65*, 424–434.

Lancaster, E., Martinez-Hernandez, E., Titulaer, M. J., Boulos, M., Weaver, S., Antoine, J. C., et al. (2011). Antibodies to metabotropic glutamate receptor 5 in the Ophelia syndrome. *Neurology*, 77, 1698–1701.

Lapteva, L., Nowak, M., Yarboro, C. H., Takada, K., Roebuck-Spencer, T., et al. (2006). Anti-N-methyl-D-aspartate receptor antibodies, cognitive dysfunction, and depression in systemic lupus erythematosus. *Arthritis and Rheumatism, 54*, 2505–2514.

Leypoldt, F., Titulaer, M. J., Aguilar, E., Walther, J., Bönstrup, M., & Havemeister, S. (2013). Herpes simplexvirus-1 encephalitis can trigger anti-NMDA receptor encephalitis: Case report. *Neurology, 81*, 1637–1639.

Lynch, D. R., & Guttmann, R. P. (2001). NMDA receptor pharmacology: Perspectives from molecular biology. *Current Drug Targets, 2*, 215–231.

Lynch, D. R., & Guttmann, R. P. (2002). Excitotoxicity: Perspectives based on N-methyl-D-aspartate receptor subtypes. *The Journal of Pharmacology and Experimental Therapeutics, 300*, 717–723.

Manto, M., Dalmau, J., Didelot, A., Rogemond, V., & Honnorat. (2010). In vivo effects of antibodies from patients with anti-NMDA receptor encephalitis: Further evidence of synaptic glutamatergic dysfunction. *Orphanet Journal of Rare Diseases, 26*, 31.

Martinez-Hernandez, E., Horvath, J., Shiloh-Malawsky, Y., Sangha, N., Martinez-Lage, M., & Dalmau, J. (2011). Analysis of complement and plasma cells in the brain of patients with anti-NMDAR encephalitis. *Neurology*, 77, 589–593.

McKeon, G. L., Robinson, G. A., Ryan, A. E., Blum, S., Gillis, D., Finke, C., et al. (2017). Cognitive outcomes following anti-N-methyl-D-aspartate receptor encephalitis: A systematic review. *Journal of Clinical and Experimental Neuropsychology, 6*, 1–19.

Mechelhoff, D., van Noort, B. M., Weschke, B., Bachmann, C. J., Wagner, C., Pfeiffer, E., et al. (2015). Anti-NMDA receptor encephalitis presenting as atypical anorexia nervosa: An adolescent case report. *European Child & Adolescent Psychiatry, 24*, 1321–1324.

Mikasova, L., De Rossi, P., Bouchet, D., Georges, F., Rogemond, V., Didelot, A., et al. (2012). Disrupted surface cross-talk between NMDA and Ephrin-B2receptors in anti-NMDA encephalitis. *Brain, 135*, 1606–1621.

Monyer, H., Sprengel, R., Schoepfer, R., Herb, A., Higuchi, M., Lomeli, H., et al. (1992). Heteromeric NMDA receptors: Molecular and functional distinction of subtypes. *Science, 256*, 1217–1221.

Moscato, E. H., Peng, X., Jain, A., Parsons, T. D., Dalmau, J., & Balice-Gordon, R. J. (2014). Acute mechanisms underlying antibody effects in anti-N-methyl-D-aspartate receptor encephalitis. *Annals of Neurology, 76*, 108–119.

Nosadini, M., Mohammad, S. S., Corazza, F., Ruga, E. M., Kothur, K., & Perilongo, G. (2017). Herpes simplex virus-induced anti-N-methyl-D-aspartate receptor encephalitis: A systematic literature review with analysis of 43 cases. *Developmental Medicine and Child Neurology*, *59*(8), 796–805.

Panzer, J. A., Gleichman, A. J., & Lynch, D. R. (2014). Glutamatergic autoencephalitides: An emerging field. *Journal of Neural Transmission*, *121*, 957–968.

Papouin, T., Ladépêche, L., Ruel, J., Sacchi, S., Labasque, M., Hanini, M., et al. (2012). Synaptic and extrasynaptic NMDA receptors are gated by different endogenous coagonists. *Cell*, *150*, 633–646.

Peng, X., Hughes, E. G., Moscato, E. H., Parsons, T. D., Dalmau, J., & Balice-Gordon, R. J. (2015). Cellular plasticity induced by anti-α-amino-3-hydroxy-5-methyl-4-isoxazolepropionic acid (AMPA) receptor encephalitis antibodies. *Annals of Neurology*, *77*, 381–398.

Petit-Pedrol, M., Armangue, T., Peng, X., Bataller, L., Cellucci, T., Davis, R., et al. (2014). Encephalitis with refractory seizures, status epilepticus, and antibodies to the GABAA receptor: A case series, characterisation of the antigen, and analysis of the effects of antibodies. *The Lancet Neurology*, *13*, 276–286.

Phan, T. G., Messacar, K., Dominguez, S. R., da Costa, A. C., Deng, X., & Delwart, E. (2016). A new densovirus in cerebrospinal fluid from a case of anti-NMDA-receptor encephalitis. *Archives of Virology*, *161*, 3231–3235.

Planagumà, J., Haselmann, H., Mannara, F., Petit-Pedrol, M., Grünewald, B., Aguilar, E., et al. (2016). Ephrin-B2 prevents N-methyl-D-aspartate receptor antibody effects on memory and neuroplasticity. *Annals of Neurology*, *80*, 388–400.

Player, B., Harmelink, M., Bordini, B., Weisgerber, M., Girolami, M., & Croix, M. (2015). Pediatric opsoclonus-myoclonus-ataxia syndrome associated with anti-N-methyl-D-aspartate receptor encephalitis. *Pediatric Neurology*, *53*, 456–458.

Pollak, T. A., McCormack, R., Peakman, M., Nicholson, T. R., & David, A. S. (2014). Prevalence of anti-N-methyl-D-aspartate (NMDA) receptor antibodies in patients with schizophrenia and related psychoses: A systematic review and meta-analysis. *Psychological Medicine*, *44*, 2475–2487.

Prüss, H., Dalmau, J., Harms, L., Höltje, M., Ahnert-Hilger, G., Borowski, K., et al. (2010). Retrospective analysis of NMDA receptor antibodies in encephalitis of unknown origin. *Neurology*, *2010*(75), 1735–1739.

Rainey, K., Gholkar, B., & Cheesman, M. (2014). Anti-NMDA receptor encephalitis: An easily missed diagnosis in older patients. *Age and Ageing*, *43*, 725–726.

Ramanathan, S., Wong, C. H., & Fung, V. S. (2013). Long duration between presentation of probable anti-N-methyl-D-aspartate receptor encephalitis and either clinical relapse or positive serum autoantibodies. *Journal of Clinical Neuroscience*, *20*, 1322–1323.

Ran, Y., Wang, L., Zhang, F., Ao, R., Dong, Z., & Yu, S. (2017). Anti-NMDAR encephalitis followed by seropositive neuromyelitis optica spectrum disorder: A case report and literature review. *Clinical Neurology and Neurosurgery*, *155*, 75–82.

Regan, M. C., Romero-Hernandez, A., & Furukawa, H. (2015). A structural biology perspective on NMDA receptor pharmacology and function. *Current Opinion in Structural Biology*, *33*, 68–75.

Rosenfeld, M. R., & Dalmau, J. (2011). Anti-NMDA-receptor encephalitis and other synaptic autoimmune disorders. *Current Treatment Options in Neurology*, *13*, 324–332.

Sans, N., Vissel, B., Petralia, R. S., Wang, Y. X., Chang, K., Royle, G. A., et al. (2003). Aberrant formation of glutamate receptor complexes in hippocampal neurons of mice lacking the GluR2 AMPA receptor subunit. *Journal of Neuroscience*, *23*, 9367–9373.

Schade, S., & Paulus, W. D. (2016). Cycloserine in neuropsychiatric diseases: A systematic review. *The International Journal of Neuropsychopharmacology*, *19*, 4.

Scheibe, F., Prüss, H., Mengel, A. M., Kohler, S., Nümann, A., & Köhnlein, M. (2017). Bortezomib for treatment of therapy-refractory anti-NMDA receptor encephalitis. *Neurology, 88*, 366–370.

Solís, N., Salazar, L., & Hasbun, R. (2016). Anti-NMDA receptor antibody encephalitis with concomitant detection of Varicella zoster virus. *Journal of Clinical Virology, 83*, 26–28.

Spatola, M., Petit-Pedrol, M., Simabukuro, M. M., Armangue, T., Castro, F. J., Barcelo Artigues, M. I., et al. (2017). Investigations in GABA(A) receptor antibody-associated encephalitis. *Neurology, 88*, 1012–1020.

Suzuki, H., Samukawa, M., Kitada, M., Ichihashi, J., Mistui, Y., & Tanaka, K. (2011). A case of anti-N-methyl-D-aspartate receptor encephalitis with systemic sclerosis. *European Journal of Neurology, 18*, e145–6.

Thomas, A., Rauschkolb, P., Gresa-Arribas, N., Schned, A., Dalmau, J. O., & Fadul, C. E. (2013). Anti-N-methyl-D-aspartate receptor encephalitis: A patient with refractory illness after 25 months of intensive immunotherapy. *JAMA Neurology, 70*, 1566–1568.

Titulaer, M. J., Höftberger, R., Iizuka, T., Leypoldt, F., McCracken, L., Cellucci, T., et al. (2014). Overlapping demyelinating syndromes and anti-N-methyl-D-aspartate receptor encephalitis. *Annals of Neurology, 75*, 411–428.

Titulaer, M. J., McCracken, L., Gabilondo, I., Armangué, T., Glaser, C., Iizuka, T., et al. (2013). Treatment and prognostic factors for long-term outcome in patients with anti-NMDA receptor encephalitis: An observational cohort study. *Lancet Neurology, 12*, 157–165.

Titulaer, M. J., McCracken, L., Gabilondo, I., Iizuka, T., Kawachi, I., Bataller, L., et al. (2013). Late-onset anti-NMDA receptor encephalitis. *Neurology, 81*, 1058–1063.

Traynelis, S. F., Wollmuth, L. P., McBain, C. J., Menniti, F. S., Vance, K. M., Ogden, K. K., et al. (2010). Glutamate receptor ion channels: Structure, regulation, and function. *Pharmacological Reviews, 62*, 405–496.

Tsutsui, K., Kanbayashi, T., Tanaka, K., Boku, S., Ito, W., Tokunaga, J., et al. (2012). Anti-NMDA-receptor antibody detected in encephalitis, schizophrenia, and narcolepsy with psychotic features. *BMC Psychiatry, 12*, 37.

Uzawa, A., Mori, M., Takahashi, Y., Ogawa, Y., Uchiyama, T., & Kuwabara, S. (2012). Anti-N-methyl D-aspartate-type glutamate receptor antibody-positive limbic encephalitis in a patient with multiple sclerosis. *Clinical Neurology and Neurosurgery, 114*(4), 402.

Wali, S. M., Cai, A., Rossor, A. M., & Clough, C. (2011). Appearance of anti-NMDAR antibodies after plasma exchange and total removal of malignant ovarian teratoma in a patient with paraneoplastic limbic encephalopathy. *BML Case Reports, 2011*, 2011.

Wenthold, R. J., Petralia, R. S., Blahos, J., II, & Niedzielski, A. S. (1996). Evidence for multiple AMPA receptor complexes in hippocampal CA1/CA2 neurons. *The Journal of Neuroscience, 16*, 1982–1989.

Wu, Y. Y., He, X. J., Zhang, M. L., Shi, Y. Y., & Zhang, J. W. (2016). Anti-N-methyl-D-aspartate receptor encephalitis with lung adenocarcinoma. *Neurological Sciences, 37*, 1573–1575.

Zekeridou, A., Karantoni, E., Viaccoz, A., Ducray, F., Gitiaux, C., Villega, F., et al. (2015). Treatment and outcome of children and adolescents with N-methyl-D-aspartate receptor encephalitis. *Journal of Neurology, 262*, 1859–1866.

Zhu, S., & Paoletti, P. (2015). Allosteric modulators of NMDA receptors: Multiple sites and mechanisms. *Current Opinion in Pharmacology, 20*, 14–23.

Zoccarato, M., Saddi, M. V., Serra, G., Pelizza, M. F., Rosellini, I., Peddone, L., et al. (2013). Aquaporin-4 antibody neuromyelitis optica following anti-NMDA receptor encephalitis. *Journal of Neurology, 260*, 3185–3187.

FURTHER READING

Schäbitz, W. R., Rogalewski, A., Hagemeister, C., & Bien, C. G. (2014). VZV brainstem encephalitis triggers NMDA receptor immunoreaction. *Neurology*, *83*, 2309–2311.

Würdemann, T., Kersten, M., Tokay, T., Guli, X., Kober, M., Rohde, M., et al. (2016). Stereotactic injection of cerebrospinal fluid from anti-NMDA receptor encephalitis into rat dentate gyrus impairs NMDA receptor function. *Brain Research*, *1633*, 10–18.

CHAPTER TWELVE

Mu Opioid Pharmacology: 40 Years to the Promised Land

Gavril W. Pasternak[1]
Memorial Sloan Kettering Cancer Center, New York, NY, United States
[1]Corresponding author: e-mail address: pasterng@mskcc.org

Contents

Abstract

Opioids continue to play a major role in medicine, but not without problems. Side effects limit their utility medically, while the potential of addiction has had a major societal impact. Pharmacologists have been trying to develop opioids lacking side effects since the first derivative, heroin, was synthesized in the 1870s. The identification of opioid receptors about 40 years ago opened up new insights into our understanding of opioid action, fueled by the molecular biology revolution of the 1980s and 1990s. A major result of these studies was the discovery that the mu opioid receptor gene, *Oprm1*, undergoes extensive alternative splicing in mice, rats, and humans. This single gene generates three sets of proteins, each containing many variants. The object of this review is to describe these variants and how they can be targeted to generate safer, effective analgesic drugs. Mu opioid receptor multiplicity was first suggested over 35 years ago based upon a series of selective antagonists and detailed binding assays. The identification of the different classes of mu opioid receptor splice variants enabled us to target one of the classes of splice variants to obtain potent analgesics lacking respiratory depression, physical dependence, and reward behavior. They also displayed no

Advances in Pharmacology, Volume 82
ISSN 1054-3589
https://doi.org/10.1016/bs.apha.2017.09.006

cross tolerance to morphine analgesia and had diminished effects on gastrointestinal transit. Forty years after the identification of opioid-binding sites in brain the promised land of safer, nonaddictive analgesics is in sight.

ABBREVIATIONS

DAMGO [D-Ala^{2},MePhe^{4},Gly(ol)^{5}]enkephalin
DPDPE [D-Pen^{2},D-Pen^{5}]enkephalin
E1 exon 1
E11 exon 11
IBNtxA 3-iodobenzoyl-6β-naloxamide
KO knockout
MOR-1 cDNA clone encoding a mu opioid receptor
Oprm1 mu opioid receptor gene
TM transmembrane domain

1. INTRODUCTION

Opium, a combination of morphine, codeine, and other alkaloids, has been used for thousands of years. The clinical utility of opioids in the management of pain, dysentery, and cough cannot be denied. However, their use comes with potential problems, including respiratory depression, physical dependence, and addiction. For over a hundred years, scientists have attempted to design more potent, selective, and safer molecules. This started with heroin (3,6-diacetylmorphine), the first semisynthetic opioid agonist synthesized in the mid-1800s and then the antagonists *N*-allylnorcodeine and nalorphine in the early 1900s. Since then, thousands of analogs have been made in an effort to dissociate analgesia from the undesirable actions. The epoxymorphinan scaffold was the starting point, with many studies dismembering or extending it. Many clinically useful drugs resulted from these efforts, but none avoided the standard side effects or abuse liability of morphine. Even the totally synthetic analogs, such as methadone, meperidone, and the fentanyl series, retained all activities. However, recent work now suggests that safer, more effective analgesics may be possible.

Understanding the mechanisms of opioid action has long been a major goal. The strict structure–activity relationships from the vast number of opioid derivatives led to the concept of the opioid receptors (Portoghese, 1965), with investigators predicting the structure of the binding pocket long before its actual demonstration. Opioid receptors were among the first neurotransmitter receptors demonstrated biochemically (Hiller, Pearson, & Simon, 1973; Pert & Snyder, 1973; Terenius, 1973) and quickly led to the identification of the endogenous opioid peptide ligands, markedly expanding our appreciation of neuropeptides (Goldstein, Tachibana, Lowney, Hunkapiller, & Hood, 1979; Hughes et al., 1975; Li, Chung, & Doneen, 1976; Pasternak, Goodman, & Snyder, 1975; Pasternak, Wilson, & Snyder, 1975; Simantov & Snyder, 1976; Terenius & Wahlstrom, 1975). Three major families were identified, each with its precursor containing multiple copies of active peptides: the enkephalins, the dynorphins, and β-endorphin. While all are potent opioid analgesics, they act through their own set of receptors (Table 1). The enkephalins are the endogenous ligands for delta receptors and the dynorphins for the kappa ones. Mu receptors have high affinity for β-endorphin, which also labels delta receptors. The endomorphins, however, are amidated tetrapeptides that are highly mu selective. Finally, it has been reported that the brain also makes it own morphine (Boettcher, Fellermeier, Boettcher, Drager, & Zenk, 2005; Gintzler, Gershon, & Spector, 1978; Goldstein et al., 1985; Weitz, Lowney, Faull, Feistner, & Goldstein, 1986).

The differentiation of agonist/antagonist binding by sodium ions (i.e., the sodium effect) was first reported with opioid receptors (Pasternak & Snyder, 1975; Pert, Pasternak, & Snyder, 1973), an observation that has now been accepted as a generalized characteristic of G-protein-coupled receptors (GPCRs). The effects of pairs of structurally related ^{3}H-labeled agonists and antagonists confirmed the generality of the effect and led us to propose interchangeable receptor conformations that could be "pushed" into an antagonist state by sodium ions and counteracted by the divalent cations magnesium and manganese, but not calcium (Fig. 1; Pasternak, Snowman, & Snyder, 1975; Pasternak & Snyder, 1975; Pasternak, Wilson, et al., 1975; Wilson, Pasternak, & Snyder, 1975). Crystallographic studies have now identified the sodium ion-binding site within a GPCR (Liu et al., 2012), while modeling studies suggested a similar localization within the mu opioid receptor (Shang et al., 2014). The ability of divalent cations to stabilize the agonist receptor conformation, countering the sodium effect, was particularly intriguing, leaving open the question of where within the receptor the divalent ions bind.

The molecular biology revolution led to the cloning of the opioid receptors (Chen, Mestek, Liu, Hurley, & Yu, 1993; Evans, Keith, Morrison, Magendzo, & Edwards, 1992; Kieffer, Befort, Gaveriaux-Ruff, & Hirth, 1992; Minami et al., 1993; Reisine & Bell, 1993; Thompson, Mansour,

Table 1 Opioid Receptor Families

		Endogenous Ligand			
Receptor	**Gene**	**Peptide**	**Precursor**	**Drug**	**Antagonist**
Mu	Oprm1	β-Endorphin	Proopiomelanocortin	Morphine	β-Funaltrexamine
		Endomorphins 1 and 2	Not known	Methadone	Naloxonazine
				Oxycodone	CTOP
		Morphine (?)		DAMGO	
Delta	Oprd1	Met-enkephalin	Preproenkephalin	DPDPE	Naltrindole
		Leu-enkephalin			
Kappa	Oprk1	Dynorphin A	Preprodynorphin	U50,488H	Norbinaltorphimine
		Dynorphin B			JDtic
		α-Neoendorphin			

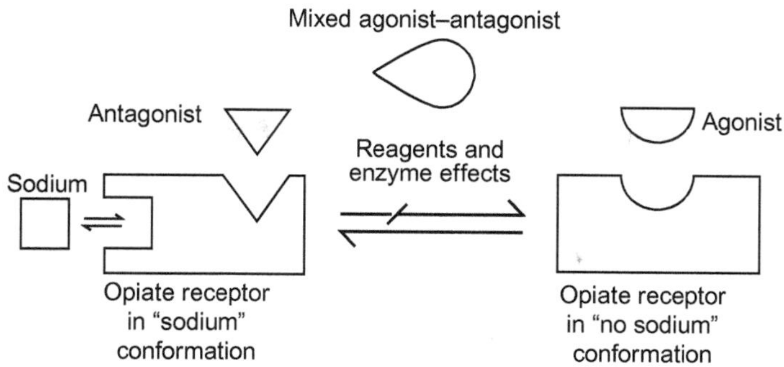

Fig. 1 Agonist–antagonist conformational changes implied by the sodium effect. The concept of interconvertible states of the mu opioid receptor modulated by sodium ions was first proposed in 1975. In addition to sodium ions, the divalent cations magnesium and manganese impacted the equilibrium between the states, as did various treatments such as protein-modifying regents and even selected enzyme digests. *From Pasternak, G. W., & Snyder, S. H. (1975). Identification of a novel high affinity opiate receptor binding in rat brain.* Nature, 253, *563–565.*

Akil, & Watson, 1993; Wang et al., 1993; Xie, Miyajima, & Goldstein, 1992), which in turn has provided extraordinary insights into their evolution and actions. They are members of the GPCR family, acting through inhibitory G-proteins. They have been crystallized in both active and inactive forms (Granier et al., 2012; Huang et al., 2015; Manglik et al., 2012; Thompson et al., 2012; Wu et al., 2012) and its transduction systems extensively studied (Bruchas & Roth, 2016). This review will integrate classical opioid pharmacology with our current understanding of opioid receptor function.

2. OVERVIEW OF OPIOID RECEPTORS

The opioid field illustrates the molecular transition of pharmacology over the past 40 years. Receptors that were first defined from classical pharmacological approaches using selective agonists/antagonists and binding assays are now defined genetically by their genes (Table 1). Early studies explored opioid actions in whole animals and bioassays and defined these receptors using various agonists and antagonists. Martin first suggested multiple classes of opioid receptors based upon the interactions of morphine and nalorphine in human subjects (Martin, 1967) and then extended the concept based upon studies in the dog (Gilbert & Martin, 1976). Today, there are three major classes of opioid receptors: mu, kappa, and delta (Table 1). The mu opioid receptors were demonstrated in binding assays in 1973

(Hiller et al., 1973; Pert & Snyder, 1973; Terenius, 1973) and the others soon followed. All three families of opioid receptors belong to the GPCR family and show marked structural homology to each other.

3. MU OPIOID RECEPTOR SUBTYPES

The initial studies attempting to demonstrate opioid-binding sites were limited by the low-specific activity of the radioligands which were insufficient to detect the very high-affinity and low-abundant sites (Goldstein, Lowney, & Pal, 1971). Higher specific activity ligands (>1–10 Ci/mmol) readily demonstrated binding sites with the appropriate high affinity for opioids corresponding to their potency, stereoselectivity, and presence in tissues known to be sensitive to opioids. These studies were greatly facilitated by the large library of ligands.

Soon afterward, a novel ultrahigh affinity site was reported (Pasternak & Snyder, 1975). The functional significance of these sites was facilitated by the synthesis of a set of antagonists, naloxonazine and naloxazone, that selectively targeted the sites both in vitro and in vivo (Hahn, Carroll-Buatti, & Pasternak, 1982; Pasternak, Childers, & Snyder, 1980a, 1980b; Pasternak & Hahn, 1980). These studies implicated the novel ultrahigh affinity site with morphine analgesia, but not respiratory depression, gastrointestinal motility, and some signs of physical dependence (Heyman, Williams, Burks, Mosberg, & Porreca, 1988; Ling, MacLeod, Lee, Lockhart, & Pasternak, 1984; Ling, Simantov, Clark, & Pasternak, 1986; Ling, Spiegel, Lockhart, & Pasternak, 1985; Pasternak et al., 1980a; Paul, Bodnar, Gistrak, & Pasternak, 1989; Paul & Pasternak, 1988). Although these early studies clearly implied the presence of mu opioid receptor subtypes (Wolozin & Pasternak, 1981), their dependence upon drug selectivity alone left many questions. The concept of multiple mu opioid receptors has now been validated at the genetic level, which revealed a complexity far beyond those initial suggestions.

4. MOLECULAR BIOLOGY OF MU OPIOID RECEPTORS

The mu opioid receptor MOR-1 was cloned in 1993 by several groups simultaneously and found to be derived from a single gene *Oprm1* (Chen et al., 1993; Thompson et al., 1993; Wang et al., 1993). It contained four exons that predicted the traditional 7 transmembrane domain (7TM) structure of GPCRs (Fig. 2). Exon 1 encoded the N-terminus and first transmembrane domain (TM1), while exons 2 and 3 each encoded TM2/3/4

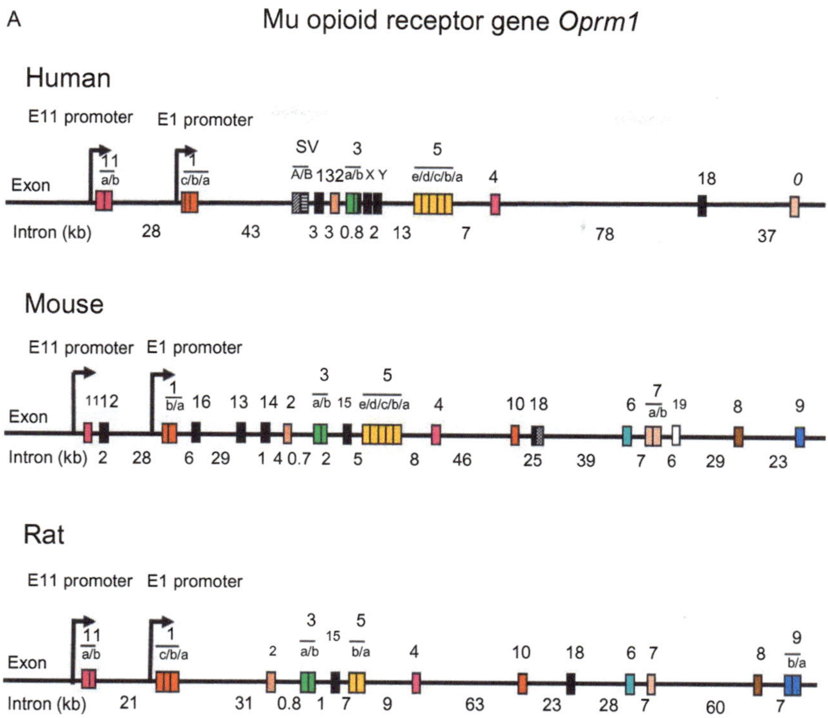

Fig. 2 *Oprm1* gene structure and splicing. (A) Oprm1 gene structure. (B) Alternative splicing of full-length variants of the mouse *Oprm1* gene. (C) Alternative splicing of truncated variants of the *Oprm1* gene. *From Pasternak, G. W., & Pan, Y.-X. (2013). Mu opioids and their receptors: Evolution of a concept.* Pharmacological Reviews, 65, *1257–1317.*

and TM5/6/7, respectively. Unlike the kappa and delta opioid receptors, the predominant mu receptor MOR-1 had a fourth exon that encoded 12 amino acids at the intracellular C-terminal. When expressed in cell lines, MOR-1 displayed the anticipated high affinity and selectivity predicted from brain membrane-binding studies. In situ hybridization studies confirmed expression in the brain that mimicked closely the distributions previously reported autoradiographically from ligand binding (Anton et al., 1994; Delfs, Yu, Reisine, & Chesselet, 1994; Grimm, Clock, & Cox, 1994; Mansour, Fox, Akil, & Watson, 1995; Mansour, Fox, Thompson, Akil, & Watson, 1994; Mansour, Watson, & Akil, 1995). Antisense models quickly confirmed the relevance of MOR-1 in morphine analgesia (Rossi, Brown, Leventhal, Yang, & Pasternak, 1996; Rossi et al., 1997; Rossi, Pan, Cheng, & Pasternak, 1994; Uhl, Childers, & Pasternak, 1994). Most

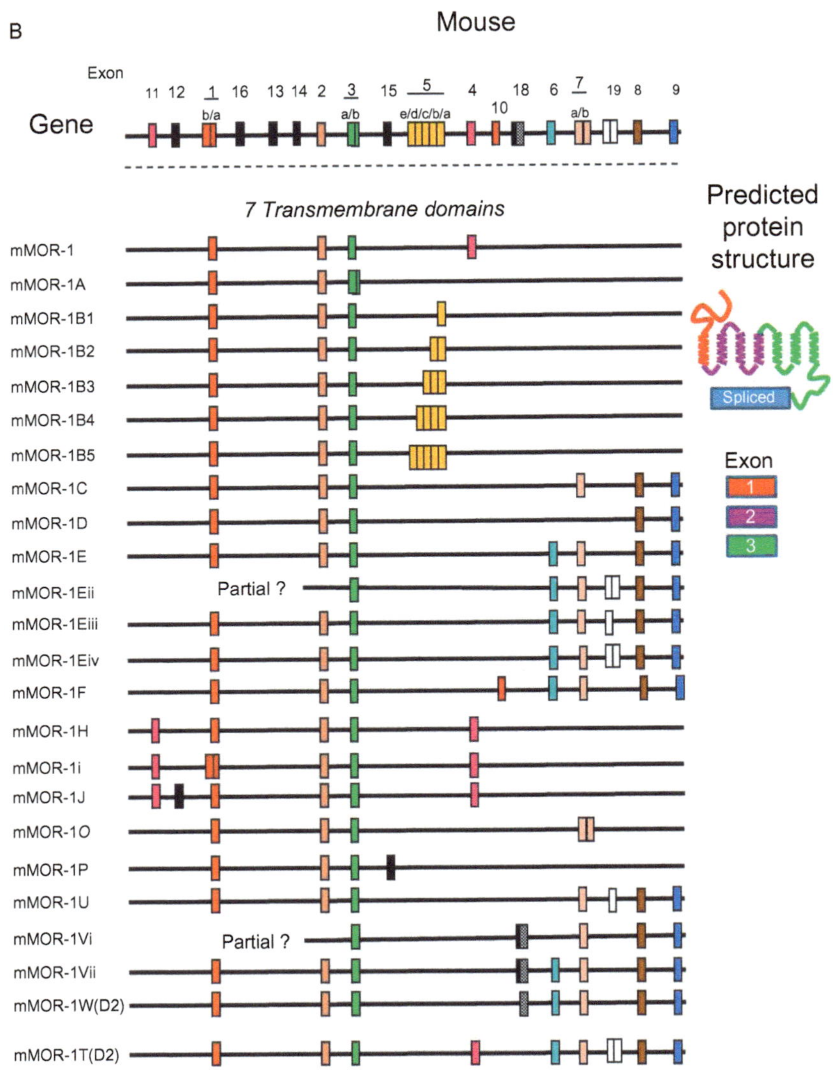

Fig. 2—Cont'd

important, elimination of MOR-1 in knockout models eliminated morphine analgesia, thereby establishing the importance of MOR-1 in morphine actions (Loh et al., 1998; Matthes et al., 1996; Rubinstein et al., 1996; Schuller et al., 1999; Sora et al., 1997).

Early on, there were suggestions that *Oprm1* expression might be complex, both functionally and at the genetic level. Antisense mapping using

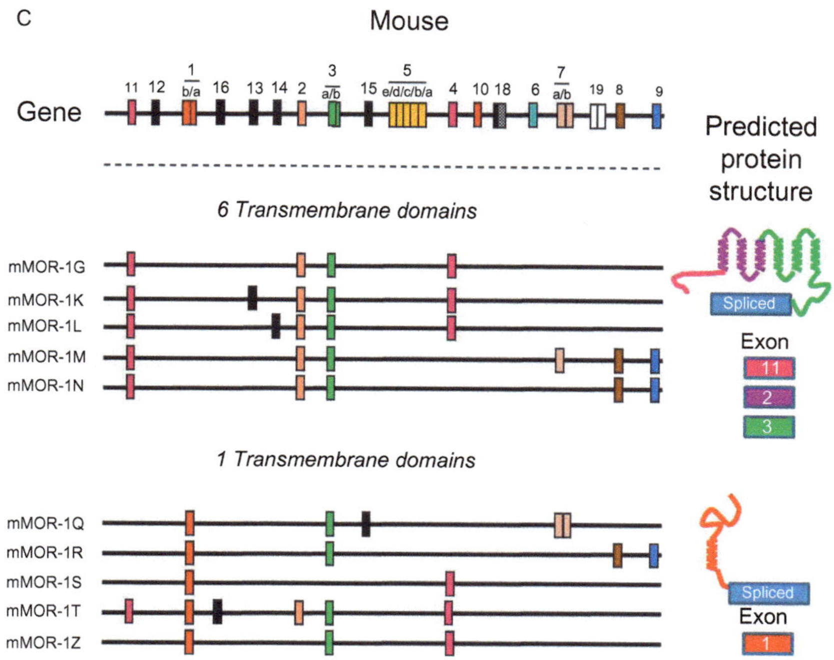

Fig. 2—Cont'd

antisense probes targeting different MOR-1 exons implied the importance of downregulating mRNA's containing exons 1 and 4 in morphine analgesia, but surprisingly targeting exon 2 or 3 had little effect. Conversely, the potent morphine metabolite morphine-6β-glucuronide was sensitive to the exons 2 and 3 probes, but not exon 1 or 4 (Rossi et al., 1996, 1997, 1994). Cloning studies identified two C-terminal splice variants of MOR-1, MOR-1A (Bare, Mansson, & Yang, 1994), and MOR-1B (Zimprich, Bacher, & Höllt, 1994). MOR-1A lacked exon 4, leading to a shortened protein, while in MOR-1B exon 4 was replaced by exon 5.

Subsequent studies from our group have established an extraordinary complexity to the *Oprm1* gene with similar splicing patterns for dozens of variants in humans, mice, and rats (Pasternak & Pan, 2013). *Oprm1* produces three classes of splice variants from two separate and distinct promoters (Fig. 2A). The traditional 7TM receptors associated with the exon 1 promoter comprise the largest group (Fig. 2B). Here, all the variants contain the same initial three exons (E1/2/3) that encode all transmembrane domains and the binding pocket, followed by distinct patters of alternative exons responsible for encoding the tip of the intracellular C-terminal. Another set of variants associated with the exon 1 promoter contain a single transmembrane domain encoded by exon 1 followed by different intracellular tails (Fig. 2C). Finally, the last set of *Oprm1* variants involve proteins generated through the exon 11 promoter, which is located approximately 30 kb upstream of exon 1 (Fig. 2C). (Note: The exon nomenclature was based upon the order of discovery, not the location on the gene.) This set of proteins is quite unusual in that they contain only 6 transmembrane domains due to skipping of exon 1. Their diversity results from both 3′ and 5′ splicing.

5. REGIONAL EXPRESSION OF *OPRM1* VARIANTS IN NAÏVE AND MORPHINE TOLERANT MICE

One initial concern regarding the splice variants was their apparent low expression levels in brain. When examined in whole brain, the abundance of MOR-1 far exceeds the other splice variants, leading to questions regarding the relevance of the others. However, a very different picture emerged when the comparisons were carried out in selected regions (Xu et al., 2015; Xu, Lu, et al., 2014). The distributions of the variants varied extensively among regions, with other 7TM splice variants predominating over MOR-1 in some (Table 2). The thalamus is associated with sensation, and opioid binding is very high in this region. Yet, when the individual variants were examined, mMOR-1 represented a very small percentage of full-length variants, with mMOR-1A and mMOR-1B1 corresponding to approximately 65% in naïve CD-1 mice. A similar situation existed in the hypothalamus. In the prefrontal cortex mMOR-1 represented a very small fraction of total 7TM expression, while the exon 7 variant mMOR-1O was approximately 40% of total 7TM expression with mMOR-1A1 (18%) and mMOR-1B1 (26%) accounting for most of the remainder. In contrast, mMOR-1 clearly predominated in the periaqueductal gray, brain stem, and spinal cord.

Early studies that failed to find major changes in *Oprm1* expression with morphine tolerance examined only MOR-1 itself after relatively short durations of morphine treatment, typically less than a week. Extending the treatment to 6 weeks had modest changes in *Oprm1* expression when we looked at whole brain (Table 3). However, select brain regions revealed dramatic changes. The greatest changes were in the striatum followed by the frontal cortex. The very modest increases in the remainder of the regions help to explain the limited increases in whole brain. In the striatum, mMOR-1D levels increased 150-fold after 6 weeks of morphine at 5 mg/kg, s.c. twice

Table 2 Estimated Levels of Selected Splice Variants as a Percentage of All Full-Length 7TM Variants in Various Brain Regions

	Percentage of the Total Full-Length 7TM Variant Levels									
	Prefrontal Cortex	**Striatum**	**Thalamus**	**Hypothalamus**	**Hippocampus**	**PAG**	**Brain Stem**	**Cerebellum**	**Spinal Cord**	**Whole Brain**
mMOR-1	<5	74	<5	<5	28	64	72	25	62	42
mMOR-1A	18	7	23	30	15	12	10	22	7	9
mMOR-1B1	26	6	41	25	<5	8	5	10	8	12
mMOR-1B4	12	<5	8	7	14	4	3	10	8	8
mMOR-1B5	5	<5	4	5	<5	<5	<5	<5	<5	<5
mMOR-1C	8	<5	6	7	3	3	3	5	5	6
mMOR-1O	41	<5	7	<5	31	<5	<5	15	<5	14

Levels of selected full-length 7TM splice variants were estimated from qPCR of the individual variants with the exception of mMOR-1. Since a specific qPCR set of primers was not available, mMOR-1 levels were determined by subtracting the levels of the other variants from the total 7TM expression to yield mMOR-1. Variants less than 5% in all regions were excluded from the table.

From Xu, J., Faskowitz, A. J., Rossi, G. C., Xu, M., Lu, Z., Pan, Y. X., et al. (2015). Stabilization of morphine tolerance with long-term dosing: Association with selective upregulation of mu-opioid receptor splice variant mRNAs. *Proceedings of the National Academy of Sciences of the United States of America, 112*, 279–284.

Table 3 Fold Change in mRNA Expression of *Oprm1* Variants Following Extended Morphine

	Prefrontal Cortex	Striatum	Thalamus	Hypothalamus	Hippocampus	PAG	Brain Stem	Cerebellum	Spinal Cord	Whole Brain
7TM										
E1-2	**21**	**18**	4	5	2	3	0	1	2	8
MOR-1A	**27**	**83**	4	2	5	5	1	1	3	5
MOR-1B1	11	**74**	4	3	14	8	1	1	1	3
MOR-1B2	7	**33**	3	3	11	7	0	1	1	3
MOR-1B3	10	**42**	6	3	1	6	0	1	1	6
MOR-1B4	10	**35**	11	5	1	10	1	1	1	3
MOR-1B5	13	**25**	4	3	5	5	0	2	1	4
MOR-1C	12	**45**	4	3	2	3	0	1	1	5
MOR-1D	10	**150**	7	7	3	11	0	1	3	7
MOR-1E	9	**29**	6	6	2	9	3	2	2	4
MOR-1F	3	**24**	6	2	4	4	1	3	5	4
MOR-1H	8	**52**	4	4	6	7	0	1	2	3
MOR-1i	6	**46**	2	2	5	5	0	0	1	2
MOR-1J	9	**56**	4	3	5	9	0	1	1	3

MOR-1O	6	**26**	6	6	1	4	2	6	1	2
MOR-1P	8	**26**	3	3	5	7	0	3	2	4
MOR-1U	8	**52**	4	2	3	7	0	1	1	3
MOR-1W	7	**46**	5	2	4	6	0	1	1	3
6TM										
MOR-1G	4	**9**	2	5	13	9	1	3	2	5
MOR-1M	5	**24**	3	4	4	8	1	3	1	5
MOR-1N	6	**32**	9	2	7	4	1	3	8	4
MOR-1K	4	**27**	7	9	1	4	0	1	1	2
MOR-1L	6	**43**	4	4	5	5	1	1	2	5
1TM										
MOR-1Q	3	1	2	3	3	4	1	4	3	4
MOR-1R	7	**44**	3	2	2	6	0	1	1	3
MOR-1S	11	**45**	5	10	1	7	2	2	2	14
MOR-1T	9	**14**	2	1	3	5	1	2	8	5
MOR-1Z	9	**41**	6	3	7	7	0.3	0.4	1	3

The abundance of the individual *Oprm1* variants was determined by qPCR and the ratio of the levels relative to naïve CD-1 mice determined and represented as the fold change in the levels of the specified variants following treatment with morphine (5 mg/kg twice a day) for 6 weeks. Results are the means of three independent determinations ±s.e.m. The numbers in bold are highly significant ($P < 0.0001$) as determined by two way ANOVA followed by Bonferroni's multiple comparisons test.

a day and over 300-fold when the morphine dose was increased to 40 mg/kg, s.c. The frontal cortex showed over a 20-fold increase in expression of all full-length receptors and of mMOR-A, with 10-fold elevations of a number of others. Thus, the regulation of *Oprm1* was region and variant specific.

The relative abundance of specific variants in various regions also changed with morphine treatment (Table 3). For example, in the striatum where mMOR-1 represented almost 75% of total full-length variants in naïve mice, its relative abundance fell to less than 30% after morphine treatment (Xu et al., 2015), reflecting a lower increase than other variants. It was particularly interesting that the expression of mMOR-1H, mMOR-1i, and mMOR-1J all increased by approximately 50-fold. While these three variants make the same protein as mMOR-1, their expression is under the control of the exon 11 promoter, illustrating the impact of morphine on both promoters. Finally, the increases in expression were not limited to the full-length variants. In the striatum many of the 6TM and 1TM variants were increased by as much as 50-fold.

6. FULL-LENGTH *OPRM1* SPLICE VARIANTS AND BIASED SIGNALING

The crystal structure of the mu opioid receptor revealed the standard 7 transmembrane domains and documented the binding pocket both in the antagonist (Manglik et al., 2012) and agonist conformations (Huang et al., 2015). All the full length, 7TM *Oprm1* splice variants share exons 1, 2, and 3, giving them all identical binding pockets (Fig. 3). With identical binding pockets, it would be expected that the variants would bind opioids with similar affinities and they do. However, functional assays reveal that the C-terminal sequence differences impact transduction. This was initially observed in assays assessing G-protein activation using ^{35}S-GTPγS binding (Bolan, Pasternak, & Pan, 2004; Pan, Xu, Bolan, et al., 2005; Pan et al., 2001; Pan, Xu, Yu, et al., 2005; Pasternak et al., 2004; Xu, Xu, et al., 2014; Xu, Xu, Hurd, Pasternak, & Pan, 2009). While the individual drugs showed similar receptor binding affinities for the variants in transfected cell lines, their EC_{50} and efficacy (i.e., maximal stimulation) varied significantly among the receptors. Furthermore, the activation patterns of the splice variants varied from drug to drug.

Initially, GPCR function was thought to be mediated through activation of G-proteins which then interacted with a range of downstream systems.

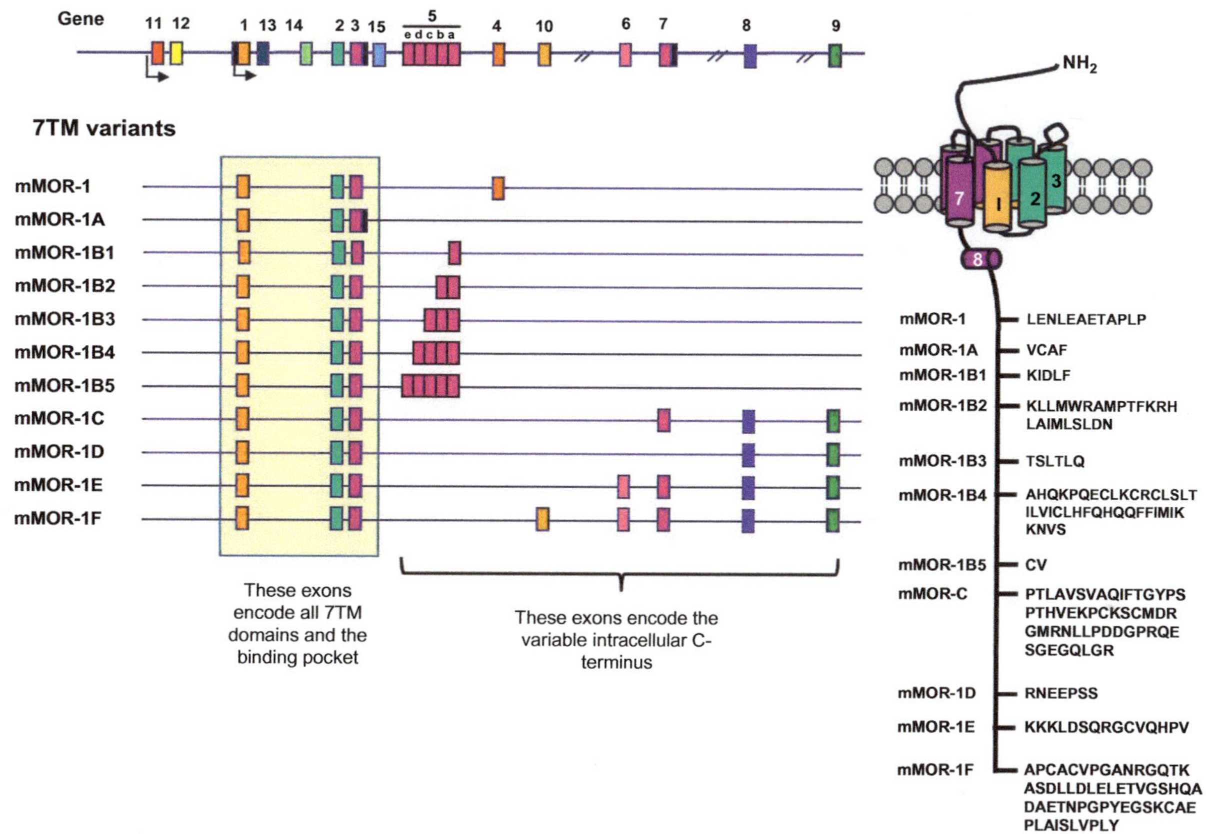

Fig. 3 C-terminal sequences. Schematic of selected mouse full-length 7TM and their C-terminal sequences.

An additional mechanism involves recruitment of β-arrestin, providing a different transduction pathway (Raehal, Schmid, Groer, & Bohn, 2011; Rankovic, Brust, & Bohn, 2016). Activation of one pathway is independent of the other, enabling drugs to show selectivity for G-protein activation or β-arrestin recruitment, a concept termed biased signaling. This is relevant to the opioids. Many of the side effects associated with morphine were attenuated in a β-arrestin knockout mouse, suggesting that G-protein-biased drugs would have advantages over current opioid analgesics (Bohn, Gainetdinov, Lin, Lefkowitz, & Caron, 2000; Bohn et al., 1999; Raehal, Walker, & Bohn, 2005). The recent development of TRV130, a G-biased opioid in clinical development, supports this concept (Dewire et al., 2013; Violin & Lefkowitz, 2007).

Like G-protein activation, β-arrestin2 recruitment among the different splice variants was variable (Fig. 4; Xu et al., 2017). When bias factors of various opioids for G-protein activation relative to β-arrestin2 recruitment were examined against a set of 7TM variants, we observed marked variability for individual opioids, indicating that the C-terminal splicing played an

Biased factor

Normalized to DAMGO at MOR-1

	MOR-1	MOR-1C	MOR-1O
DAMGO	1.0	−2.0	−10.2
Morphine	−1.5	−1.3	−5.0
Fentanyl	−4.4	−10.2	−44.3

Normalized to drug at variant

	MOR-1	MOR-1C	MOR-1O
DAMGO	1.0	−2.0	−10.2
Morphine	1.0	−1.2	−3.3
Fentanyl	1.0	−2.3	−10.0

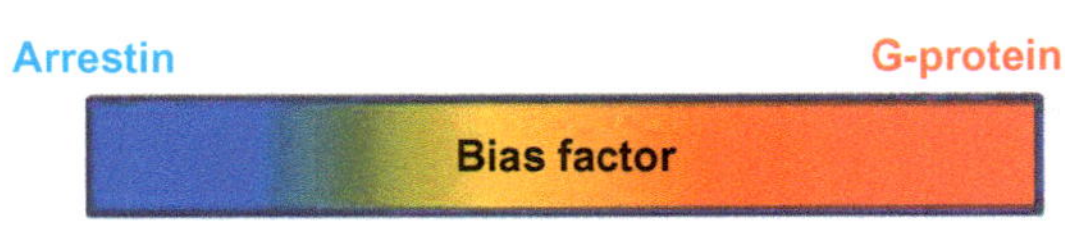

Fig. 4 Bias factors of various opioids for selected *Oprm1* full-length variants. Bias factors were determine based upon stimulation of ^{35}S-GTPγS binding and β-arrestin2 recruitment. *From Xu, J., Lu, Z., Narayan, A., Le Rouzic, V. P., Xu, M., Hunkele, A., et al. (2017). Alternatively spliced mu opioid receptor C termini impact the diverse actions of morphine.* The Journal of Clinical Investigation, 127, *1561–1573.*

important role in the functional characteristics of the drug. Bias factors showed different patterns among the splice variants for different drugs. It was particularly interesting to note that drugs commonly showed greater β-arrestin bias toward mMOR-1O than the other variants tested. Since opioids show similar binding affinities for the full-length 7TM splice variants, their in vivo pharmacological profile will reflect the summation of the simultaneous activation of all the 7TM variants. The transduction patterns that differ from drug to drug may lead to subtle, but important, differences in their overall actions and may contribute to the clinically observed differences among the opioids.

7. PHARMACOLOGICAL CHARACTERIZATION OF *OPRM1* SPLICE VARIANTS

Much of the evidence regarding the functional relevance of these receptors has come from in vivo approaches. All three sets of *Oprm1* splice variants are functionally active and relevant. Antisense knockdown provided many of the initial observations, but the most definitive results were obtained from sets of knockout (KO) mice (Table 4). A number of laboratories generated KO mice lacking traditional 7TM receptors by targeting different regions of the *Oprm1* gene, but the full extent of the disruption

Table 4 *Oprm1* Knockout Models

	Knockout Target		
	Exon 1[a]	**Exon 11[b]**	**Exons 1 and 11[c]**
Mu Receptor			
7TM	Lost	Retained	Lost
6TM	Retained	Lost	Lost
1TM	Lost	Retained	Lost
Analgesia			
Morphine	Lost	Retained	Lost
IBNtxA	Retained	Lost	Lost

[a]Schuller et al. (1999).
[b]Pan et al. (2009).
[c]Lu et al. (2015).
Summary of three knockout models used to classify opioid actions. A number of other knockout mice targeting the *Oprm1* gene have been generated. However, the extent of disruption with regards to the various classes of splice variants was not reported, making the interpretation of their pharmacology in the context of subtypes difficult.

of the *Oprm1* gene in most of these animals has not been fully defined (Kieffer, 1999; Loh et al., 1998; Matthes et al., 1996; Roy, Barke, & Loh, 1998; Schuller et al., 1999; Sora et al., 1997). Morphine analgesia was lost in all these mice, consistent with the importance of 7TM mu opioid receptors in morphine action. One model has proven quite informative (Schuller et al., 1999). This model targeted exon 1, selectively removing 7TM and 1TM variants and leaving expression of the exon 11-associated 6TM receptors intact. Like the others, this E1 KO mouse was insensitive to morphine analgesia. However, the retention of heroin and morphine-6β-glucuronide activity in the mice distinguished it from other models and raised the question of whether the 6TM variants may be involved.

Selectively removing the 6TM variants by targeting exon 11 provided additional insights into mu pharmacology (Pan et al., 2009). Although these animals lack 6TM variants, they still express 7TM and 1TM variants. Loss of 6TM variants did not affect morphine and methadone analgesia, which remained fully intact, although several other morphine actions were impacted. For example, morphine hyperalgesia and hyperlocomotion were both lost in the E11 KO (Marrone et al., 2017). Some opioids were sensitive to the loss of 6TM variants, best illustrated by buprenorphine, which lost all analgesic activity in the E11 KO mice (Grinnell et al., 2016).

A recent *Oprm1* knockout targeted both exons 1 and 11 (E1/E11 KO), eliminating all *Oprm1* expression (Lu et al., 2015). This is not necessarily the case with the earlier ones. Indeed, the initial MOR-1 KO generated by the Kieffer group (Matthes et al., 1996) disrupted the gene by inserting a neomycin cassette into exon 2. This mouse still expresses *Oprm1* transcripts and generates 1TM variants, which is not generally appreciated. A different model targeting exons 2 and 3 (Loh et al., 1998) presumably will also continue to produce 1TM variants, although this has not been examined directly. The E1 mouse produced by the Pintar group (Schuller et al., 1999) targeted exon 1 and its promoter, but left intact the E11 promoter, explaining the persistent expression of the 6TM variants. Another mouse targeting exon 1 (Sora et al., 1997) showed differences from the Pintar mouse, which might be explained by its larger deletion that extended further upstream and may have disrupted splicing overall. Unfortunately, a full description of *Oprm1* gene expression in this model has not been described. Thus, determining the potential involvement of a mu opioid receptor in a behavior is best carried out in a fully evaluated, complete knockout that lacks any Oprm1 expression, such as the E1/E11 KO mice (Fig. 5). The analgesic actions of morphine and other classical mu opioids are totally lost in the E1/E11 KO mice (Lu et al., 2015).

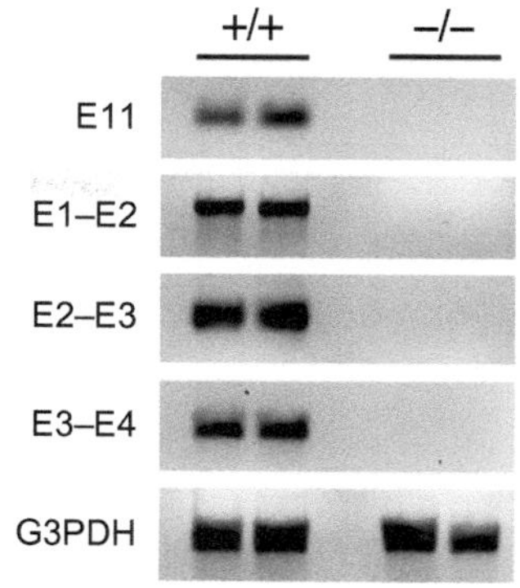

Fig. 5 mRNA expression levels in E1/E11 *Oprm1* knockout mice. mRNA levels were determined by qPCR of the full-length splice variants. Individual variants were assessed independently, with the exception of mMOR-1 for which no selective primers were available. Total expression of all 7TM variants was defined as the levels from the exons 2–3 primers since they were common to all. Levels of mMOR-1 expression were calculated by subtracting expression of all other 7TM variants from the total levels. *From Xu, J., Faskowitz, A. J., Rossi, G. C., Xu, M., Lu, Z., Pan, Y. X., et al. (2015). Stabilization of morphine tolerance with long-term dosing: Association with selective upregulation of mu-opioid receptor splice variant mRNAs.* Proceedings of the National Academy of Sciences of the United States of America, 112, *279–284.*

8. PHARMACOLOGICAL CHARACTERIZATION OF C-TERMINAL *OPRM1* SPLICE VARIANTS

One problem with the earlier KO mice was their focus upon 5′ splicing—i.e., exon 1-associated variants or exon 11-associated ones. They did not address the role of 3′ splicing of the C-terminal sequences. This is important with regards to their impact on signaling pathways and bias, as discussed earlier. We addressed this question by generating a novel set of genetically engineered mice (Fig. 6A; Xu et al., 2017). In these animals, we maintained the *Oprm1* gene architecture but inserted stop codons at the end of exon 3 in one mouse and at the beginning of exon 4 or the beginning of exon 7 in two others. These modifications resulted in truncations that were selective for the variants containing the specific exons. These mutations provided a means of exploring whether the spliced sequences downstream of exon 3 were pharmacologically relevant. However, it should be noted that these truncations were manifest in both full-length 7TM and in 6TM variants since the exons were shared by both.

The most interesting results were from the exons 4 and 7 truncations. Truncation of exon 4 facilitated morphine tolerance, while truncation of

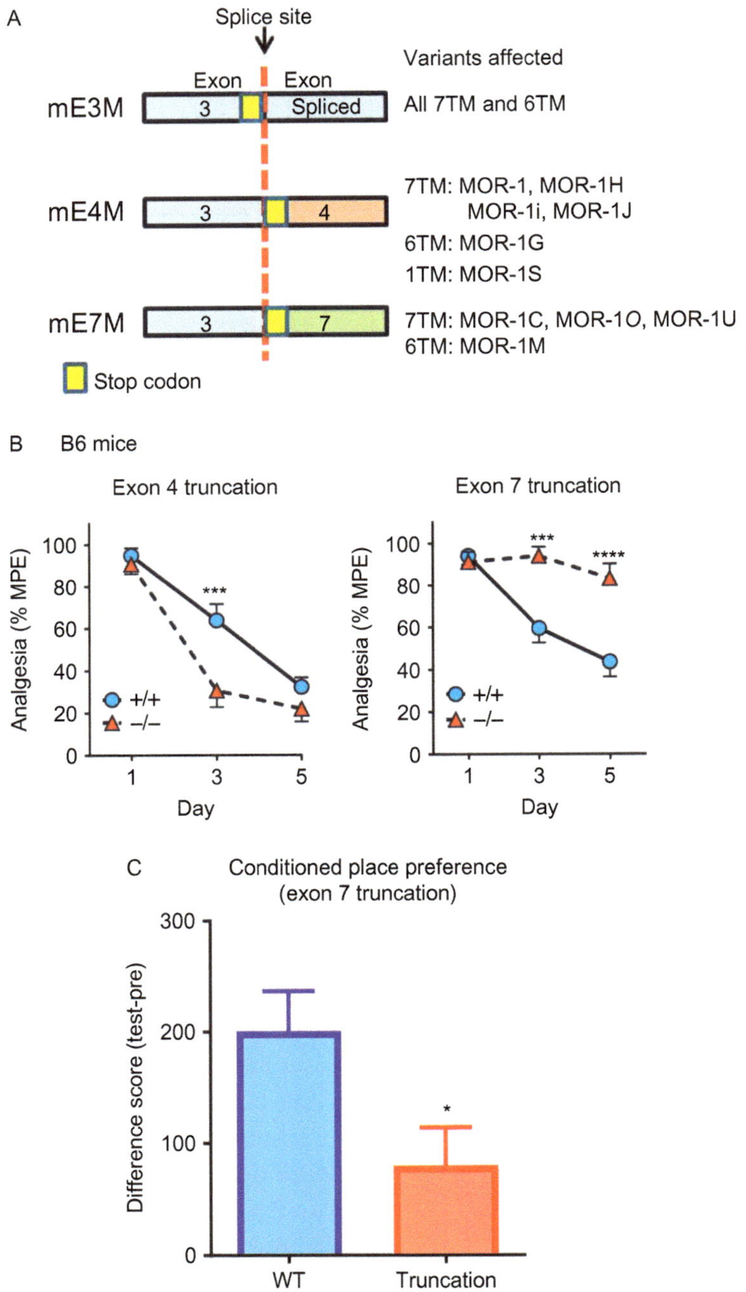

Fig. 6 Functional consequences of C-terminal truncated transgenic mice and morphine tolerance. (A) Schematic showing the location of the placement of the stop codons. (B) Effects of exons 4 and 7 truncations on morphine tolerance. (C) Effects of exon 4 truncation on conditioned place preference. *From Xu, J., Lu, Z., Narayan, A., Le Rouzic, V. P., Xu, M., Hunkele, A., et al. (2017). Alternatively spliced mu opioid receptor C termini impact the diverse actions of morphine.* The Journal of Clinical Investigation, 127, *1561–1573.*

exon 7 inhibited it (Fig. 6B). This implies that exon 4-containing variants minimize tolerance in wild-type mice, while exon 7 variants facilitate it. The exon 4 actions may be related to a specific protein sequence within exon 4 identified by von Zastrow that is responsible for trafficking the internalized receptor back to the cell surface, thereby replenishing surface receptor expression (Tanowitz, Hislop, & Von Zastrow, 2008). Conversely, the exon 7 variants may enhance due to their greater bias toward β-arrestin2 than the other variants, as shown by mMOR-1O (Fig. 4).

9. CHAPERONE EFFECTS OF 1TM VARIANTS

Single transmembrane *Oprm1* variants have been identified in mice, rats, and humans (Pasternak & Pan, 2013; Xu et al., 2013). While it is tempting to consider them aberrant and of no relevance, evidence now shows that they are pharmacologically important. Based upon gene structure, it is possible that as many as 10% of GPCRs may produce variants containing a single TM. In the opioid system, they result from skipping exon 2, leading to frameshifts and intracellular tails of different lengths with unique intracellular amino acid sequences downstream from the single transmembrane domain. With only a single transmembrane domain, it is highly unlikely that the protein is capable of binding ligands. However, when coexpressed, the 1TM variants increase expression of stably expressing traditional 7TM variants at the protein level without altering 7TM mRNA expression (Xu et al., 2013). In vitro studies revealed that the 1TM variants physically associate with the 7TM variants, stabilizing them in the membrane and thereby increasing their abundance. In vivo studies confirmed their functional significance. Selectively downregulating 1TM variants in vivo diminished morphine analgesia, implicating the protein in morphine function. Here, an antisense probe spanning the splice site between exons 1 and 4 to selectively downregulated expression of the 1TM variant mMOR-1S and diminished in morphine analgesia. Thus, the 1TM variants have a modulatory role on the actions of the 7TM variants.

10. 6TM AND IBNtxA PHARMACOLOGY

The 6TM variants represent a truncated class of receptor in which the first transmembrane domain present in the 7TM is missing due to exon skipping of exon 1. These variants are generated by the exon 11 promoter, which is located approximately 30 kb upstream of exon 1. (Note: Exons were named based upon their time of their identification and not by location on the gene.) As with the other classes, the 6TM variants also undergo 3′ splicing to yield variants with alternative C-terminal sequences. Our understanding of this group of variants has depended heavily upon a knockout mouse in which we targeted exon 11 to eliminate the 6TM variants (E11 KO) (Table 4; Pan et al., 2009) and IBNtxA (3-iodobenzoyl-6β-naltrexamide) (Lu et al., 2015; Majumdar et al., 2011, 2012; Wieskopf et al., 2014). While targeting exon 11 eliminated it and the 6TM variants, expression from the exon 1 promoter was minimally affected, leaving little change in the expression of the 7TM variant mRNAs or full-length mu receptor binding which explains why morphine and methadone analgesia was unaffected in this E11 KO.

The epoxymorphinan IBNtxA (3-iodobenzoyl-6β-naltrexamide) (Fig. 7) has a broad range of analgesic activity that is dependent upon 6TM variants (Table 5; Majumdar et al., 2011; Wieskopf et al., 2014). IBNtxA analgesia was lost in the E11 KO mouse, but it retained full analgesic activity in the E1 KO that still expressed 6TM variants. This residual analgesia was not due to cross labeling delta or kappa opioid receptors since IBNtxA still was active in a "tripe KO" mouse which was generated by crossing the E1 KO with a delta and kappa KO animal (Table 4). Thus, IBNtxA analgesia required 6TM variants and was independent of all the classical mu, delta, and kappa opioid receptors. This association between IBNtxA and 6TM variants was validated in a series of rescue studies (Lu et al., 2015). As expected, IBNtxA was inactive in E1/E11 KO mice. Reconstituting expression of the 6TM

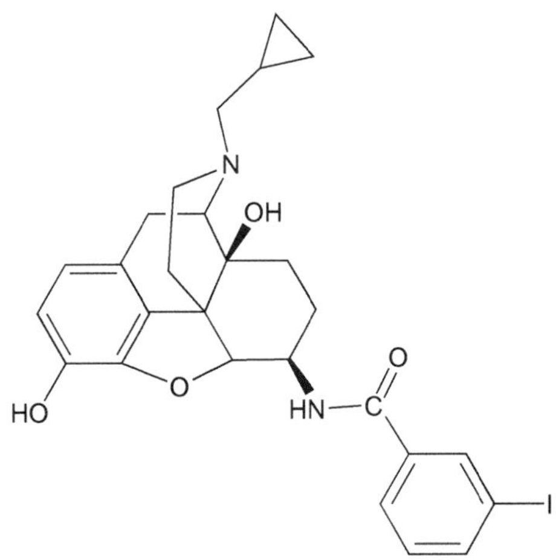

Fig. 7 IBNtxA.

Table 5 Analgesic Activity of IBNtxA

Assay	ED_{50} (mg/kg, s.c.)
Tail withdrawal (49°C)	0.78
Hot plate (54°C)	0.53
Paw withdrawal	0.27
Formalin (late phase)	0.32
Spared nerve injury (mechanical allodynia)	0.35
Complete Freunds adjuvant	0.35

Mice were administered IBNtxA and tested in the indicated assay. Results are from the literature (Wieskopf et al., 2014).

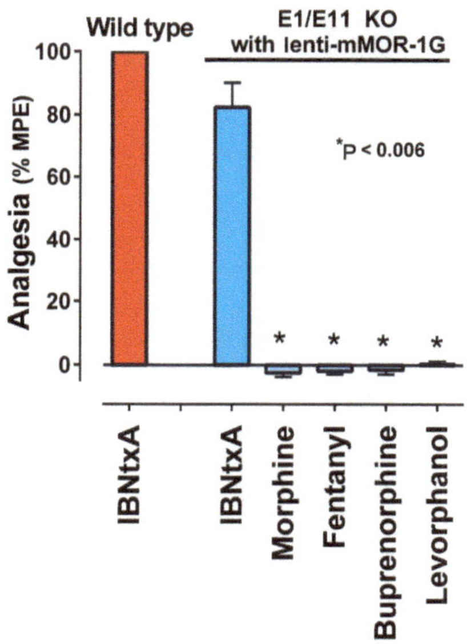

Fig. 8 Rescue of IBNtxA analgesia in an E1/E11 KO mouse. Lentivirus expressing the 6TM variant mMOR-1 were administered intrathecally into E1/E11 knockout mice, which were then tested for analgesia with the indicated opioid at least 6 weeks later. No analgesic responses were observed in controls injected with lentivirus lacking the mMOR-1. The response of IBNtxA in wild-type mice is shown on the far left for comparison. *From Lu, Z., Xu, J., Rossi, G. C., Majumdar, S., Pasternak, G. W., & Pan, Y. X. (2015). Mediation of opioid analgesia by a truncated 6-transmembrane GPCR.* The Journal of Clinical Investigation, 125, *2626–2630.*

variant mMOR-1G by lentiviral transfection into E1/E11 KO mice rescued IBNtxA analgesia, firmly establishing that 6TM variants were both necessary and sufficient for IBNtxA analgesia (Fig. 8).

The overall profile of IBNtxA was quite unusual (Fig. 9). As noted, it had wide spectrum of activity in a range of nociceptive assays. Equally important,

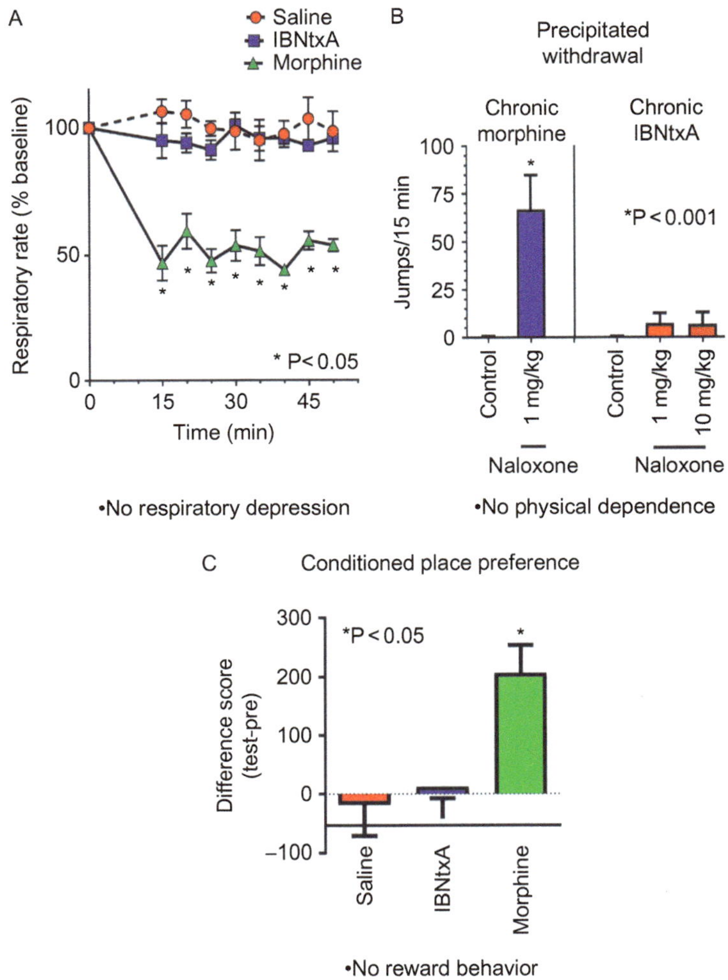

Fig. 9 Pharmacology of IBNtxA. IBNtxA actions in assays of (A) respiratory depression, as assessed by respiratory rate, (B) physical dependence, and (C) reward, as assessed with conditioned place preference. (A) Equianalgesic doses of morphine and IBNtxA (fivefold their respective ED_{50} values) were administered and respiratory rate monitored. In contrast to morphine, which significantly lowered respiratory rate at all time points after drug, IBNtxA was indistinguishable from saline. (B) Mice were administered equianalgesic doses of either morphine or IBNtxA chronically for 10 days and were then challenged with naloxone (morphine) or both naloxone and levallorphan (IBNtxA). Antagonist challenge induced marked jumping in the morphine animals but was without effect in the IBNtxA-treated mice. (C) Mice were assayed in a two-compartment conditioned place preference apparatus using equianalgesic doses of either morphine, IBNtxA, or saline. *From Majumdar, S., Grinnell, S., Le, R. V., Burgman, M., Polikar, L., Ansonoff, M., et al. (2011). Truncated G protein-coupled mu opioid receptor MOR-1 splice variants are targets for highly potent opioid analgesics lacking side effects.* Proceedings of the National Academy of Sciences of the United States of America, 108, *19776–19783.*

IBNtxA lacked respiratory depression at doses up to fivefold greater than its analgesic dose as well as reward behavior in the conditioned place preference paradigm and physical dependence following chronic administration, showing no signs of withdrawal with antagonist challenge. While it produced tolerance with repeated administration, it failed to show cross tolerance to morphine. Thus, compared to traditional opioids, IBNtxA is a potent analgesic with broader range of activity and a safer pharmacological profile.

11. CONCLUSION

The demonstration of opioid receptors a little over 40 years ago transformed neuropharmacology in many ways and gave new hope to the ultimate goal in opioid pharmacology, the development of safe, nonaddicting analgesics. It has been a journey. Much like the biblical story, it required a period of maturation and the appearance of a new generation of ideas and technologies that strengthened our ability to tackle the problem, led by the molecular biology revolution. The advances in the past decade have been transformative, with the elucidation of the structure of the receptors of both inactive and active conformations at the atomic level. It has seen the discovery of multitudes of receptors generated by splicing of the mu opioid receptor gene *Oprm1*, some with novel and unique structures that may provide insight into GPCR pharmacology in general. We now have the tools to truly address the goal of opioid research since the isolation of morphine by Serturner (1805). The concept of biased agonism and targeting novel *Oprm1* targets has provided major steps forward, giving confidence that we soon will reach the promised land.

CONFLICT OF INTEREST

G.W.P. reports no conflicts of interest in this research review. He consults with a number of pharmaceutical companies, but does not discuss any products or companies.

ACKNOWLEDGMENTS

The work described in this review was supported, in part, by grants from the National Institute on Drug Abuse (DA02615, DA07242, and DA06241), the Peter F. McManus Charitable Trust, and The Mayday Foundation to GWP and a core grant to MSKCC from the National Cancer Institute (CA08748).

REFERENCES

Anton, B., Husain, M., Kaufman, D., Stickney, E., Keith, D., Jr., Evans, C. J., et al. (1994). Localization of mu, delta and kappa opioid receptor mRNAs in human brain. *Regulatory Peptides*, *54*, 11–12.

Bare, L. A., Mansson, E., & Yang, D. (1994). Expression of two variants of the human μ opioid receptor mRNA in SK-N-SH cells and human brain. *FEBS Letters*, *354*, 213–216.

Boettcher, C., Fellermeier, M., Boettcher, C., Drager, B., & Zenk, M. H. (2005). How human neuroblastoma cells make morphine. *Proceedings of the National Academy of Sciences of the United States of America*, *102*, 8495–8500.

Bohn, L. M., Gainetdinov, R. R., Lin, F. T., Lefkowitz, R. J., & Caron, M. G. (2000). Mu-opioid receptor desensitization by beta-arrestin-2 determines morphine tolerance but not dependence. *Nature*, *408*, 720–723.

Bohn, L. M., Lefkowitz, R. J., Gainetdinov, R. R., Peppel, K., Caron, M. G., & Lin, F. T. (1999). Enhanced morphine analgesia in mice lacking β-arrestin 2. *Science*, *286*, 2495–2498.

Bolan, E. A., Pasternak, G. W., & Pan, Y.-X. (2004). Functional analysis of MOR-1 splice variants of the mu opioid receptor gene, *Oprm. Synapse*, *51*, 11–18.

Bruchas, M. R., & Roth, B. L. (2016). New technologies for elucidating opioid receptor function. *Trends in Pharmacological Sciences*, *37*, 279–289.

Chen, Y., Mestek, A., Liu, J., Hurley, J. A., & Yu, L. (1993). Molecular cloning and functional expression of a μ-opioid receptor from rat brain. *Molecular Pharmacology*, *44*, 8–12.

Delfs, J. M., Yu, L., Reisine, T., & Chesselet, M.-F. (1994). The distribution and regulation of mu opioid receptor mRNA in rat basal ganglia. *Regulatory Peptides*, *54*, 79–80.

Dewire, S. M., Yamashita, D. S., Rominger, D. H., Liu, G., Cowan, C. L., Graczyk, T. M., et al. (2013). A G protein-biased ligand at the mu-opioid receptor is potently analgesic with reduced gastrointestinal and respiratory dysfunction compared with morphine. *The Journal of Pharmacology and Experimental Therapeutics*, *344*, 708–717.

Evans, C. J., Keith, D. E., Jr., Morrison, H., Magendzo, K., & Edwards, R. H. (1992). Cloning of a delta opioid receptor by functional expression. *Science*, *258*, 1952–1955.

Gilbert, P. E., & Martin, W. R. (1976). The effects of morphine and nalorphine-like drugs in the nondependent, morphine-dependent and cyclazocine-dependent chronic spinal dog. *The Journal of Pharmacology and Experimental Therapeutics*, *198*, 66–82.

Gintzler, A. R., Gershon, M. D., & Spector, S. (1978). A nonpeptide morphine-like compound: Immunocytochemical localization in the mouse brain. *Science*, *199*, 447–448.

Goldstein, A., Barrett, R. W., James, I. F., Lowney, L. I., Weitz, C. J., Knipmeyer, L. L., et al. (1985). Morphine and other opiates from beef brain and adrenal. *Proceedings of the National Academy of Sciences of the United States of America*, *82*, 5203–5207.

Goldstein, A., Lowney, L. I., & Pal, B. K. (1971). Stereospecific and nonspecific interactions of the morphine congener levorphanol in subcellular fractions of mouse brain. *Proceedings of the National Academy of Sciences of the United States of America*, *68*, 1742–1747.

Goldstein, A., Tachibana, S., Lowney, L. I., Hunkapiller, M., & Hood, L. (1979). Dynorphin-(1-13), an extraordinarily potent opioid peptide. *Proceedings of the National Academy of Sciences of the United States of America*, *76*, 6666–6670.

Granier, S., Manglik, A., Kruse, A. C., Kobilka, T. S., Thian, F. S., Weis, W. I., et al. (2012). Structure of the delta-opioid receptor bound to naltrindole. *Nature*, *485*, 400–404.

Grimm, L. J., Clock, B. J., & Cox, B. M. (1994). Comparison of the distribution of mu and delta opiate receptor mRNAs in rat and mouse brain by in situ hybridization. *Regulatory Peptides*, *54*, 111–112.

Grinnell, S. G., Ansonoff, M., Marrone, G. F., Lu, Z., Narayan, A., Xu, J., et al. (2016). Mediation of buprenorphine analgesia by a combination of traditional and truncated mu opioid receptor splice variants. *Synapse, 70*, 395–407.

Hahn, E. F., Carroll-Buatti, M., & Pasternak, G. W. (1982). Irreversible opiate agonists and antagonists: The 14-hydroxydihydromorphinone azines. *The Journal of Neuroscience, 2*, 572–576.

Heyman, J. S., Williams, C. L., Burks, T. F., Mosberg, H. I., & Porreca, F. (1988). Dissociation of opioid antinociception and central gastrointestinal propulsion in the mouse: Studies with naloxonazine. *The Journal of Pharmacology and Experimental Therapeutics, 245*, 238–243.

Hiller, J. M., Pearson, J., & Simon, E. J. (1973). Distribution of stereospecific binding of the potent narcotic analgesic etorphine in the human brain: Predominance in the limbic system. *Research Communications in Chemical Pathology and Pharmacology, 6*, 1052–1062.

Huang, W., Manglik, A., Venkatakrishnan, A. J., Laeremans, T., Feinberg, E. N., Sanborn, A. L., et al. (2015). Structural insights into micro-opioid receptor activation. *Nature, 524*, 315–321.

Hughes, J., Smith, T. W., Kosterlitz, H. W., Fothergill, L. A., Morgan, B. A., & Morris, H. R. (1975). Identification of two related pentapeptides from the brain with potent opiate agonist activity. *Nature, 258*, 577–579.

Kieffer, B. L. (1999). Opioids: First lessons from knockout mice. *Trends in Pharmacological Sciences, 20*, 19–26.

Kieffer, B. L., Befort, K., Gaveriaux-Ruff, C., & Hirth, C. G. (1992). The δ-opioid receptor: Isolation of a cDNA by expression cloning and pharmacological characterization. *Proceedings of the National Academy of Sciences of the United States of America, 89*, 12048–12052.

Li, C. H., Chung, D., & Doneen, B. A. (1976). Isolation, characterization and opiate activity of beta-endorphin from human pituitary glands. *Biochemical and Biophysical Research Communications, 72*, 1542–1547.

Ling, G. S. F., MacLeod, J. M., Lee, S., Lockhart, S. H., & Pasternak, G. W. (1984). Separation of morphine analgesia from physical dependence. *Science, 226*, 462–464.

Ling, G. S. F., Simantov, R., Clark, J. A., & Pasternak, G. W. (1986). Naloxonazine actions in vivo. *European Journal of Pharmacology, 129*, 33–38.

Ling, G. S. F., Spiegel, K., Lockhart, S. H., & Pasternak, G. W. (1985). Separation of opioid analgesia from respiratory depression: Evidence for different receptor mechanisms. *The Journal of Pharmacology and Experimental Therapeutics, 232*, 149–155.

Liu, W., Chun, E., Thompson, A., Chubukov, P., Xu, F., Katritch, V., et al. (2012). Structural basis for allosteric regulation of GPCRs by sodium ions. *Science, 337*, 232–236.

Loh, H. H., Liu, H. C., Cavalli, A., Yang, W. L., Chen, Y. F., & Wei, L. N. (1998). Mu opioid receptor knockout in mice: Effects on ligand-induced analgesia and morphine lethality. *Molecular Brain Research, 54*, 321–326.

Lu, Z., Xu, J., Rossi, G. C., Majumdar, S., Pasternak, G. W., & Pan, Y. X. (2015). Mediation of opioid analgesia by a truncated 6-transmembrane GPCR. *The Journal of Clinical Investigation, 125*, 2626–2630.

Majumdar, S., Grinnell, S., Le, R. V., Burgman, M., Polikar, L., Ansonoff, M., et al. (2011). Truncated G protein-coupled mu opioid receptor MOR-1 splice variants are targets for highly potent opioid analgesics lacking side effects. *Proceedings of the National Academy of Sciences of the United States of America, 108*, 19776–19783.

Majumdar, S., Subrath, J., Le Rouzic, V., Polikar, L., Burgman, M., Nagakura, K., et al. (2012). Synthesis and evaluation of aryl-naloxamide opiate analgesics targeting truncated exon 11-associated mu opioid receptor (MOR-1) splice variants. *Journal of Medicinal Chemistry, 55*, 6352–6362.

Manglik, A., Kruse, A. C., Kobilka, T. S., Thian, F. S., Mathiesen, J. M., Sunahara, R. K., et al. (2012). Crystal structure of the mu-opioid receptor bound to a morphinan antagonist. *Nature*, *485*, 321–326.

Mansour, A., Fox, C. A., Akil, H., & Watson, S. J. (1995). Opioid-receptor mRNA expression in the rat CNS: Anatomical and functional implications. *Trends in Neurosciences*, *18*, 22–29.

Mansour, A., Fox, C. A., Thompson, R. C., Akil, H., & Watson, S. J. (1994). μ-Opioid receptor mRNA expression in the rat CNS: Comparison to μ-receptor binding. *Brain Research*, *643*, 245–265.

Mansour, A., Watson, S. J., & Akil, H. (1995). Opioid receptors: Past, present and future. *Trends in Neurosciences*, *18*, 69–70.

Marrone, G. F., Le Rouzic, V., Varadi, A., Xu, J., Rajadhyaksha, A. M., Majumdar, S., et al. (2017). Genetic dissociation of morphine analgesia from hyperalgesia in mice. *Psychopharmacology (Berl)*, *234*, 1891–1900.

Martin, W. R. (1967). Opioid antagonists. *Pharmacological Reviews*, *19*, 463–521.

Matthes, H. W., Maldonado, R., Simonin, F., Valverde, O., Slowe, S., Kitchen, I., et al. (1996). Loss of morphine-induced analgesia, reward effect and withdrawal symptoms in mice lacking the μ-opioid-receptor gene. *Nature*, *383*, 819–823.

Minami, M., Toya, T., Katao, Y., Maekawa, K., Nakamura, S., Onogi, T., et al. (1993). Cloning and expression of a cDNA for the rat kappa-opioid receptor. *FEBS Letters*, *329*, 291–295.

Pan, Y. X., Xu, J., Bolan, E., Moskowitz, H. S., Xu, M., & Pasternak, G. W. (2005). Identification of four novel exon 5 splice variants of the mouse mu-opioid receptor gene: Functional consequences of C-terminal splicing. *Molecular Pharmacology*, *68*, 866–875.

Pan, Y.-X., Xu, J., Mahurter, L., Bolan, E. A., Xu, M. M., & Pasternak, G. W. (2001). Generation of the mu opioid receptor (MOR-1) protein by three new splice variants of the *Oprm* gene. *Proceedings of the National Academy of Sciences of the United States of America*, *98*, 14084–14089.

Pan, Y. X., Xu, J., Xu, M., Rossi, G. C., Matulonis, J. E., & Pasternak, G. W. (2009). Involvement of exon 11-associated variants of the mu opioid receptor MOR-1 in heroin, but not morphine, actions. *Proceedings of the National Academy of Sciences of the United States of America*, *106*, 4917–4922.

Pan, L., Xu, J., Yu, R., MM, X., Pan, Y. X., & Pasternak, G. W. (2005). Identification and characterization of six new alternatively spliced variants of the human mu opioid receptor gene, Oprm. *Neuroscience*, *133*, 209–220.

Pasternak, G. W., Childers, S. R., & Snyder, S. H. (1980a). Naloxazone, a long-acting opiate antagonist: Effects on analgesia in intact animals and on opiate receptor binding in vitro. *The Journal of Pharmacology and Experimental Therapeutics*, *214*, 455–462.

Pasternak, G. W., Childers, S. R., & Snyder, S. H. (1980b). Opiate analgesia: Evidence for mediation by a subpopulation of opiate receptors. *Science*, *208*, 514–516.

Pasternak, G. W., Goodman, R., & Snyder, S. H. (1975). An endogenous morphine like factor in mammalian brain. *Life Sciences*, *16*, 1765–1769.

Pasternak, G. W., & Hahn, E. F. (1980). Long-acting opiate agonists and antagonists: 14-Hydroxydihydromorphinone hydrazones. *Journal of Medicinal Chemistry*, *23*, 674–677.

Pasternak, G. W., & Pan, Y.-X. (2013). Mu opioids and their receptors: Evolution of a concept. *Pharmacological Reviews*, *65*, 1257–1317.

Pasternak, D. A., Pan, L., Xu, J., Yu, R., Xu, M. M., Pasternak, G. W., et al. (2004). Identification of three new alternatively spliced variants of the rat mu opioid receptor gene: Dissociation of affinity and efficacy. *Journal of Neurochemistry*, *91*, 881–890.

Pasternak, G. W., Snowman, A. S., & Snyder, S. H. (1975). Selective enhancement of [^{3}H] opiate agonist binding by divalent cations. *Molecular Pharmacology*, *11*, 478–484.

Pasternak, G. W., & Snyder, S. H. (1975). Identification of a novel high affinity opiate receptor binding in rat brain. *Nature*, *253*, 563–565.

Pasternak, G. W., Wilson, H. A., & Snyder, S. H. (1975). Differential effects of protein-modifying reagents on receptor binding of opiate agonists and antagonists. *Molecular Pharmacology*, *11*, 340–351.

Paul, D., Bodnar, R. J., Gistrak, M. A., & Pasternak, G. W. (1989). Different μ receptor subtypes mediate spinal and supraspinal analgesia in mice. *European Journal of Pharmacology*, *168*, 307–314.

Paul, D., & Pasternak, G. W. (1988). Differential blockade by naloxonazine of two μ opiate actions: Analgesia and inhibition of gastrointestinal transit. *European Journal of Pharmacology*, *149*, 403–404.

Pert, C. B., Pasternak, G. W., & Snyder, S. H. (1973). Opiate agonists and antagonists discriminated by receptor binding in brain. *Science*, *182*, 1359–1361.

Pert, C. B., & Snyder, S. H. (1973). Opiate receptor: Demonstration in nervous tissue. *Science*, *179*, 1011–1014.

Portoghese, P. S. (1965). A new concept on the mode of interaction of narcotic analgesics with receptors. *Journal of Medicinal Chemistry*, *8*, 609–616.

Raehal, K. M., Schmid, C. L., Groer, C. E., & Bohn, L. M. (2011). Functional selectivity at the mu-opioid receptor: Implications for understanding opioid analgesia and tolerance. *Pharmacological Reviews*, *63*, 1001–1019.

Raehal, K. M., Walker, J. K., & Bohn, L. M. (2005). Morphine side effects in beta-arrestin 2 knockout mice. *The Journal of Pharmacology and Experimental Therapeutics*, *314*, 1195–1201.

Rankovic, Z., Brust, T. F., & Bohn, L. M. (2016). Biased agonism: An emerging paradigm in GPCR drug discovery. *Bioorganic & Medicinal Chemistry Letters*, *26*, 241–250.

Reisine, T., & Bell, G. I. (1993). Molecular biology of opioid receptors. *Trends in Neurosciences*, *16*, 506–510.

Rossi, G. C., Brown, G. P., Leventhal, L., Yang, K., & Pasternak, G. W. (1996). Novel receptor mechanisms for heroin and morphine-6β-glucuronide analgesia. *Neuroscience Letters*, *216*, 1–4.

Rossi, G. C., Leventhal, L., Pan, Y. X., Cole, J., Su, W., Bodnar, R. J., et al. (1997). Antisense mapping of MOR-1 in rats: Distinguishing between morphine and morphine-6beta-glucuronide antinociception. *The Journal of Pharmacology and Experimental Therapeutics*, *281*, 109–114.

Rossi, G. C., Pan, Y.-X., Cheng, J., & Pasternak, G. W. (1994). Blockade of morphine analgesia by an antisense oligodeoxynucleotide against the mu receptor. *Life Sciences*, *54*, L375–L379.

Roy, S., Barke, R. A., & Loh, H. H. (1998). MU-opioid receptor-knockout mice: Role of μ-opioid receptor in morphine mediated immune functions. *Molecular Brain Research*, *61*, 190–194.

Rubinstein, M., Mogil, J. S., Japón, M., Chan, E. C., Allen, R. G., & Low, M. J. (1996). Absence of opioid stress-induced analgesia in mice lacking β-endorphin by site-directed mutagenesis. *Proceedings of the National Academy of Sciences of the United States of America*, *93*, 3995–4000.

Schuller, A. G., King, M. A., Zhang, J., Bolan, E., Pan, Y. X., Morgan, D. J., et al. (1999). Retention of heroin and morphine-6 beta-glucuronide analgesia in a new line of mice lacking exon 1 of MOR-1. *Nature Neuroscience*, *2*, 151–156.

Serturner, F. W. A. (1805). *Trommsdorff's Journal der Pharmacie*, *13*, 229–235.

Shang, Y., LeRouzic, V., Schneider, S., Bisignano, P., Pasternak, G. W., & Filizola, M. (2014). Mechanistic insights into the allosteric modulation of opioid receptors by sodium ions. *Biochemistry*, *53*, 5140–5149.

Simantov, R., & Snyder, S. H. (1976). Isolation and structure identification of a morphine-like peptide "enkephalin" in bovine brain. *Life Sciences*, *18*, 781–788.

Sora, I., Takahashi, N., Funada, M., Ujike, H., Revay, R. S., Donovan, D. M., et al. (1997). Opiate receptor knockout mice define μ receptor roles in endogenous nociceptive responses and morphine-induced analgesia. *Proceedings of the National Academy of Sciences of the United States of America*, *94*, 1544–1549.

Tanowitz, M., Hislop, J. N., & Von Zastrow, M. (2008). Alternative splicing determines the post-endocytic sorting fate of G-protein-coupled receptors. *The Journal of Biological Chemistry*, *283*, 35614–35621.

Terenius, L. (1973). Stereospecific interaction between narcotic analgesics and a synaptic plasma membrane fraction of rat cerebral cortex. *Acta Pharmacologica et Toxicologica*, *32*, 317–320.

Terenius, L., & Wahlstrom, A. (1975). Search for an endogenous ligand for the opiate receptor. *Acta Physiologica Scandinavica*, *94*, 74–81.

Thompson, A. A., Liu, W., Chun, E., Katritch, V., Wu, H., Vardy, E., et al. (2012). Structure of the nociceptin/orphanin FQ receptor in complex with a peptide mimetic. *Nature*, *485*, 395–399.

Thompson, R. C., Mansour, A., Akil, H., & Watson, S. J. (1993). Cloning and pharmacological characterization of a rat μ opioid receptor. *Neuron*, *11*, 903–913.

Uhl, G. R., Childers, S., & Pasternak, G. W. (1994). An opiate-receptor gene family reunion. *Trends in Neurosciences*, *17*, 89–93.

Violin, J. D., & Lefkowitz, R. J. (2007). Beta-arrestin-biased ligands at seven-transmembrane receptors. *Trends in Pharmacological Sciences*, *28*, 416–422.

Wang, J. B., Imai, Y., Eppler, C. M., Gregor, P., Spivak, C. E., & Uhl, G. R. (1993). μ Opiate receptor: cDNA cloning and expression. *Proceedings of the National Academy of Sciences of the United States of America*, *90*, 10230–10234.

Weitz, C. J., Lowney, L. I., Faull, K. F., Feistner, G., & Goldstein, A. (1986). Morphine and codeine from mammalian brain. *Proceedings of the National Academy of Sciences of the United States of America*, *83*, 9784–9788.

Wieskopf, J. S., Pan, Y. X., Marcovitz, J., Tuttle, A. H., Majumdar, S., Pidakala, J., et al. (2014). Broad-spectrum analgesic efficacy of IBNtxA is mediated by exon 11-associated splice variants of the mu-opioid receptor gene. *Pain*, *155*, 2063–2070.

Wilson, H. A., Pasternak, G. W., & Snyder, S. H. (1975). Differentiation of opiate agonist and antagonist receptor binding by protein modifying reagents. *Nature*, *253*, 448–450.

Wolozin, B. L., & Pasternak, G. W. (1981). Classification of multiple morphine and enkephalin binding sites in the central nervous system. *Proceedings of the National Academy of Sciences of the United States of America*, *78*, 6181–6185.

Wu, H., Wacker, D., Mileni, M., Katritch, V., Han, G. W., Vardy, E., et al. (2012). Structure of the human kappa-opioid receptor in complex with JDTic. *Nature*, *485*, 327–332.

Xie, G.-X., Miyajima, A., & Goldstein, A. (1992). Expression cloning of cDNA encoding a seven-helix receptor from human placenta with affinity for opioid ligands. *Proceedings of the National Academy of Sciences of the United States of America*, *89*, 4124–4128.

Xu, J., Faskowitz, A. J., Rossi, G. C., Xu, M., Lu, Z., Pan, Y. X., et al. (2015). Stabilization of morphine tolerance with long-term dosing: Association with selective upregulation of mu-opioid receptor splice variant mRNAs. *Proceedings of the National Academy of Sciences of the United States of America*, *112*, 279–284.

Xu, J., Lu, Z., Narayan, A., Le Rouzic, V. P., Xu, M., Hunkele, A., et al. (2017). Alternatively spliced mu opioid receptor C termini impact the diverse actions of morphine. *The Journal of Clinical Investigation*, *127*, 1561–1573.

Xu, J., Lu, Z., Xu, M., Rossi, G. C., Kest, B., Waxman, A. R., et al. (2014). Differential expressions of the alternatively spliced variant mRNAs of the mu opioid receptor gene, OPRM1, in brain regions of four inbred mouse strains. *PLoS One*, *9*, e111267.

Xu, J., Xu, M., Bolan, E., Gilbert, A. K., Pasternak, G. W., & Pan, Y. X. (2014). Isolating and characterizing three alternatively spliced mu opioid receptor variants: mMOR-1A, mMOR-1O, and mMOR-1P. *Synapse*, *68*, 144–152.

Xu, J., Xu, M., Brown, T., Rossi, G. C., Hurd, Y. L., Inturrisi, C. E., et al. (2013). Stabilization of the mu opioid receptor by truncated single transmembrane splice variants through a chaperone-like action. *The Journal of Biological Chemistry*, *288*, 21211–21227.

Xu, J., Xu, M., Hurd, Y. L., Pasternak, G. W., & Pan, Y. X. (2009). Isolation and characterization of new exon 11-associated N-terminal splice variants of the human mu opioid receptor gene. *Journal of Neurochemistry*, *108*, 962–972.

Zimprich, A., Bacher, B., & Höllt, V. (1994). Cloning and expression of an isoform of the rmu-opioid receptor (rmuOR1B). *Regulatory Peptides*, *54*, 347–348.

CHAPTER THIRTEEN

Synaptotoxic Signaling by Amyloid Beta Oligomers in Alzheimer's Disease Through Prion Protein and mGluR5

A. Harrison Brody*,†, Stephen M. Strittmatter*,†,1
*Program in Cellular Neuroscience, Neurodegeneration & Repair, Yale University School of Medicine, New Haven, CT, United States
†Yale University, New Haven, CT, United States
[1]Corresponding author: e-mail address: stephen.strittmatter@yale.edu

Contents

Abstract

Alzheimer's disease (AD) represents an impending global health crisis, yet the complexity of AD pathophysiology has so far precluded the development of any interventions to successfully slow or halt AD progression. It is clear that accumulation of Amyloid-beta (Aβ) peptide triggers progressive synapse loss to cause AD symptoms. Once initiated by Aβ, disease progression is complicated and accelerated by inflammation and by tau pathology. The recognition that Aβ peptide assumes multiple distinct states and that soluble oligomeric species (Aβo) are critical for synaptic damage is central to molecular

Advances in Pharmacology, Volume 82
ISSN 1054-3589
https://doi.org/10.1016/bs.apha.2017.09.007

understanding of AD. This knowledge has led to the identification of specific Aβo receptors, such as cellular prion protein (PrP^C), mediating synaptic toxicity and neuronal dysfunction. The identification of PrP^C as an Aβo receptor has illuminated an Aβo-induced signaling cascade involving mGluR5, Fyn, and Pyk2 that links Aβ and tau pathologies. This pathway provides novel potential therapeutic targets for disease-modifying AD therapy. Here, we discuss the methods by which several putative Aβo receptors were identified. We also offer an in-depth examination of the known molecular mechanisms believed to mediate Aβo-induced synaptic dysfunction, toxicity, and memory dysfunction.

ABBREVIATIONS

3×Tg	triple transgenic
Aβ	amyloid beta
AD	Alzheimer's disease
ADNI	Alzheimer's Disease Neuroimaging Initiative
AMPA	α-amino-3-hydroxy-5-methyl-4-isoxazolepropionic acid
AMPAR	α-amino-3-hydroxy-5-methyl-4-isoxazolepropionic acid receptor
APP	amyloid precursor protein
CamKII	Ca2+/calmodulin-dependent protein kinase II
CNS	central nervous system
CSF	cerebrospinal fluid
DHPG	(*S*)-3,5-dihydroxyphenylglycine
EGFR	epidermal growth factor receptor
ERK2	extracellular signal-regulated kinase 2
FcγRIIB	Fc gamma receptor IIB
GPI	glycosylphosphatidylinositol
HEK293T	human embryonic kidney cells 293 with SV40 large T antigen
IR	insulin receptor
LGI1	leucine-rich, glioma-inactivated 1
LilRB2	leukocyte immunoglobulin-like receptor B2
LOAD	late-onset Alzheimer's disease
LTD	long-term depression
LTP	long-term potentiation
MAG	myelin-associated glycoprotein
mGluR5	metabotropic glutamate receptor 5
MHC	major histocompatibility complex
MLA	recombinant histone H3K79me3
MPEP	2-methyl-6-(phenylethynyl)pyridine
MPMQ	6-methoxy-*N*-(4-methoxyphenyl)-4-quinazolinamine
MTEP	3-((2-methyl-4-thiazolyl)ethynyl)pyridine
NFT	neurofibrillary tangle
NgR1	Nogo receptor 1
NMDA	*N*-methyl-D-aspartate
NMDAR	*N*-methyl-D-aspartate receptor
NR2B	*N*-methyl D-aspartate receptor subtype 2B

PET	positron emission tomography
PGRN	progranulin
PP2B	protein phosphatase 2B
PrP^C	cellular prion protein
PS1	presenilin 1
PS2	presenilin 2
PSD	postsynaptic density
PSD-95	postsynaptic density protein 95
Pyk2	protein tyrosine kinase 2
RAGE	receptor for advanced glycation end products
RGM	repulsive guidance molecule A
SAM	silent allosteric modulator
STEP	striatally enriched phosphatase
α7nAChR α7	nicotinic acetylcholine receptor
σ2R/PGRMC1	sigma 2 receptor/progesterone receptor membrane component 1

1. INTRODUCTION

Alzheimer's disease (AD) is the most common cause of dementia and the sixth leading cause of death in the United States, where there are an estimated 5.5 million individuals currently living with the disease. While AD is now the fifth leading cause of death in Americans 65 and older, the number of individuals who will succumb to AD or AD-related complications is expected to rise as deaths from heart disease and prostate cancer continue to fall Alzheimer's Association (2017). While no dollar amount can accurately represent the pain and suffering AD inflicts on patients and their families, an estimated 236 billion US dollars were spent on health care and long-term care services for patients with AD in 2016, while an additional 230 billion US dollars were lost due to unearned wages and opportunity costs (Alzheimer's Association, 2016; Hurd, Martorell, Delavande, Mullen, & Langa, 2013), a total figure representing approximately 2.5% of US gross domestic product in 2016. AD's rapidly increasing prevalence along with the current lack of therapeutic interventions to successfully slow or halt disease progression makes AD an impending global health crisis.

AD is classically characterized by both the extracellular accumulation of senile plaques composed of amyloid beta (Aβ) and the intracellular deposition of neurofibrillary tangles (NFTs) composed of hyperphosphorylated tau (Grundke-Iqbal et al., 1986). While Alois Alzheimer first described these senile plaques and NFTs in the brains patients who had suffered from dementia over a century ago (Alzheimer's Association, 1907), it would take more than three-quarters of a century for the protein constituents of senile plaques and NFTs to finally be purified and identified (reviewed by Haass & Selkoe, 2007). In addition to the hallmark appearance of these two lesion types, AD is also characterized by the appearance of neuropil threads, dystrophic neurites, and cerebral amyloid angiopathy as well as neuroinflammation, synapse loss, neuronal cell death, and cortical atrophy (Holtzman, Morris, & Goate, 2011; Serrano-Pozo, Frosch, Masliah, & Hyman, 2011). As the disease progresses, characteristic symptoms such as impairments in episodic memory and olfactory deficits eventually transition into severe dementia and ultimately death (Murphy, Gilmore, Seery, Salmon, & Lasker, 1990). The molecular mechanisms that mediate the progression of AD pathophysiology and associated symptomatology are the focus of this review.

2. THE AMYLOID HYPOTHESIS AND ITS CRITIQUES

Despite the prerequisite coincidence of both Aβ and hyperphosphorylated tau aggregation in AD pathology, a number of observations led to the development of and widespread focus on the "amyloid cascade hypothesis," which highlights Aβ accumulation as the primary causative factor of AD (Hardy & Higgins, 1992). The first line of evidence to support the amyloid cascade hypothesis comes from genomic data of patients with rare forms of familial, early-onset AD. Apart from their early-onset and dominant inheritance, the pathology and symptoms of these cases are indistinguishable from common late-onset AD (LOAD). Most of the identified genetic mutations known to be associated with familial AD involve mechanisms that result in the pathogenic processing and increased aggregation of Aβ itself (Bertram, Lill, & Tanzi, 2010). In fact, the first early-onset AD-associated mutations identified were found in the gene that encodes amyloid-precursor protein (APP), a single-transmembrane protein that when cleaved by the protease γ-secretase liberates Aβ peptide extracellularly (Levy et al., 1990). Every known familial mutation of APP associated with AD either occurs in or immediately flanks the Aβ domain of APP (reviewed by Haass & Selkoe, 2007).

Additional early-onset AD-associated mutations have been identified in the genes of both presenilin 1 (PS1) and presenilin 2 (PS2), either of which can form a catalytic subunit of γ-secretase (Bertram et al., 2010). It is widely believed that these autosomal dominant mutations lead to an amyloidogenic shift in the cleavage of APP resulting in the favored generation of the $A\beta_{42}$ isoform over the smaller, less hydrophobic $A\beta_{40}$ isoform (reviewed by Haass & Selkoe, 2007).

Second, changes in cerebrospinal fluid (CSF) concentrations of $A\beta_{42}$, the suspected pathological isoform of Aβ that most readily oligomerizes to form protein aggregates (Bitan et al., 2003), precede changes in CSF concentrations of tau (Jack et al., 2013). A characteristic biomarker of AD is a reduction in CSF $A\beta_{42}$ levels (Fagan et al., 2006). In fact, an analysis of data collected from the Alzheimer's Disease Neuroimaging Initiative (ADNI) revealed CSF $A\beta_{42}$ concentration to be the most sensitive biomarker for the detection of AD (Shaw et al., 2009). Coincident with decreased CSF $A\beta_{42}$, the peptide is deposited in Aβ plaques. The presence of plaque can be detected by positron emission tomography (PET) imaging with ligands such as Pittsburgh compound B (PiB), a radioactive label which binds selectively to Aβ plaque. The detection of Aβ plaque by PET and decreased CSF Aβ levels are contemporaneous and observed well before the emergence of AD symptomology (Fagan et al., 2009; McKhann et al., 2011; Sperling et al., 2011; reviewed by Karran, Mercken, & De Strooper, 2011). Thus, the earliest signs of clinical AD validate Aβ as a trigger for the ensuing decades-long disease process that ends in severe dementia and death.

Experimental validation of the amyloid hypothesis derives from the repeated demonstration that transgenic mice overexpressing human mutant APP with or without mutated forms of presenilin (corresponding to mutations seen in familial AD) develop both senile plaques and age-dependent AD-like phenotypes including synapse loss and impaired memory and cognition (Citron et al., 1997; Games et al., 1995; Oakley et al., 2006; Oddo, Caccamo, Kitazawa, Tseng, & LaFerla, 2003; Oddo, Caccamo, Shepherd, et al., 2003; Puolivali et al., 2002).

Despite these multiple findings, there have been substantial challenges to the amyloid cascade hypothesis, prompting continued reevaluation. First, the degree of plaque burden observed in AD brains correlates with neither the degree of patient cognitive impairment nor the duration of patient illness (Ingelsson et al., 2004). This may be related to Aβ functioning as a trigger of a process which becomes much more complicated over time, involving the immune system, metabolism, and tau. Thus, one hypothesis does not explain all phenomena in AD. Second, there exist a considerable number of documented cases in which appreciable senile plaque burden is observed in brains collected from healthy individuals with no presentation of dementia

(Perez-Nievas et al., 2013; Shankar et al., 2008). This may suggest that these individuals died during the presymptomatic stage of AD and were destined to develop AD if they had survived, though this must remain unproven. Finally, while immunotherapy with antibodies raised against Aβ has been shown to reduce plaque burden in AD patients, such interventions have failed to improve patient outcome (Doody et al., 2013, 2014; Holmes et al., 2008; Salloway et al., 2014; reviewed by Spires-Jones & Hyman, 2014). Caveats have been provided that anti-Aβ interventions were too late or at too low dose in these instances, and ongoing trails explore these possibilities.

3. SOLUBLE, OLIGOMERIC Aβ TOXICITY AS KEY TO AMYLOID CASCADE HYPOTHESIS

A key shift for the AD field came after observations that transgenic mice overexpressing a disease-causing mutant form of human APP showed a reduced density of presynaptic terminals paired with severe impairments in synaptic transmission in the hippocampus months *before* the appearance of amyloid plaques (Hsia et al., 1999). These results strongly suggest that some component of mutated APP could be leading to synapse loss in early stages of the disease through a mechanism independent of senile plaque accumulation. Around the same time Lambert and colleagues demonstrated that soluble Aβo could inhibit long-term potentiation (LTP) in mouse hippocampal slices, suggesting that a soluble, oligomerized form of Aβ might represent the species that triggers synapse loss and memory impairment in AD (Lambert et al., 1998). Immunological studies, in particular those of Glabe and colleagues, provided clear evidence for antigenically distinct conformations of Aβ peptide as monomer, oligomer, and fibril (Kayed et al., 2003). Soon after, Gong and colleagues discovered that patient-derived soluble Aβo bound to dendrites in cultured mouse hippocampal neurons with high, "ligand-like" specificity (Gong et al., 2003).

Further support for the Aβ oligomer hypothesis came from experiments conducted by Selkoe and colleagues demonstrating that acute administration of soluble Aβo (but not Aβ monomers or insoluble amyloid plaque cores) derived from AD brains could inhibit LTP (an electrophysiological enhancement mechanism believed to contribute to memory formation) and enhance long-term depression (LTD, a mechanism that mediates a stable reduction in postsynaptic response) in hippocampal slices. The authors additionally showed that 10-day incubation with patient-derived Aβo significantly reduced spine density in cultured rat pyramidal cells (Shankar et al., 2008).

Although amyloid plaque burden does not correlate with memory loss, astrocyte inflammatory response, or neuronal loss in transgenic AD animals, the level of oligomeric Aβ in the brain does (DaRocha-Souto et al., 2011; Kostylev et al., 2015; Lue et al., 1999; McLean et al., 1999). Similarly, while increases in the amount of Aβ monomers and Aβ plaque burden are indeed pathological hallmarks of AD, Aβo represents the species of Aβ that correlates most strongly with the severity of dementia in humans (Esparza et al., 2013; Haass & Selkoe, 2007; Koffie et al., 2009; Reiman et al., 2009; Savage et al., 2014; Yang et al., 2013). Taken together, these results suggest that soluble Aβo likely represents the most synaptotoxic and pathophysiologically relevant form of Aβ to AD. A caveat remains that Aβo is a generic term for a collection of heterogeneous Aβ oligomer states, and the relative role of different oligomer species is ill defined (Benilova, Karran, & De Strooper, 2012; Kostylev et al., 2015).

4. MECHANISMS OF Aβ OLIGOMER TOXICITY AT THE SYNAPSE

Synapse loss is the strongest pathological correlate of cognitive deficits in AD (Lansbury, 1999) and can be observed in the earliest stage of AD progression (Scheff, Price, Schmitt, DeKosky, & Mufson, 2007). Further physiological evidence of Aβ-induced synapse loss comes from the observation that the degree of synapse loss is greatest surrounding amyloid plaques (Lanz, Carter, & Merchant, 2003). In AD transgenic animals, Aβo has been found to colocalize with synaptic puncta, and this degree of colocalization correlates positively with the loss of excitatory synapses (Koffie et al., 2009).

The mechanisms of Aβo-induced disruption of synaptic transmission and subsequent synapse loss are obviously key to explaining AD, but have only recently begun to be elucidated (Heiss et al., 2016) (Fig. 1). Considering the importance of glutamatergic signaling in synaptic transmission and plasticity, it is unsurprising that Aβo treatment reduces the expression of both AMPA and NMDA receptors as well as PSD-95, a membrane-associated scaffolding protein and a common marker of postsynaptic densities, in glutamatergic synapses (Almeida et al., 2005; Jurgensen et al., 2011; Roselli et al., 2005; reviewed by Jurgensen & Ferreira, 2010). However, the mechanism by which extracellular Aβo signals to affect synaptic plasticity was absent of molecular understanding prior to the last 10 years.

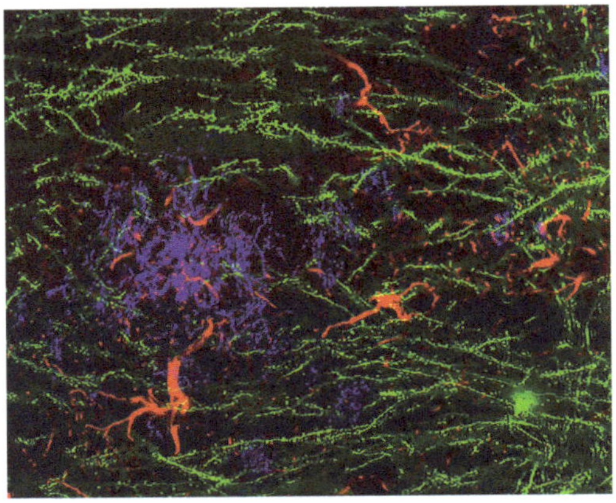

Fig. 1 Synaptic structures and amyloid plaques in Alzheimer model mice. Image of cerebral cortical tissue from a transgenic Alzheimer model mouse, expressing human mutant APP and PS1. This mouse also carries a Thy1-EGFP transgene to sparsely fill individual neurons in the cerebral cortex (*green*). The amyloid plaque stain is *blue*, and reactive astrocytes are revealed by anti-GFAP staining in *red*. *Derived from experimental system described previously (Heiss, J. K., Barrett, J., Yu, Z., Haas, L. T., Kostylev, M. A., & Strittmatter, S. M. (2016). Early activation of experience-independent dendritic spine turnover in a mouse model of Alzheimer's disease.* Cerebral Cortex 27:*3660–3674. (https://doi.org/10.1093/cercor/bhw188).*

5. NEURONAL RECEPTOR AS CENTRAL MEDIATOR OF Aβo SYNAPSE DAMAGE

The evidence that Aβo action to impair synapses is central to AD pathophysiology focuses attention on the initial molecular mechanisms that trigger these toxicities. One hypothesis is that Aβo interacts with phospholipid bilayers directly to alter conductance nonspecifically. While there is evidence for such membrane-disrupting activity at high Aβ concentration, it is unclear how this might explain the selectivity in AD for the CNS and for specific pathways within the brain, or for synapses. Instead, the potent, selective, and rapid effects of Aβo on synaptic function suggest that specific polypeptide cell surface receptors for their action exist. Certain effects on synaptic function may be noncell autonomous. For example, Aβo may trigger microglial- and/or complement-mediated attack on the synapse (Hong et al., 2016). Especially, in late stages of disease as inflammation and cellular reaction becomes prominent, the cellular environment around neuronal synapses and noncell autonomous synapse damage may be key. However, at the first triggering stages of AD, direct interaction of Aβo with neuronal synaptic receptors to mediate dysregulation and synapse loss appear most consistent with the phenomena described earlier.

What characteristics might be expected of a neuronal receptor-mediating Aβo synaptic dysfunction and loss? The relevant binding site is expected to be oligomer specific, rather than monomer specific, of high affinity and present at adult synapses. Monomers of Aβ are present in all individuals and their levels do not substantially change with disease, so any binding site that does not distinguish between monomers and oligomers is likely irrelevant to AD pathophysiology. Evidence for a role requires demonstration not only of binding but also protection from the deleterious effects of Aβo in cells and slices, as well as AD transgenes in experimental animal models. While assessment of human genetic risk for AD might bolster the case for specific receptor function, none of the currently identified human genetic risk genes can be classified as a synaptic receptor protein, implying that the relevant proteins may not exhibit substantial polymorphisms. The biochemical basis for discovery of a potential Aβo receptor is strongest when unbiased genome-wide methods are utilized, and receptor expression cloning has been applied to a number of systems. In our studies of neuronal receptors for Semaphorins (Kolodkin et al., 1997; Nakamura, Tanaka, Takahashi, Kalb, & Strittmatter, 1998; Takahashi et al., 1999; Takahashi, Nakamura, & Strittmatter, 1997), Nogo (Fournier, GrandPre, & Strittmatter, 2001), MAG (Liu, Fournier, GrandPre, & Strittmatter, 2002), LGI1 (Owuor et al., 2009), RGM (Rajagopalan et al., 2004), and PGRN (Hu et al., 2010), we utilized tagged recombinant protein ligands to screen brain cDNA libraries expressed in nonneuronal cell lines. In each case, receptors relevant to physiological and pathological functions were discovered. Therefore, the expression cloning method is predicted to be of utility for identification of Aβo receptors.

6. IDENTIFICATION OF PrP^C AS A RECEPTOR FOR Aβo

Using an adult mouse brain library of 225,000 cDNA clones expressed in Cos-7 cells, cellular prion protein (PrP^C), a membrane-anchored glycoprotein, was identified in a screen for Aβo binding (Lauren, Gimbel, Nygaard, Gilbert, & Strittmatter, 2009). Cos-7 cells expressing PrP^C were found to have a substantially higher affinity for Aβo compared to low-molecular weight Aβ and a dissociation constant identical to that of Aβo for cultured hippocampal neurons, observations that, respectively, reveal both PrP^C's oligomeric specificity and high affinity for Aβo (Balducci et al., 2010; Calella et al., 2010;

Chen, Yadav, & Surewicz, 2010; Lauren et al., 2009; Rushworth, Griffiths, Watt, & Hooper, 2013). While LTP is inhibited in wild-type mouse hippocampal slices treated with Aβo, no such Aβo-induced LTP inhibition is detected in hippocampal slices from mice in which PrP^C was genetically deleted, thereby supporting PrP^C's role as a pathophysiologically relevant Aβo receptor (Lauren et al., 2009). Similarly, Aβo-induced LTP inhibition in wild-type hippocampal slices could be rescued through pretreatment with an anti-PrP^C antibody. While one study did not observe a requirement for PrP^C in Aβo inhibition (Kessels, Nguyen, Nabavi, & Malinow, 2010), this key observation has been confirmed now in multiple studies (Barry et al., 2011; Haas et al., 2016; Hu et al., 2014; Nicoll et al., 2013; Scott-McKean et al., 2016; Zhang et al., 2017).

Subsequent work has corroborated PrP^C's role as a pathophysiologically relevant receptor for Aβo. PrP^C has been shown to be required for Aβo-induced loss of synapses (Bate & Williams, 2011; Kudo et al., 2012; Ostapchenko et al., 2013), memory impairment and cognitive deficits (Chung et al., 2010; Gimbel et al., 2010), dendritic spine turnover in vivo (Heiss et al., 2016), and the early mortality phenotype of APP/PS1 transgenic mice (Gimbel et al., 2010; Haas et al., 2016). The role of PrP^C as a human disease relevant receptor for $A\beta_{42}$ has also been confirmed; $A\beta_{42}$ has been shown to bind specifically to immobilized PrP^C in brain homogenates from AD patients but not in homogenates derived from healthy controls, an effect that is dependent on the significantly higher concentration of $A\beta_{42}$ present in AD brains (Dohler et al., 2014; Kostylev et al., 2015; Um et al., 2012).

Thus, a preponderance of evidence suggests that for Aβo, PrP^C meets typical requirements for a putative receptor: high affinity, specificity, saturability, reversibility, and the ability to mediate biologically relevant, downstream, intracellular signaling events (Creese, Burt, & Snyder, 1976). However, it is important to note that while PrP^C was the only positive hit identified in the unbiased genome-wide screen, the genetic deletion of PrP^C in cultured mouse neurons only reduced Aβo binding by 50%, suggesting the contribution of other Aβo-binding cell-surface molecules in addition to PrP^C (Lauren et al., 2009).

While the necessity of PrP^C to mediate Aβo-induced reduction in synaptic density, LTP inhibition, and synaptotoxicity has been well documented (Barry et al., 2011; Bate & Williams, 2011; Chung et al., 2010; Fluharty et al., 2013; Freir et al., 2011; Gimbel et al., 2010; Kostylev et al., 2015; Lauren et al., 2009; Resenberger et al., 2011), certain

Aβ-induced phenotypes, including neural network dysfunction and in vitro dendritic spine loss after longer periods of high-concentration Aβo incubation, appear to be independent of PrP^C, suggesting that these phenotypes may be mediated by alternative Aβo receptors or possibly distinct species of oligomeric Aβ (Balducci et al., 2010; Calella et al., 2010; Cisse et al., 2011; Kessels et al., 2010). However, since PrP^C is the only putative Aβ receptor shown to bind specifically to Aβo, the identity of additional Aβo receptors requires further investigation (reviewed by Smith & Strittmatter, 2017).

7. IDENTIFICATION OF mGluR5 AS AN Aβo CORECEPTOR

The activation of intracellular Fyn kinase and its subsequent phosphorylation of NMDARs has been shown to be triggered by the Aβo–PrP^C complex (Larson et al., 2012; Rushworth et al., 2013; Um et al., 2012). A requirement for this signaling pathway was employed to identify a transmembrane coreceptor that might link the GPI-anchored PrP^C to the cytoplasmic Fyn kinase, both of which are enriched in the postsynaptic density (PSD) (Collins et al., 2006; Um et al., 2013, 2012). A screen of 61-transmembrane PSD-enriched proteins expressed in HEK293T cells identified mGluR5 as the only candidate to mediate Aβo-induced Fyn phosphorylation in a PrP^C-dependent manner (Um et al., 2013) (Fig. 2). In cultured cortical neurons, Aβo-induced Fyn activation is eliminated with the application of mGluR5 antagonists MPEP and MTEP (but not the mGluR1 antagonist MPMQ) and through the genetic deletion of mGluR5. Notably, while mGluR5 associates with both PrP^C and Fyn, mGluR5 does not bind directly to Aβo. Additionally, the interaction between Aβo–PrP^C is independent of mGluR5 expression, suggesting the existence of direct, pairwise associations between Aβo and PrP^C, PrP^C and mGluR5, and mGluR5 and Fyn.

In high-density cortical cultures, Aβo administration (but not Aβ monomers) increased levels of intracellular calcium through a mechanism dependent on the expression of both mGluR5 and PrP^C (Um et al., 2013). Although Fyn is also activated through Aβo–PrP^C–mGluR5 signaling, the administration of saracatinib to inhibit Fyn failed to eliminate Aβo-induced increases in intracellular calcium in high-density cortical cultures. Conversely, while Aβo-induced calcium increases were abolished after pretreatment with thapsigargin to deplete endoplasmic reticulum calcium stores, thapsigargin pretreatment failed to inhibit Aβo-induced Fyn

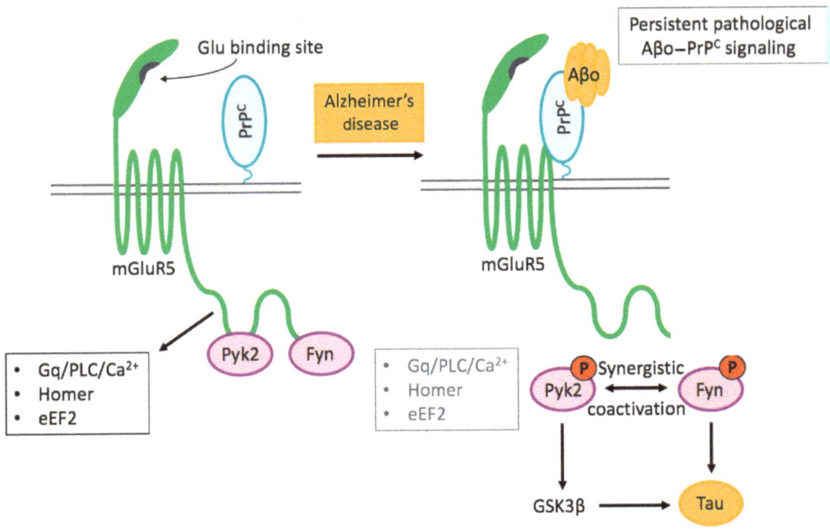

Fig. 2 Receptor signaling cascade mediating Alzheimer's disease synapse damage by Aβ oligomers. Schematic illustrates the role of mGluR5 in linking cell surface Aβo–PrP^C complexes to intracellular Fyn/Pyk2 and synaptic loss. Proteins are clustered in the PSD and alter NMDARs, calcium, and protein translation. Pyk2(PTK2B) variation is a verified genetic risk for late-onset AD. Tau plays a role in localizing Fyn. Aberrant PrP^C–mGluR5–Fyn–Tau signaling leads to synaptic malfunction and loss.

activation. Since the pharmacological inhibition of Fyn has been shown to rescue memory deficits and spine loss in APPswe/PS1ΔE9 transgenic mice, these results suggest the existence of at least two pharmacologically divergent Aβo–PrP^C–mGluR5 signaling pathways (Kaufman et al., 2015).

8. Aβo-INDUCED DISRUPTION OF THE mGluR5–Homer1b/c–Pyk2–CamKII COMPLEX

In lysates extracted from acute mouse brain slices, anti-PrP^C coimmunoprecipitation reveals that the PrP^C–mGluR5 complex associates with Homer1b/c, Pyk2, and CamKII (Haas et al., 2016, 2017; Haas & Strittmatter, 2016) (Fig. 2). Moreover, the mGluR5–Homer1b/c–Pyk2–CamKII complex is modulated by Aβo. While acute (*S*)-3,5-dihydroxyphenylglycine (DHPG) administration enhances the indirect association between PrP^C and Homer1b/c and reduces PrP^C's association with Pyk2 and CamKII, acute Aβo administration enhances not only the association between PrP^C and mGluR5 but also the association between PrP^C and CamKII. Conversely, through mGluR5, acute Aβo administration reduces

PrP^C's indirect association with Homer1b/c and Pyk2, suggesting that normal glutamatergic signaling mediated by mGluR5 is aberrantly disrupted by Aβo. Furthermore, pretreatment of brain slices with Aβo blocks DHPG's normal ability to modulate mGluR5's interactions with Homer1b/c and CamKII.

Since Aβo levels are chronically elevated in the AD brain and correlate with disease severity, the disruption of normal mGluR5 signaling would be persistent, and worsening as the disease progresses. In brain slices from APPswe/PS1ΔE9 transgenic mice, DHPG-induced changes in the behavior of the mGluR5–Homer1b/c–Pyk2-CamKII complex are completely abolished (Haas & Strittmatter, 2016). Additionally, DHPG-induced activation of Pyk2 and CamKII is absent in brain slices from APPswe/PS1ΔE9 animals, suggesting that chronic exposure to pathologically high levels of Aβo disrupts glutamate's ability to regulate Pyk2 and CamKII signaling through mGluR5. Interestingly, DHPG and Aβo's ability to activate Pyk2 activity is dependent on Fyn, since pharmacological inhibition of Fyn abolishes DHPG and Aβo-induced Pyk2 phosphorylation at Tyr402.

Since it has been previously demonstrated that mGluR-dependent synaptic plasticity is dependent on the interaction between Homer and mGluR proteins (Ronesi & Huber, 2008), and that CamKII's dissociation from mGluR is associated with LTP (Jin et al., 2011), it is quite possible that Aβo's ability to disrupt synaptic plasticity is at least partially explained by the Aβo-induced disruption of these two synaptic proteins. Whatever role Pyk2 may have in mediating Aβo-induced disruption of synaptic plasticity has yet to be fully elucidated, but Fyn signaling is likely to be implicated in such a mechanism.

9. TARGETING THE Aβo–PrP^C–mGluR5 COMPLEX

The role of mGluR5 in mediating Aβo-induced synaptic dysfunction and memory impairment has been repeatedly demonstrated (Beraldo et al., 2016; Hamilton, Esseltine, DeVries, Cregan, & Ferguson, 2014; Hu et al., 2014; Overk et al., 2014; Raka et al., 2015; Renner et al., 2010; Um et al., 2013; Wang, Walsh, Rowan, Selkoe, & Anwyl, 2004; Zhang et al., 2015). However, since the inhibition of glutamatergic signaling via mGluR5 disrupts normal learning and memory, any therapeutic intervention designed to disrupt Aβo–PrP^C signaling through mGluR5 would ideally leave physiological glutamatergic signaling intact (Abou Farha, Bruggeman, & Balje-Volkers, 2014; Campbell et al., 2004; Lu et al., 1997;

Porter et al., 2005; Rodriguez et al., 2010; Um et al., 2013; Xu, Zhu, Contractor, & Heinemann, 2009).

Our group recently demonstrated that the silent allosteric modulator (SAM) of mGluR5 BMS-984923 selectively inhibits Aβo-induced inhibition of LTP in mouse hippocampal slices, memory deficits and synaptic loss in APP/PS1 transgenic mice, and tau pathology in triple transgenic (3 × Tg) mice-expressing APP, PS1, and human mutant tau while preserving normal mGluR5-mediated glutamatergic signaling (Haas et al., 2017). Thus, BMS-984923 may represent a potentially effective disease-modifying therapy for AD.

10. ADDITIONAL RECEPTORS FOR Aβ: LilRB2, α7nAChR, AND OTHERS

While PrP^{C}'s interaction with Aβo was discovered via a genome-wide unbiased screen, a number of other receptors for Aβo have been proposed from selected candidate studies, and we have reviewed these in detail (reviewed by Smith & Strittmatter, 2017). The relative roles of these different receptor mechanisms require further investigation. Here, we briefly describe a few of these pathways.

Shatz and colleagues started with physiological studies showing that LilRB2 is a receptor for both MHC proteins and myelin inhibitor proteins, which titrates synaptic plasticity (Atwal et al., 2008; Bochner et al., 2014; Syken, Grandpre, Kanold, & Shatz, 2006). Based on this background, they considered whether it might also bind Aβo and modify synapse function and stability. Their studies demonstrated a role for LilRB2 in mediating Aβo action to inhibit LTP in slices and to mediate impairments in AD transgenic mice (Kim et al., 2013). The interplay of Aβo with endogenous ligands at different development stages has not yet been clarified.

In 2000, Wang and colleagues proposed α7nAChR, a homomeric, ionotropic acetylcholine receptor with high Ca^{2+} permeability as a receptor for monomeric $Aβ_{42}$, a proposal that was in part informed by the loss of cholinergic neurons commonly observed in AD (Hogg, Raggenbass, & Bertrand, 2003; Wang et al., 2000). Subsequent work by Dineley and colleagues demonstrated that in brain slices both nicotine and $Aβ_{42}$ administration could stimulate the activation of extracellular signal-regulated kinase 2 (ERK2), an effect that could be reversed with the application of MLA, an α7nAChR antagonist (Dineley et al., 2001). Conversely, pretreatment of slices with $Aβ_{42}$ prevented nicotine-induced activation of ERK2 in a manner that reflects Aβo's ability to impair DHPG-induced regulation of the mGluR5–Homer1b/c–Pyk2–CamKII complex. Furthermore, the authors showed that the degree of α7nAChR brain expression in mice correlated positively with memory deficits in a Morris water maze task.

Additional research conducted by Greengard's team in the mid-2000s demonstrated that soluble Aβ treatment induced the endocytosis of NMDA receptors in cultured cortical neurons through a mechanism involving the binding of Aβ to α7nAChR and the subsequent activation of the striatally enriched phosphatase (STEP) via dephosphorylation by the Ca^{2+}-sensitive phosphatase PP2B, also known as calcineurin (Snyder et al., 2005). The authors hypothesized that the activation of α7nAChR by soluble Aβ could promote calcium influx and the activation of calcineurin (mirroring Aβo's previously discussed ability to stimulate the release of calcium from intracellular stores, a mechanism dependent on the formation of the Aβo–PrP^C–mGluR5 complex). Once activated, calcineurin could then dephosphorylate and thus activate STEP. Activated STEP would then promote the dephosphorylation of the NMDA receptor subunit NR2B at Tyr1472, a residue whose phosphorylation state regulates the activity and endocytosis of NMDA receptors.

Other experiments have confirmed that Aβo treatment reduces NMDA receptor Ca^{2+} conductance, which consequently leads to a reduction in the activity of CamKII, the inhibition of LTP and the promotion of LTD (Mulkey, Endo, Shenolikar, & Malenka, 1994; reviewed by Koffie, Hyman, & Spires-Jones, 2011). Aβo-induced calcineurin activation has also been shown to be mediated by the activation of mGluRs, initiating a cascade that ultimately leads to the endocytosis of AMPA receptors (Mulkey et al., 1994; Zhang et al., 2008).

It is clear that NMDAR contributes to Aβo-induced dysfunction as a downstream mediator, but there is also some evidence that there is a direct interaction of Aβo with NMDAR that contributes to AD pathophysiology. De Felice et al. demonstrated that binding of Aβo to cultured hippocampal neurons could be substantially reduced with an antibody raised against the extracellular N-terminal of NMDAR (De Felice et al., 2007). Disrupting the interaction between Aβo and NMDAR with this antibody also helped prevent Aβo-induced increases in intracellular calcium levels and the generation of reactive oxygen species (ROS). The same group subsequently found that knocking down NMDAR in cultured hippocampal neurons dramatically reduced dendritic Aβo-binding and Aβo-induced ROS generation. However, since the authors observed no difference in NMDAR expression between oligomer-bound and nonbound neurons and observed no reduction in NMDAR expression after insulin-induced disruption of Aβo binding, the authors conclude that additional sites likely mediate direct dendritic Aβo binding (Decker et al., 2010).

11. Tau AND Aβ IN CONCERT: THE ROLE OF Fyn AND Pyk2

A possible link between Aβ and tau pathology is elucidated by considering Aβo's ability to activate Fyn, since Fyn has previously been shown to both physically associate with tau and to phosphorylate tyrosine residues of tau (Bhaskar, Hobbs, Yen, & Lee, 2010; Lee et al., 2004). The phosphorylation of tau by Fyn depends on the upstream formation of the Aβo–PrP^C complex (Larson et al., 2012), and the endogenous expression of PrP^C correlates positively with the expression of tau in a transgenic APP/PS1 mice (Vergara et al., 2015). Notably, extracts from human AD brains have been shown to activate Fyn in cultured mouse cortical neurons (Um et al., 2012).

While the role of hyperphosphorylated tau in neuronal cell death has traditionally been thought to occur through the physical impedance of axonal trafficking, more recent work suggests a mechanistic relationship between Aβ and tau that mediates synaptic dysfunction and neuronal toxicity. Hyperphosphorylated tau has been shown to abnormally localize to dendrites (Zempel, Thies, Mandelkow, & Mandelkow, 2010). Aβo also promotes downstream phosphorylation of tau (Jin et al., 2011). Conversely, it has also been demonstrated that Aβ-induced memory impairment and neuronal hyperexcitability in transgenic mice overexpressing mutant human APP depend on the expression of endogenous tau (Roberson et al., 2007). Additionally, the pathological localization of Fyn to the postsynaptic site and its subsequent binding to NMDA receptors intracellularly are also dependent on the expression of tau (Ittner et al., 2010).

The pathological relationship between tau and Fyn is bidirectional; while activated Fyn can phosphorylate tau, phosphorylated tau has a higher propensity to bind with Fyn, increasing the likelihood of Fyn's aberrant localization into dendrites (Mondragon-Rodriguez et al., 2012). Specifically, tau delivers Fyn preferentially to NMDA receptors, where Fyn readily promotes the phosphorylation of the NMDA receptor subunit NR2B at Tyr1472 (Roche et al., 2001). The phosphorylation of NR2B at Tyr1472 has been shown to both inhibit NMDA receptor endocytosis and increase NMDA receptor current (Roche et al., 2001; Snyder et al., 2005).

The role of Fyn in linking Aβ and tau pathologies implicates it as a potential therapeutic target for AD treatment. As mentioned previously, inhibiting Fyn pharmacologically with the Src family kinase inhibitor AZD0530 rescues both memory impairment and synapse loss in APP/PS1 mice (Kaufman et al., 2015). As such, AZD0530 is currently being evaluated as a candidate for disease-modifying therapy in a multicenter NIH-funded Phase2a clinical trial (ClinicalTrials.gov NCT02167256) (Nygaard et al., 2015).

Evidence suggest that Fyn and Pyk2 may function together to mediate pathological Aβo signaling. Pyk2 was identified as a LOAD risk gene in the largest Genome Wide Association Study yet conducted to assess AD risk, and Pyk2 was separately identified as a non-ApoE4 genetic risk loci for AD (Beecham et al., 2014; Lambert et al., 2013). Additionally, Pyk2 has been identified as a node for differential gene expression in both ApoE4 allele carriers and in patients with early-onset AD (Rhinn et al., 2013).

Pyk2, like Fyn, is enriched in PSDs and has been shown to play a mechanistic role in regulating synaptic plasticity (Bartos et al., 2010; Heidinger et al., 2002; Huang et al., 2001; Park, Avraham, & Avraham, 2004; Seabold, Burette, Lim, Weinberg, & Hell, 2003). Bartos and colleagues showed that NMDAR-mediated Ca^{2+} influx induced Pyk2 autophosphorylation and binding to PSD-95, a process that is necessary for LTP induction in hippocampal slices. More recently, Giralt and colleagues showed that genetic deletion of Pyk2 in mice impaired performance on hippocampal-dependent behavioral tasks as well as the induction of LTP in hippocampal slices (Giralt et al., 2017). Conversely, Hsin and colleagues demonstrated that Pyk2 was required for LTD induction, and that Pyk2 overexpression also blocked LTP (Hsin, Kim, Wang, & Sheng, 2010).

As mentioned previously, Pyk2's association with mGluR5 is disrupted in the presence of Aβo (Haas et al., 2016). Pyk2 has also been shown to interact directly with Fyn, which phosphorylates and thus fully activates Pyk2 (Collins, Bartelt, & Houtman, 2010; Collins, Tremblay, et al., 2010; Park et al., 2004). While Fyn has been shown to phosphorylate residues of tau, Pyk2 has been shown to interact with and phosphorylate GSK3β (Hartigan, Xiong, & Johnson, 2001; Sayas, Ariaens, Ponsioen, & Moolenaar, 2006), a kinase thought to be involved in the hyperphosphorylation of tau (reviewed by Hooper, Killick, & Lovestone, 2008). Taken together, these results suggest that Pyk2 may play a critical role in mediating Aβ-induced synaptic dysregulation through a process involving Fyn. However, the specifics of this mechanism have yet to be elucidated.

12. Aβ AND DISRUPTED HOMEOSTATIC EQUILIBRIUM

It may appear as if different studies of Aβo on NMDA receptor activity were contradictory with one another. On the one hand, the phosphorylation of NR2B at Tyr1472 via Fyn increases NMDA receptor net activity (Um et al., 2012). On the other hand, NR2B dephosphorylation by STEP promotes the endocytosis of NMDA receptors, which would reasonably lead to a net reduction in NMDA receptor-mediated currents (Snyder et al., 2005). However, it would also appear that this pathological system includes redundancies that promote NR2B dephosphorization; while STEP dephosphorylates NR2B directly, it also dephosphorylates and inactivates Fyn (Nguyen, Liu, & Lombroso, 2002). Because mGluR5 activation triggers the localization of STEP into dendrites (Zhang et al., 2008) and because Aβo has been shown to activate mGluR5, Aβo would also have the dual effect of both activating Fyn and promoting its inactivation through recruitment of STEP at different time points (Um et al., 2012). The system is further complicated by the previously discussed observation that Aβo also leads to tau phosphorylation and thus the activation and recruitment of Fyn to the PSD.

Nevertheless, it is highly probable that this system would result in an overall shift toward NMDA receptor dysregulation in such a way that contributes to neuronal toxicity. Given the necessity of stable NMDA receptor expression for the maintenance of LTP, which would be precluded by chronic STEP activation, the net result of NR2B phosphorylation by Fyn might solely be to disrupt calcium homeostasis within the cell. Indeed, Aβo administration has been shown to disrupt Ca^{2+} homeostasis through a mechanism dependent on NR2B activation (Ferreira et al., 2012). Promisingly, and in support of this theory, an uncompetitive NMDA receptor channel blocker memantine has shown modest effectiveness in symptomatically improving memory in AD patients (Reisberg, Doody, & Mobius, 2003; reviewed by Mota, Ferreira, & Rego, 2014).

13. FUTURE DIRECTIONS

There remain many unanswered questions regarding the mechanisms of oligomeric Aβ-induced neurotoxicity and its contribution to the pathophysiology of AD. For example, the precise Aβo species that are the most pathologically relevant forms require better definition. While, Shankar and colleagues initially determined Aβ dimers to be the neurotoxic species, other groups have subsequently reached conflicting conclusions (Kostylev et al., 2015; Shankar et al., 2008; reviewed by Haass & Selkoe, 2007). Considering the existence of Aβo-induced phenotypes that appear to be independent of PrP^C, it is likely that a number of additional receptors are mediating these phenotypes. Indeed, a number of other teams have identified Aβ receptors in addition to PrP^C, LilRB2, α7nAChR, and NMDAR including RAGE (Yan et al., 1996), $p75^{NTR}$ (Kuner, Schubenel, & Hertel, 1998; Yaar et al., 1997), NgR1 (Park et al., 2006), EphB2 (Cisse et al., 2011) and EphA4 (Fu et al., 2014), FcγRIIB (Kam et al., 2013), Sortilin (Carlo et al., 2013), IR (Xie et al., 2002), EGFR (Wang et al., 2012), and σ_2R/PGRMC1 (Izzo, Staniszewski, et al., 2014; Izzo, Xu, et al., 2014; reviewed by Smith & Strittmatter, 2017). It is possible that these additional Aβ receptors may demonstrate distinct specificities for monomeric or particular oligomeric Aβ species, each potentially signaling through distinct molecular pathways. Indeed, work from Sergio Ferreira's group suggests that high- and low-molecular weight Aβo produce aberrant phenotypes in vitro and in vivo through separate molecular mechanisms (Figueiredo et al., 2013). Notably, Selkoe, Walsh, and colleagues have shown that human AD brains contain high-molecular weight oligomers which can interconvert into more bioactive, low-molecular weight oligomers under certain buffer conditions (Yang, Li, Xu, Walsh, & Selkoe, 2017). Further studies are required to elucidate the specificity of each proposed Aβo receptor and the downstream signaling pathways that are subsequently disrupted by Aβ. In addition, the connections between Aβo neuronal receptor-signaling, glial and immune response, and the progression to tau pathology remain to be elucidated.

14. CONCLUSION

A collection of evidence supports the hypothesis that accumulation of misfolded forms of Aβ peptide trigger the Alzheimer's disease cascade. Synapse damage is an early and critical phenomenon in the progression of the disease with increasing complexity involving cellular inflammation, tau accumulation, and cell death. Receptors for Aβo at the synapse initiate this toxic cascade. Here, we have reviewed a collection of data showing that Aβo interacts with PrP^C to trigger mGluR5 signaling at the synapse, a mechanism that involves Fyn and Pyk2 kinases. For experimental AD transgenic mouse models, this pathway is required for synapse loss and memory dysfunction. Clinical tests of the role of this pathway are underway now.

CONFLICT OF INTEREST

None.

ACKNOWLEDGMENTS

This work was supported by Grants from NIH and the Falk Medical Research Trust to S.M.S.

REFERENCES

Abou Farha, K., Bruggeman, R., & Balje-Volkers, C. (2014). Metabotropic glutamate receptor 5 negative modulation in phase I clinical trial: Potential impact of circadian rhythm on the neuropsychiatric adverse reactions—Do hallucinations matter? *ISRN Psychiatry, 2014*, 652750. https://doi.org/10.1155/2014/652750.

Almeida, C. G., Tampellini, D., Takahashi, R. H., Greengard, P., Lin, M. T., Snyder, E. M., et al. (2005). Beta-amyloid accumulation in APP mutant neurons reduces PSD-95 and GluR1 in synapses. *Neurobiology of Disease, 20*(2), 187–198. https://doi.org/10.1016/j.nbd.2005.02.008.

Alzheimer's Association. (1907). Über eine eigenartige Erkrankung der Hirnrinde. *Allgemeine Zeitschrift fur Psychiatrie und Psychisch-gerichtliche Medizin, 64*, 146–148.

Alzheimer's Association. (2016). Alzheimer's disease facts and figures. *Alzheimer's & Dementia, 12*, 459–509.

Alzheimer's Association. (2017). Alzheimer's disease facts and figures. *Alzheimer's & Dementia, 13*, 325–373.

Atwal, J. K., Pinkston-Gosse, J., Syken, J., Stawicki, S., Wu, Y., Shatz, C., et al. (2008). PirB is a functional receptor for myelin inhibitors of axonal regeneration. *Science, 322*(5903), 967–970. https://doi.org/10.1126/science.1161151.

Balducci, C., Beeg, M., Stravalaci, M., Bastone, A., Sclip, A., Biasini, E., et al. (2010). Synthetic amyloid-beta oligomers impair long-term memory independently of cellular prion protein. *Proceedings of the National Academy of Sciences of the United States of America, 107*(5), 2295–2300. https://doi.org/10.1073/pnas.0911829107.

Barry, A. E., Klyubin, I., Mc Donald, J. M., Mably, A. J., Farrell, M. A., Scott, M., et al. (2011). Alzheimer's disease brain-derived amyloid-beta-mediated inhibition of LTP in vivo is prevented by immunotargeting cellular prion protein. *The Journal of Neuroscience, 31*(20), 7259–7263. https://doi.org/10.1523/JNEUROSCI.6500-10.2011.

Bartos, J. A., Ulrich, J. D., Li, H., Beazely, M. A., Chen, Y., Macdonald, J. F., et al. (2010). Postsynaptic clustering and activation of Pyk2 by PSD-95. *The Journal of Neuroscience, 30*(2), 449–463. https://doi.org/10.1523/JNEUROSCI.4992-08.2010.

Bate, C., & Williams, A. (2011). Amyloid-beta-induced synapse damage is mediated via cross-linkage of cellular prion proteins. *Journal of Biological Chemistry, 286*(44), 37955–37963. https://doi.org/10.1074/jbc.M111.248724.

Beecham, G. W., Hamilton, K., Naj, A. C., Martin, E. R., Huentelman, M., Myers, A. J., et al. (2014). Genome-wide association meta-analysis of neuropathologic features of Alzheimer's disease and related dementias. *PLoS Genetics, 10*(9), e1004606. https://doi.org/10.1371/journal.pgen.1004606.

Benilova, I., Karran, E., & De Strooper, B. (2012). The toxic Abeta oligomer and Alzheimer's disease: An emperor in need of clothes. *Nature Neuroscience, 15*(3), 349–357. https://doi.org/10.1038/nn.3028.

Beraldo, F. H., Ostapchenko, V. G., Caetano, F. A., Guimaraes, A. L., Ferretti, G. D., Daude, N., et al. (2016). Regulation of amyloid beta oligomer binding to neurons and neurotoxicity by the prion protein-mGluR5 complex. *Journal of Biological Chemistry, 291*(42), 21945–21955. https://doi.org/10.1074/jbc.M116.738286.

Bertram, L., Lill, C. M., & Tanzi, R. E. (2010). The genetics of Alzheimer disease: Back to the future. *Neuron, 68*(2), 270–281. https://doi.org/10.1016/j.neuron.2010.10.013.

Bhaskar, K., Hobbs, G. A., Yen, S. H., & Lee, G. (2010). Tyrosine phosphorylation of tau accompanies disease progression in transgenic mouse models of tauopathy. *Neuropathology and Applied Neurobiology, 36*(6), 462–477. https://doi.org/10.1111/j.1365-2990.2010.01103.x.

Bitan, G., Kirkitadze, M. D., Lomakin, A., Vollers, S. S., Benedek, G. B., & Teplow, D. B. (2003). Amyloid beta-protein (Abeta) assembly: Abeta 40 and Abeta 42 oligomerize through distinct pathways. *Proceedings of the National Academy of Sciences of the United States of America, 100*(1), 330–335. https://doi.org/10.1073/pnas.222681699.

Bochner, D. N., Sapp, R. W., Adelson, J. D., Zhang, S., Lee, H., Djurisic, M., et al. (2014). Blocking PirB up-regulates spines and functional synapses to unlock visual cortical plasticity and facilitate recovery from amblyopia. *Science Translational Medicine, 6*(258), 258ra140. https://doi.org/10.1126/scitranslmed.3010157.

Calella, A. M., Farinelli, M., Nuvolone, M., Mirante, O., Moos, R., Falsig, J., et al. (2010). Prion protein and Abeta-related synaptic toxicity impairment. *EMBO Molecular Medicine, 2*(8), 306–314. https://doi.org/10.1002/emmm.201000082.

Campbell, U. C., Lalwani, K., Hernandez, L., Kinney, G. G., Conn, P. J., & Bristow, L. J. (2004). The mGluR5 antagonist 2-methyl-6-(phenylethynyl)-pyridine (MPEP) potentiates PCP-induced cognitive deficits in rats. *Psychopharmacology, 175*(3), 310–318. https://doi.org/10.1007/s00213-004-1827-5.

Carlo, A. S., Gustafsen, C., Mastrobuoni, G., Nielsen, M. S., Burgert, T., Hartl, D., et al. (2013). The pro-neurotrophin receptor sortilin is a major neuronal apolipoprotein E receptor for catabolism of amyloid-beta peptide in the brain. *The Journal of Neuroscience, 33*(1), 358–370. https://doi.org/10.1523/JNEUROSCI.2425-12.2013.

Chen, S., Yadav, S. P., & Surewicz, W. K. (2010). Interaction between human prion protein and amyloid-beta (Abeta) oligomers: Role OF N-terminal residues. *Journal of Biological Chemistry, 285*(34), 26377–26383. https://doi.org/10.1074/jbc.M110.145516.

Chung, E., Ji, Y., Sun, Y., Kascsak, R. J., Kascsak, R. B., Mehta, P. D., et al. (2010). Anti-PrPC monoclonal antibody infusion as a novel treatment for cognitive deficits in an Alzheimer's disease model mouse. *BMC Neuroscience, 11*, 130. https://doi.org/10.1186/1471-2202-11-130.

Cisse, M., Halabisky, B., Harris, J., Devidze, N., Dubal, D. B., Sun, B., et al. (2011). Reversing EphB2 depletion rescues cognitive functions in Alzheimer model. *Nature, 469*(7328), 47–52. https://doi.org/10.1038/nature09635.

Citron, M., Westaway, D., Xia, W., Carlson, G., Diehl, T., Levesque, G., et al. (1997). Mutant presenilins of Alzheimer's disease increase production of 42-residue amyloid β-protein in both transfected cells and transgenic mice. *Nature Medicine, 3*(1), 67–72. https://doi.org/10.1038/nm0197-67.

Collins, M., Bartelt, R. R., & Houtman, J. C. (2010). T cell receptor activation leads to two distinct phases of Pyk2 activation and actin cytoskeletal rearrangement in human T cells. *Molecular Immunology, 47*(9), 1665–1674. https://doi.org/10.1016/j.molimm.2010.03.009.

Collins, M. O., Husi, H., Yu, L., Brandon, J. M., Anderson, C. N., Blackstock, W. P., et al. (2006). Molecular characterization and comparison of the components and multiprotein complexes in the postsynaptic proteome. *Journal of Neurochemistry, 97*(Suppl. 1), 16–23. https://doi.org/10.1111/j.1471-4159.2005.03507.x.

Collins, M., Tremblay, M., Chapman, N., Curtiss, M., Rothman, P. B., & Houtman, J. C. (2010). The T cell receptor-mediated phosphorylation of Pyk2 tyrosines 402 and 580

occurs via a distinct mechanism than other receptor systems. *Journal of Leukocyte Biology, 87*(4), 691–701. https://doi.org/10.1189/jlb.0409227.
Creese, I., Burt, D. R., & Snyder, S. H. (1976). Dopamine receptor binding predicts clinical and pharmacological potencies of antischizophrenic drugs. *Science, 192*(4238), 481–483.
DaRocha-Souto, B., Scotton, T. C., Coma, M., Serrano-Pozo, A., Hashimoto, T., Sereno, L., et al. (2011). Brain oligomeric beta-amyloid but not total amyloid plaque burden correlates with neuronal loss and astrocyte inflammatory response in amyloid precursor protein/tau transgenic mice. *Journal of Neuropathology and Experimental Neurology, 70*(5), 360–376. https://doi.org/10.1097/NEN.0b013e318217a118.
De Felice, F. G., Velasco, P. T., Lambert, M. P., Viola, K., Fernandez, S. J., Ferreira, S. T., et al. (2007). Abeta oligomers induce neuronal oxidative stress through an N-methyl-D-aspartate receptor-dependent mechanism that is blocked by the Alzheimer drug memantine. *Journal of Biological Chemistry, 282*(15), 11590–11601. https://doi.org/10.1074/jbc.M607483200.
Decker, H., Jurgensen, S., Adrover, M. F., Brito-Moreira, J., Bomfim, T. R., Klein, W. L., et al. (2010). N-methyl-D-aspartate receptors are required for synaptic targeting of Alzheimer's toxic amyloid-beta peptide oligomers. *Journal of Neurochemistry, 115*(6), 1520–1529. https://doi.org/10.1111/j.1471-4159.2010.07058.x.
Dineley, K. T., Westerman, M., Bui, D., Bell, K., Ashe, K. H., & Sweatt, J. D. (2001). Beta-amyloid activates the mitogen-activated protein kinase cascade via hippocampal alpha 7 nicotinic acetylcholine receptors: In vitro and in vivo mechanisms related to Alzheimer's disease. *Journal of Neuroscience, 21*(12), 4125–4133.
Dohler, F., Sepulveda-Falla, D., Krasemann, S., Altmeppen, H., Schluter, H., Hildebrand, D., et al. (2014). High molecular mass assemblies of amyloid-beta oligomers bind prion protein in patients with Alzheimer's disease. *Brain, 137*(Pt. 3), 873–886. https://doi.org/10.1093/brain/awt375.
Doody, R. S., Raman, R., Farlow, M., Iwatsubo, T., Vellas, B., Joffe, S., et al. (2013). A phase 3 trial of semagacestat for treatment of Alzheimer's disease. *The New England Journal of Medicine, 369*(4), 341–350. https://doi.org/10.1056/NEJMoa1210951.
Doody, R. S., Thomas, R. G., Farlow, M., Iwatsubo, T., Vellas, B., Joffe, S., et al. (2014). Phase 3 trials of solanezumab for mild-to-moderate Alzheimer's disease. *The New England Journal of Medicine, 370*(4), 311–321. https://doi.org/10.1056/NEJMoa1312889.
Esparza, T. J., Zhao, H., Cirrito, J. R., Cairns, N. J., Bateman, R. J., Holtzman, D. M., et al. (2013). Amyloid-beta oligomerization in Alzheimer dementia versus high-pathology controls. *Annals of Neurology, 73*(1), 104–119. https://doi.org/10.1002/ana.23748.
Fagan, A. M., Mintun, M. A., Mach, R. H., Lee, S. Y., Dence, C. S., Shah, A. R., et al. (2006). Inverse relation between in vivo amyloid imaging load and cerebrospinal fluid Abeta42 in humans. *Annals of Neurology, 59*(3), 512–519. https://doi.org/10.1002/ana.20730.
Fagan, A. M., Mintun, M. A., Shah, A. R., Aldea, P., Roe, C. M., Mach, R. H., et al. (2009). Cerebrospinal fluid tau and ptau(181) increase with cortical amyloid deposition in cognitively normal individuals: Implications for future clinical trials of Alzheimer's disease. *EMBO Molecular Medicine, 1*(8–9), 371–380. https://doi.org/10.1002/emmm.200900048.
Ferreira, I. L., Bajouco, L. M., Mota, S. I., Auberson, Y. P., Oliveira, C. R., & Rego, A. C. (2012). Amyloid beta peptide 1-42 disturbs intracellular calcium homeostasis through activation of GluN2B-containing N-methyl-D-aspartate receptors in cortical cultures. *Cell Calcium, 51*(2), 95–106. https://doi.org/10.1016/j.ceca.2011.11.008.
Figueiredo, C. P., Clarke, J. R., Ledo, J. H., Ribeiro, F. C., Costa, C. V., Melo, H. M., et al. (2013). Memantine rescues transient cognitive impairment caused by high-molecular-weight abeta oligomers but not the persistent impairment induced by low-molecular-

weight oligomers. *The Journal of Neuroscience*, *33*(23), 9626–9634. https://doi.org/10.1523/JNEUROSCI.0482-13.2013.

Fluharty, B. R., Biasini, E., Stravalaci, M., Sclip, A., Diomede, L., Balducci, C., et al. (2013). An N-terminal fragment of the prion protein binds to amyloid-beta oligomers and inhibits their neurotoxicity in vivo. *Journal of Biological Chemistry*, *288*(11), 7857–7866. https://doi.org/10.1074/jbc.M112.423954.

Fournier, A. E., GrandPre, T., & Strittmatter, S. M. (2001). Identification of a receptor mediating Nogo-66 inhibition of axonal regeneration. *Nature*, *409*(6818), 341–346. https://doi.org/10.1038/35053072.

Freir, D. B., Nicoll, A. J., Klyubin, I., Panico, S., Mc Donald, J. M., Risse, E., et al. (2011). Interaction between prion protein and toxic amyloid beta assemblies can be therapeutically targeted at multiple sites. *Nature Communications*, *2*, 336. https://doi.org/10.1038/ncomms1341.

Fu, A. K., Hung, K. W., Huang, H., Gu, S., Shen, Y., Cheng, E. Y., et al. (2014). Blockade of EphA4 signaling ameliorates hippocampal synaptic dysfunctions in mouse models of Alzheimer's disease. *Proceedings of the National Academy of Sciences of the United States of America*, *111*(27), 9959–9964. https://doi.org/10.1073/pnas.1405803111.

Games, D., Adams, D., Alessandrini, R., Barbour, R., Berthelette, P., Blackwell, C., et al. (1995). Alzheimer-type neuropathology in transgenic mice overexpressing V717F beta-amyloid precursor protein. *Nature*, *373*(6514), 523–527. https://doi.org/10.1038/373523a0.

Gimbel, D. A., Nygaard, H. B., Coffey, E. E., Gunther, E. C., Lauren, J., Gimbel, Z. A., et al. (2010). Memory impairment in transgenic Alzheimer mice requires cellular prion protein. *The Journal of Neuroscience*, *30*(18), 6367–6374. https://doi.org/10.1523/JNEUROSCI.0395-10.2010.

Giralt, A., Brito, V., Chevy, Q., Simonnet, C., Otsu, Y., Cifuentes-Diaz, C., et al. (2017). Pyk2 modulates hippocampal excitatory synapses and contributes to cognitive deficits in a Huntington's disease model. *Nature Communications*, *8*, 15592. https://doi.org/10.1038/ncomms15592.

Gong, Y., Chang, L., Viola, K. L., Lacor, P. N., Lambert, M. P., Finch, C. E., et al. (2003). Alzheimer's disease-affected brain: Presence of oligomeric A beta ligands (ADDLs) suggests a molecular basis for reversible memory loss. *Proceedings of the National Academy of Sciences of the United States of America*, *100*(18), 10417–10422. https://doi.org/10.1073/pnas.1834302100.

Grundke-Iqbal, I., Iqbal, K., Tung, Y. C., Quinlan, M., Wisniewski, H. M., & Binder, L. I. (1986). Abnormal phosphorylation of the microtubule-associated protein tau (tau) in Alzheimer cytoskeletal pathology. *Proceedings of the National Academy of Sciences of the United States of America*, *83*(13), 4913–4917. https://doi.org/10.1073/pnas.83.13.4913.

Haas, L. T., Salazar, S. V., Kostylev, M. A., Um, J. W., Kaufman, A. C., & Strittmatter, S. M. (2016). Metabotropic glutamate receptor 5 couples cellular prion protein to intracellular signalling in Alzheimer's disease. *Brain*, *139*(Pt. 2), 526–546. https://doi.org/10.1093/brain/awv356.

Haas, L. T., Salazar, S. V., Smith, L. M., Zhao, H. R., Cox, T. O., Herber, C. S., et al. (2017). Silent allosteric modulation of mGluR5 maintains glutamate signaling while rescuing Alzheimer's mouse phenotypes. *Cell Reports*, *20*(1), 76–88. https://doi.org/10.1016/j.celrep.2017.06.023.

Haas, L. T., & Strittmatter, S. M. (2016). Oligomers of amyloid beta prevent physiological activation of the cellular prion protein-metabotropic glutamate receptor 5 complex by glutamate in Alzheimer disease. *Journal of Biological Chemistry*, *291*(33), 17112–17121. https://doi.org/10.1074/jbc.M116.720664.

Haass, C., & Selkoe, D. J. (2007). Soluble protein oligomers in neurodegeneration: Lessons from the Alzheimer's amyloid beta-peptide. *Nature Reviews. Molecular Cell Biology*, *8*(2), 101–112. https://doi.org/10.1038/nrm2101.

Hamilton, A., Esseltine, J. L., DeVries, R. A., Cregan, S. P., & Ferguson, S. S. (2014). Metabotropic glutamate receptor 5 knockout reduces cognitive impairment and pathogenesis in a mouse model of Alzheimer's disease. *Molecular Brain*, *7*, 40. https://doi.org/10.1186/1756-6606-7-40.

Hardy, J. A., & Higgins, G. A. (1992). Alzheimer's disease: The amyloid cascade hypothesis. *Science*, *256*(5054), 184–185.

Hartigan, J. A., Xiong, W. C., & Johnson, G. V. (2001). Glycogen synthase kinase 3beta is tyrosine phosphorylated by PYK2. *Biochemical and Biophysical Research Communications*, *284*(2), 485–489. https://doi.org/10.1006/bbrc.2001.4986.

Heidinger, V., Manzerra, P., Wang, X. Q., Strasser, U., Yu, S. P., Choi, D. W., et al. (2002). Metabotropic glutamate receptor 1-induced upregulation of NMDA receptor current: Mediation through the Pyk2/Src-family kinase pathway in cortical neurons. *Journal of Neuroscience*, *22*(13), 5452–5461.

Heiss, J. K., Barrett, J., Yu, Z., Haas, L. T., Kostylev, M. A., & Strittmatter, S. M. (2016). Early activation of experience-independent dendritic spine turnover in a mouse model of Alzheimer's disease. *Cerebral Cortex*, *27*, 3660–3674. https://doi.org/10.1093/cercor/bhw188.

Hogg, R. C., Raggenbass, M., & Bertrand, D. (2003). Nicotinic acetylcholine receptors: From structure to brain function. *Reviews of Physiology, Biochemistry and Pharmacology*, *147*, 1–46. https://doi.org/10.1007/s10254-003-0005-1.

Holmes, C., Boche, D., Wilkinson, D., Yadegarfar, G., Hopkins, V., Bayer, A., et al. (2008). Long-term effects of Aβ42 immunisation in Alzheimer's disease: Follow-up of a randomised, placebo-controlled phase I trial. *The Lancet*, *372*(9634), 216–223. https://doi.org/10.1016/s0140-6736(08)61075-2.

Holtzman, D. M., Morris, J. C., & Goate, A. M. (2011). Alzheimer's disease: The challenge of the second century. *Science Translational Medicine*, *3*(77). 77sr71. https://doi.org/10.1126/scitranslmed.3002369.

Hong, S., Beja-Glasser, V. F., Nfonoyim, B. M., Frouin, A., Li, S., Ramakrishnan, S., et al. (2016). Complement and microglia mediate early synapse loss in Alzheimer mouse models. *Science*, *352*(6286), 712–716. https://doi.org/10.1126/science.aad8373.

Hooper, C., Killick, R., & Lovestone, S. (2008). The GSK3 hypothesis of Alzheimer's disease. *Journal of Neurochemistry*, *104*(6), 1433–1439. https://doi.org/10.1111/j.1471-4159.2007.05194.x.

Hsia, A. Y., Masliah, E., McConlogue, L., Yu, G. Q., Tatsuno, G., Hu, K., et al. (1999). Plaque-independent disruption of neural circuits in Alzheimer's disease mouse models. *Proceedings of the National Academy of Sciences of the United States of America*, *96*(6), 3228–3233. https://doi.org/10.1073/pnas.96.6.3228.

Hsin, H., Kim, M. J., Wang, C. F., & Sheng, M. (2010). Proline-rich tyrosine kinase 2 regulates hippocampal long-term depression. *The Journal of Neuroscience*, *30*(36), 11983–11993. https://doi.org/10.1523/JNEUROSCI.1029-10.2010.

Hu, N. W., Nicoll, A. J., Zhang, D., Mably, A. J., O'Malley, T., Purro, S. A., et al. (2014). mGlu5 Receptors and cellular prion protein mediate amyloid-beta-facilitated synaptic long-term depression in vivo. *Nature Communications*, *5*, 3374. https://doi.org/10.1038/ncomms4374.

Hu, F., Padukkavidana, T., Vaegter, C. B., Brady, O. A., Zheng, Y., Mackenzie, I. R., et al. (2010). Sortilin-mediated endocytosis determines levels of the frontotemporal dementia protein, progranulin. *Neuron*, *68*(4), 654–667. https://doi.org/10.1016/j.neuron.2010.09.034.

Huang, Y.-Q., Lu, W.-Y., Ali, D. W., Pelkey, K. A., Pitcher, G. M., Lu, Y. M., et al. (2001). CAKβ/Pyk2 kinase is a signaling link for induction of long-term potentiation in CA1 hippocampus. *Neuron*, *29*(2), 485–496. https://doi.org/10.1016/s0896-6273(01)00220-3.

Hurd, M. D., Martorell, P., Delavande, A., Mullen, K. J., & Langa, K. M. (2013). Monetary costs of dementia in the United States. *The New England Journal of Medicine*, *368*(14), 1326–1334. https://doi.org/10.1056/NEJMsa1204629.

Ingelsson, M., Fukumoto, H., Newell, K. L., Growdon, J. H., Hedley-Whyte, E. T., Frosch, M. P., et al. (2004). Early A beta accumulation and progressive synaptic loss, gliosis, and tangle formation in AD brain. *Neurology*, *62*(6), 925–931.

Ittner, L. M., Ke, Y. D., Delerue, F., Bi, M., Gladbach, A., van Eersel, J., et al. (2010). Dendritic function of tau mediates amyloid-beta toxicity in Alzheimer's disease mouse models. *Cell*, *142*(3), 387–397. https://doi.org/10.1016/j.cell.2010.06.036.

Izzo, N. J., Staniszewski, A., To, L., Fa, M., Teich, A. F., Saeed, F., et al. (2014). Alzheimer's therapeutics targeting amyloid beta 1-42 oligomers I: Abeta 42 oligomer binding to specific neuronal receptors is displaced by drug candidates that improve cognitive deficits. *PLoS One*, *9*(11), e111898. https://doi.org/10.1371/journal.pone.0111898.

Izzo, N. J., Xu, J., Zeng, C., Kirk, M. J., Mozzoni, K., Silky, C., et al. (2014). Alzheimer's therapeutics targeting amyloid beta 1-42 oligomers II: Sigma-2/PGRMC1 receptors mediate Abeta 42 oligomer binding and synaptotoxicity. *PLoS One*, *9*(11), e111899. https://doi.org/10.1371/journal.pone.0111899.

Jack, C. R., Jr., Knopman, D. S., Jagust, W. J., Petersen, R. C., Weiner, M. W., Aisen, P. S., et al. (2013). Tracking pathophysiological processes in Alzheimer's disease: An updated hypothetical model of dynamic biomarkers. *Lancet Neurology*, *12*(2), 207–216. https://doi.org/10.1016/S1474-4422(12)70291-0.

Jin, M., Shepardson, N., Yang, T., Chen, G., Walsh, D., & Selkoe, D. J. (2011). Soluble amyloid beta-protein dimers isolated from Alzheimer cortex directly induce Tau hyperphosphorylation and neuritic degeneration. *Proceedings of the National Academy of Sciences of the United States of America*, *108*(14), 5819–5824. https://doi.org/10.1073/pnas.1017033108.

Jurgensen, S., Antonio, L. L., Mussi, G. E., Brito-Moreira, J., Bomfim, T. R., De Felice, F. G., et al. (2011). Activation of D1/D5 dopamine receptors protects neurons from synapse dysfunction induced by amyloid-beta oligomers. *Journal of Biological Chemistry*, *286*(5), 3270–3276. https://doi.org/10.1074/jbc.M110.177790.

Jurgensen, S., & Ferreira, S. T. (2010). Nicotinic receptors, amyloid-beta, and synaptic failure in Alzheimer's disease. *Journal of Molecular Neuroscience*, *40*(1–2), 221–229. https://doi.org/10.1007/s12031-009-9237-0.

Kam, T. I., Song, S., Gwon, Y., Park, H., Yan, J. J., Im, I., et al. (2013). FcgammaRIIb mediates amyloid-beta neurotoxicity and memory impairment in Alzheimer's disease. *Journal of Clinical Investigation*, *123*(7), 2791–2802. https://doi.org/10.1172/JCI66827.

Karran, E., Mercken, M., & De Strooper, B. (2011). The amyloid cascade hypothesis for Alzheimer's disease: An appraisal for the development of therapeutics. *Nature Reviews Drug Discovery*, *10*(9), 698–712. https://doi.org/10.1038/nrd3505.

Kaufman, A. C., Salazar, S. V., Haas, L. T., Yang, J., Kostylev, M. A., Jeng, A. T., et al. (2015). Fyn inhibition rescues established memory and synapse loss in Alzheimer mice. *Annals of Neurology*, 77(6), 953–971. https://doi.org/10.1002/ana.24394.

Kayed, R., Head, E., Thompson, J. L., McIntire, T. M., Milton, S. C., Cotman, C. W., et al. (2003). Common structure of soluble amyloid oligomers implies common mechanism of pathogenesis. *Science*, *300*(5618), 486–489. https://doi.org/10.1126/science.1079469.

Kessels, H. W., Nguyen, L. N., Nabavi, S., & Malinow, R. (2010). The prion protein as a receptor for amyloid-beta. *Nature*, *466*(7308). E3-4; discussion E4-5. https://doi.org/10.1038/nature09217.

Kim, T., Vidal, G. S., Djurisic, M., William, C. M., Birnbaum, M. E., Garcia, K. C., et al. (2013). Human LilrB2 is a beta-amyloid receptor and its murine homolog PirB regulates synaptic plasticity in an Alzheimer's model. *Science*, *341*(6152), 1399–1404. https://doi.org/10.1126/science.1242077.

Koffie, R. M., Hyman, B. T., & Spires-Jones, T. L. (2011). Alzheimer's disease: Synapses gone cold. *Molecular Neurodegeneration*, *6*(1), 63. https://doi.org/10.1186/1750-1326-6-63.

Koffie, R. M., Meyer-Luehmann, M., Hashimoto, T., Adams, K. W., Mielke, M. L., Garcia-Alloza, M., et al. (2009). Oligomeric amyloid beta associates with postsynaptic densities and correlates with excitatory synapse loss near senile plaques. *Proceedings of the National Academy of Sciences of the United States of America*, *106*(10), 4012–4017. https://doi.org/10.1073/pnas.0811698106.

Kolodkin, A. L., Levengood, D. V., Rowe, E. G., Tai, Y. T., Giger, R. J., & Ginty, D. D. (1997). Neuropilin is a semaphorin III receptor. *Cell*, *90*(4), 753–762. https://doi.org/10.1016/S0092-8674(00)80535-8.

Kostylev, M. A., Kaufman, A. C., Nygaard, H. B., Patel, P., Haas, L. T., Gunther, E. C., et al. (2015). Prion-protein-interacting amyloid-beta oligomers of high molecular weight are tightly correlated with memory impairment in multiple Alzheimer mouse models. *Journal of Biological Chemistry*, *290*(28), 17415–17438. https://doi.org/10.1074/jbc.M115.643577.

Kudo, W., Lee, H. P., Zou, W. Q., Wang, X., Perry, G., Zhu, X., et al. (2012). Cellular prion protein is essential for oligomeric amyloid-beta-induced neuronal cell death. *Human Molecular Genetics*, *21*(5), 1138–1144. https://doi.org/10.1093/hmg/ddr542.

Kuner, P., Schubenel, R., & Hertel, C. (1998). β-Amyloid binds to p75NTR and activates NFκB in human neuroblastoma cells. *Journal of Neuroscience Research*, *54*(6), 798–804. https://doi.org/10.1002/(SICI)1097-4547(19981215)54:6<798::AID-JNR7>3.0.CO;2-T/abstract.

Lambert, M. P., Barlow, A. K., Chromy, B. A., Edwards, C., Freed, R., Liosatos, M., et al. (1998). Diffusible, nonfibrillar ligands derived from A 1-42 are potent central nervous system neurotoxins. *Proceedings of the National Academy of Sciences of the United States of America*, *95*(11), 6448–6453. https://doi.org/10.1073/pnas.95.11.6448.

Lambert, J. C., Ibrahim-Verbaas, C. A., Harold, D., Naj, A. C., Sims, R., Bellenguez, C., et al. (2013). Meta-analysis of 74,046 individuals identifies 11 new susceptibility loci for Alzheimer's disease. *Nature Genetics*, *45*(12), 1452–1458. https://doi.org/10.1038/ng.2802.

Lansbury, P. T. (1999). Evolution of amyloid: What normal protein folding may tell us about fibrillogenesis and disease. *Proceedings of the National Academy of Sciences of the United States of America*, *96*(7), 3342–3344. https://doi.org/10.1073/pnas.96.7.3342.

Lanz, T. A., Carter, D. B., & Merchant, K. M. (2003). Dendritic spine loss in the hippocampus of young PDAPP and Tg2576 mice and its prevention by the ApoE2 genotype. *Neurobiology of Disease*, *13*(3), 246–253. https://doi.org/10.1016/S0969-9961(03)00079-2.

Larson, M., Sherman, M. A., Amar, F., Nuvolone, M., Schneider, J. A., Bennett, D. A., et al. (2012). The complex PrP(c)-Fyn couples human oligomeric Abeta with pathological tau changes in Alzheimer's disease. *The Journal of Neuroscience*, *32*(47), 16857–16871a. https://doi.org/10.1523/JNEUROSCI.1858-12.2012.

Lauren, J., Gimbel, D. A., Nygaard, H. B., Gilbert, J. W., & Strittmatter, S. M. (2009). Cellular prion protein mediates impairment of synaptic plasticity by amyloid-beta oligomers. *Nature*, *457*(7233), 1128–1132. https://doi.org/10.1038/nature07761.

Lee, G., Thangavel, R., Sharma, V. M., Litersky, J. M., Bhaskar, K., Fang, S. M., et al. (2004). Phosphorylation of tau by fyn: Implications for Alzheimer's disease. *The Journal of Neuroscience*, *24*(9), 2304–2312. https://doi.org/10.1523/JNEUROSCI.4162-03.2004.

Levy, E., Carman, M., Fernandez-Madrid, I., Power, M., Lieberburg, I., van Duinen, S., et al. (1990). Mutation of the Alzheimer's disease amyloid gene in hereditary cerebral hemorrhage, Dutch type. *Science*, *248*(4959), 1124–1126. https://doi.org/10.1126/science.2111584.

Liu, B. P., Fournier, A., GrandPre, T., & Strittmatter, S. M. (2002). Myelin-associated glycoprotein as a functional ligand for the Nogo-66 receptor. *Science*, *297*(5584), 1190–1193. https://doi.org/10.1126/science.1073031.

Lu, Y. M., Jia, Z. P., Janus, C., Henderson, J. T., Gerlai, R., Wojtowicz, J. M., et al. (1997). Mice lacking metabotropic glutamate receptor 5 show impaired learning and reduced CA1 long-term potentiation (LTP) but normal CA3 LTP. *Journal of Neuroscience*, *17*(13), 5196–5205.

Lue, L. F., Kuo, Y. M., Roher, A. E., Brachova, L., Shen, Y., Sue, L., et al. (1999). Soluble amyloid beta peptide concentration as a predictor of synaptic change in Alzheimer's disease. *The American Journal of Pathology*, *155*(3), 853–862.

McKhann, G. M., Knopman, D. S., Chertkow, H., Hyman, B. T., Jack, C. R., Jr., Kawas, C. H., et al. (2011). The diagnosis of dementia due to Alzheimer's disease: Recommendations from the National Institute on Aging-Alzheimer's Association workgroups on diagnostic guidelines for Alzheimer's disease. *Alzheimer's & Dementia*, 7(3), 263–269. https://doi.org/10.1016/j.jalz.2011.03.005.

McLean, C. A., Cherny, R. A., Fraser, F. W., Fuller, S. J., Smith, M. J., Beyreuther, K., et al. (1999). Soluble pool of Abeta amyloid as a determinant of severity of neurodegeneration in Alzheimer's disease. *Annals of Neurology*, *46*(6), 860–866.

Mondragon-Rodriguez, S., Trillaud-Doppia, E., Dudilot, A., Bourgeois, C., Lauzon, M., Leclerc, N., et al. (2012). Interaction of endogenous tau protein with synaptic proteins is regulated by N-methyl-D-aspartate receptor-dependent tau phosphorylation. *Journal of Biological Chemistry*, *287*(38), 32040–32053. https://doi.org/10.1074/jbc.M112.401240.

Mota, S. I., Ferreira, I. L., & Rego, A. C. (2014). Dysfunctional synapse in Alzheimer's disease—A focus on NMDA receptors. *Neuropharmacology*, *76*(Pt. A), 16–26. https://doi.org/10.1016/j.neuropharm.2013.08.013.

Mulkey, R. M., Endo, S., Shenolikar, S., & Malenka, R. C. (1994). Involvement of a calcineurin/inhibitor-1 phosphatase cascade in hippocampal long-term depression. *Nature*, *369*(6480), 486–488. https://doi.org/10.1038/369486a0.

Murphy, C., Gilmore, N. M., Seery, C. S., Salmon, D. P., & Lasker, B. R. (1990). Olfactory thresholds are associated with degree of dementia in Alzheimer's disease. *Neurobiology of Aging*, *11*(4), 465–469. https://doi.org/10.1016/0197-4580(90)90014-Q.

Nakamura, F., Tanaka, M., Takahashi, T., Kalb, R. G., & Strittmatter, S. M. (1998). Neuropilin-1 extracellular domains mediate semaphorin D/III-induced growth cone collapse. *Neuron*, *21*(5), 1093–1100. https://doi.org/10.1016/S0896-6273(00)80626-1.

Nguyen, T. H., Liu, J., & Lombroso, P. J. (2002). Striatal enriched phosphatase 61 dephosphorylates Fyn at phosphotyrosine 420. *Journal of Biological Chemistry*, *277*(27), 24274–24279. https://doi.org/10.1074/jbc.M111683200.

Nicoll, A. J., Panico, S., Freir, D. B., Wright, D., Terry, C., Risse, E., et al. (2013). Amyloid-beta nanotubes are associated with prion protein-dependent synaptotoxicity. *Nature Communications*, *4*, 2416. https://doi.org/10.1038/ncomms3416.

Nygaard, H. B., Wagner, A. F., Bowen, G. S., Good, S. P., MacAvoy, M. G., Strittmatter, K. A., et al. (2015). A phase Ib multiple ascending dose study of the safety, tolerability, and central nervous system availability of AZD0530 (saracatinib) in Alzheimer's disease. *Alzheimer's Research & Therapy*, 7(1), 35. https://doi.org/10.1186/s13195-015-0119-0.

Oakley, H., Cole, S. L., Logan, S., Maus, E., Shao, P., Craft, J., et al. (2006). Intraneuronal beta-amyloid aggregates, neurodegeneration, and neuron loss in transgenic mice with five familial Alzheimer's disease mutations: Potential factors in amyloid plaque formation. *The Journal of Neuroscience, 26*(40), 10129–10140. https://doi.org/10.1523/JNEUROSCI.1202-06.2006.

Oddo, S., Caccamo, A., Kitazawa, M., Tseng, B. P., & LaFerla, F. M. (2003). Amyloid deposition precedes tangle formation in a triple transgenic model of Alzheimer's disease. *Neurobiology of Aging, 24*(8), 1063–1070. https://doi.org/10.1016/j.neurobiolaging.2003.08.012.

Oddo, S., Caccamo, A., Shepherd, J. D., Murphy, M. P., Golde, T. E., Kayed, R., et al. (2003). Triple-transgenic model of Alzheimer's disease with plaques and tangles. *Neuron, 39*(3), 409–421. https://doi.org/10.1016/s0896-6273(03)00434-3.

Ostapchenko, V. G., Beraldo, F. H., Mohammad, A. H., Xie, Y. F., Hirata, P. H., Magalhaes, A. C., et al. (2013). The prion protein ligand, stress-inducible phosphoprotein 1, regulates amyloid-beta oligomer toxicity. *The Journal of Neuroscience, 33*(42), 16552–16564. https://doi.org/10.1523/JNEUROSCI.3214-13.2013.

Overk, C. R., Cartier, A., Shaked, G., Rockenstein, E., Ubhi, K., Spencer, B., et al. (2014). Hippocampal neuronal cells that accumulate alpha-synuclein fragments are more vulnerable to Abeta oligomer toxicity via mGluR5—Implications for dementia with Lewy bodies. *Molecular Neurodegeneration, 9*, 18. https://doi.org/10.1186/1750-1326-9-18.

Owuor, K., Harel, N. Y., Englot, D. J., Hisama, F., Blumenfeld, H., & Strittmatter, S. M. (2009). LGI1-associated epilepsy through altered ADAM23-dependent neuronal morphology. *Molecular and Cellular Neurosciences, 42*(4), 448–457. https://doi.org/10.1016/j.mcn.2009.09.008.

Park, S. Y., Avraham, H. K., & Avraham, S. (2004). RAFTK/Pyk2 activation is mediated by trans-acting autophosphorylation in a Src-independent manner. *Journal of Biological Chemistry, 279*(32), 33315–33322. https://doi.org/10.1074/jbc.M313527200.

Park, J. H., Gimbel, D. A., GrandPre, T., Lee, J. K., Kim, J. E., Li, W., et al. (2006). Alzheimer precursor protein interaction with the Nogo-66 receptor reduces amyloid-beta plaque deposition. *The Journal of Neuroscience, 26*(5), 1386–1395. https://doi.org/10.1523/JNEUROSCI.3291-05.2006.

Perez-Nievas, B. G., Stein, T. D., Tai, H. C., Dols-Icardo, O., Scotton, T. C., Barroeta-Espar, I., et al. (2013). Dissecting phenotypic traits linked to human resilience to Alzheimer's pathology. *Brain, 136*(Pt. 8), 2510–2526. https://doi.org/10.1093/brain/awt171.

Porter, R. H., Jaeschke, G., Spooren, W., Ballard, T. M., Buttelmann, B., Kolczewski, S., et al. (2005). Fenobam: A clinically validated nonbenzodiazepine anxiolytic is a potent, selective, and noncompetitive mGlu5 receptor antagonist with inverse agonist activity. *Journal of Pharmacology and Experimental Therapeutics, 315*(2), 711–721. https://doi.org/10.1124/jpet.105.089839.

Puolivali, J., Wang, J., Heikkinen, T., Heikkila, M., Tapiola, T., van Groen, T., et al. (2002). Hippocampal A beta 42 levels correlate with spatial memory deficit in APP and PS1 double transgenic mice. *Neurobiology of Disease, 9*(3), 339–347. https://doi.org/10.1006/nbdi.2002.0481.

Rajagopalan, S., Deitinghoff, L., Davis, D., Conrad, S., Skutella, T., Chedotal, A., et al. (2004). Neogenin mediates the action of repulsive guidance molecule. *Nature Cell Biology, 6*(8), 756–762. https://doi.org/10.1038/ncb1156.

Raka, F., Di Sebastiano, A. R., Kulhawy, S. C., Ribeiro, F. M., Godin, C. M., Caetano, F. A., et al. (2015). Ca(2+)/calmodulin-dependent protein kinase II interacts with group I metabotropic glutamate and facilitates receptor endocytosis and ERK1/2 signaling: Role of beta-amyloid. *Molecular Brain, 8*, 21. https://doi.org/10.1186/s13041-015-0111-4.

Reiman, E. M., Chen, K., Liu, X., Bandy, D., Yu, M., Lee, W., et al. (2009). Fibrillar amyloid-beta burden in cognitively normal people at 3 levels of genetic risk for

Alzheimer's disease. *Proceedings of the National Academy of Sciences of the United States of America, 106*(16), 6820–6825. https://doi.org/10.1073/pnas.0900345106.
Reisberg, B., Doody, R., & Mobius, H. J. (2003). Memantine in moderate-to-severe Alzheimer's disease—Reply. *New England Journal of Medicine, 349*(6), 610.
Renner, M., Lacor, P. N., Velasco, P. T., Xu, J., Contractor, A., Klein, W. L., et al. (2010). Deleterious effects of amyloid beta oligomers acting as an extracellular scaffold for mGluR5. *Neuron, 66*(5), 739–754. https://doi.org/10.1016/j.neuron.2010.04.029.
Resenberger, U. K., Harmeier, A., Woerner, A. C., Goodman, J. L., Muller, V., Krishnan, R., et al. (2011). The cellular prion protein mediates neurotoxic signalling of beta-sheet-rich conformers independent of prion replication. *EMBO Journal, 30*(10), 2057–2070. https://doi.org/10.1038/emboj.2011.86.
Rhinn, H., Fujita, R., Qiang, L., Cheng, R., Lee, J. H., & Abeliovich, A. (2013). Integrative genomics identifies APOE epsilon4 effectors in Alzheimer's disease. *Nature, 500*(7460), 45–50. https://doi.org/10.1038/nature12415.
Roberson, E. D., Scearce-Levie, K., Palop, J. J., Yan, F., Cheng, I. H., Wu, T., et al. (2007). Reducing endogenous tau ameliorates amyloid beta-induced deficits in an Alzheimer's disease mouse model. *Science, 316*(5825), 750–754. https://doi.org/10.1126/science.1141736.
Roche, K. W., Standley, S., McCallum, J., Dune Ly, C., Ehlers, M. D., & Wenthold, R. J. (2001). Molecular determinants of NMDA receptor internalization. *Nature Neuroscience, 4*(8), 794–802. https://doi.org/10.1038/90498.
Rodriguez, A. L., Grier, M. D., Jones, C. K., Herman, E. J., Kane, A. S., Smith, R. L., et al. (2010). Discovery of novel allosteric modulators of metabotropic glutamate receptor subtype 5 reveals chemical and functional diversity and in vivo activity in rat behavioral models of anxiolytic and antipsychotic activity. *Molecular Pharmacology, 78*(6), 1105–1123. https://doi.org/10.1124/mol.110.067207.
Ronesi, J. A., & Huber, K. M. (2008). Homer interactions are necessary for metabotropic glutamate receptor-induced long-term depression and translational activation. *The Journal of Neuroscience, 28*(2), 543–547. https://doi.org/10.1523/JNEUROSCI.5019-07.2008.
Roselli, F., Tirard, M., Lu, J., Hutzler, P., Lamberti, P., Livrea, P., et al. (2005). Soluble beta-amyloid1-40 induces NMDA-dependent degradation of postsynaptic density-95 at glutamatergic synapses. *The Journal of Neuroscience, 25*(48), 11061–11070. https://doi.org/10.1523/JNEUROSCI.3034-05.2005.
Rushworth, J. V., Griffiths, H. H., Watt, N. T., & Hooper, N. M. (2013). Prion protein-mediated toxicity of amyloid-beta oligomers requires lipid rafts and the transmembrane LRP1. *Journal of Biological Chemistry, 288*(13), 8935–8951. https://doi.org/10.1074/jbc.M112.400358.
Salloway, S., Sperling, R., Fox, N. C., Blennow, K., Klunk, W., Raskind, M., et al. (2014). Two phase 3 trials of bapineuzumab in mild-to-moderate Alzheimer's disease. *The New England Journal of Medicine, 370*(4), 322–333. https://doi.org/10.1056/NEJMoa1304839.
Savage, M. J., Kalinina, J., Wolfe, A., Tugusheva, K., Korn, R., Cash-Mason, T., et al. (2014). A sensitive abeta oligomer assay discriminates Alzheimer's and aged control cerebrospinal fluid. *The Journal of Neuroscience, 34*(8), 2884–2897. https://doi.org/10.1523/JNEUROSCI.1675-13.2014.
Sayas, C. L., Ariaens, A., Ponsioen, B., & Moolenaar, W. H. (2006). GSK-3 is activated by the tyrosine kinase Pyk2 during LPA1-mediated neurite retraction. *Molecular Biology of the Cell, 17*(4), 1834–1844.
Scheff, S. W., Price, D. A., Schmitt, F. A., DeKosky, S. T., & Mufson, E. J. (2007). Synaptic alterations in CA1 in mild Alzheimer disease and mild cognitive impairment. *Neurology, 68*(18), 1501–1508. https://doi.org/10.1212/01.wnl.0000260698.46517.8f.
Scott-McKean, J. J., Surewicz, K., Choi, J. K., Ruffin, V. A., Salameh, A. I., Nieznanski, K., et al. (2016). Soluble prion protein and its N-terminal fragment prevent impairment of

synaptic plasticity by Abeta oligomers: Implications for novel therapeutic strategy in Alzheimer's disease. *Neurobiology of Disease*, *91*, 124–131. https://doi.org/10.1016/j.nbd.2016.03.001.

Seabold, G. K., Burette, A., Lim, I. A., Weinberg, R. J., & Hell, J. W. (2003). Interaction of the tyrosine kinase Pyk2 with the N-methyl-D-aspartate receptor complex via the Src homology 3 domains of PSD-95 and SAP102. *Journal of Biological Chemistry*, *278*(17), 15040–15048. https://doi.org/10.1074/jbc.M212825200.

Serrano-Pozo, A., Frosch, M. P., Masliah, E., & Hyman, B. T. (2011). Neuropathological alterations in Alzheimer disease. *Cold Spring Harbor Perspectives in Medicine*, *1*(1), a006189. https://doi.org/10.1101/cshperspect.a006189.

Shankar, G. M., Li, S., Mehta, T. H., Garcia-Munoz, A., Shepardson, N. E., Smith, I., et al. (2008). Amyloid-beta protein dimers isolated directly from Alzheimer's brains impair synaptic plasticity and memory. *Nature Medicine*, *14*(8), 837–842. https://doi.org/10.1038/nm1782.

Shaw, L. M., Vanderstichele, H., Knapik-Czajka, M., Clark, C. M., Aisen, P. S., Petersen, R. C., et al. (2009). Cerebrospinal fluid biomarker signature in Alzheimer's disease neuroimaging initiative subjects. *Annals of Neurology*, *65*(4), 403–413. https://doi.org/10.1002/ana.21610.

Smith, L. M., & Strittmatter, S. M. (2017). Binding sites for amyloid-beta oligomers and synaptic toxicity. *Cold Spring Harbor Perspectives in Medicine*, 7(5). https://doi.org/10.1101/cshperspect.a024075.

Snyder, E. M., Nong, Y., Almeida, C. G., Paul, S., Moran, T., Choi, E. Y., et al. (2005). Regulation of NMDA receptor trafficking by amyloid-beta. *Nature Neuroscience*, *8*(8), 1051–1058. https://doi.org/10.1038/nn1503.

Sperling, R. A., Aisen, P. S., Beckett, L. A., Bennett, D. A., Craft, S., Fagan, A. M., et al. (2011). Toward defining the preclinical stages of Alzheimer's disease: Recommendations from the National Institute on Aging-Alzheimer's Association workgroups on diagnostic guidelines for Alzheimer's disease. *Alzheimer's & Dementia*, 7(3), 280–292. https://doi.org/10.1016/j.jalz.2011.03.003.

Spires-Jones, T. L., & Hyman, B. T. (2014). The intersection of amyloid beta and tau at synapses in Alzheimer's disease. *Neuron*, *82*(4), 756–771. https://doi.org/10.1016/j.neuron.2014.05.004.

Syken, J., Grandpre, T., Kanold, P. O., & Shatz, C. J. (2006). PirB restricts ocular-dominance plasticity in visual cortex. *Science*, *313*(5794), 1795–1800. https://doi.org/10.1126/science.1128232.

Takahashi, T., Fournier, A., Nakamura, F., Wang, L. H., Murakami, Y., Kalb, R. G., et al. (1999). Plexin-neuropilin-1 complexes form functional semaphorin-3A receptors. *Cell*, *99*(1), 59–69. https://doi.org/10.1016/S0092-8674(00)80062-8.

Takahashi, T., Nakamura, F., & Strittmatter, S. M. (1997). Neuronal and non-neuronal collapsin-1 binding sites in developing chick are distinct from other semaphorin binding sites. *The Journal of Neuroscience*, *17*(23), 9183–9193.

Um, J. W., Kaufman, A. C., Kostylev, M., Heiss, J. K., Stagi, M., Takahashi, H., et al. (2013). Metabotropic glutamate receptor 5 is a coreceptor for Alzheimer abeta oligomer bound to cellular prion protein. *Neuron*, *79*(5), 887–902. https://doi.org/10.1016/j.neuron.2013.06.036.

Um, J. W., Nygaard, H. B., Heiss, J. K., Kostylev, M. A., Stagi, M., Vortmeyer, A., et al. (2012). Alzheimer amyloid-beta oligomer bound to postsynaptic prion protein activates Fyn to impair neurons. *Nature Neuroscience*, *15*(9), 1227–1235. https://doi.org/10.1038/nn.3178.

Vergara, C., Ordonez-Gutierrez, L., Wandosell, F., Ferrer, I., del Rio, J. A., & Gavin, R. (2015). Role of PrP(C) expression in tau protein levels and phosphorylation in Alzheimer's disease evolution. *Molecular Neurobiology*, *51*(3), 1206–1220. https://doi.org/10.1007/s12035-014-8793-7.

Wang, L., Chiang, H. C., Wu, W., Liang, B., Xie, Z., Yao, X., et al. (2012). Epidermal growth factor receptor is a preferred target for treating amyloid-beta-induced memory loss. *Proceedings of the National Academy of Sciences of the United States of America, 109*(41), 16743–16748. https://doi.org/10.1073/pnas.1208011109.

Wang, H.-Y., Lee, D. H. S., D'Andrea, M. R., Peterson, P. A., Shank, R. P., & Reitz, A. B. (2000). β-Amyloid1–42 binds to α7 nicotinic acetylcholine receptor with high affinity. *Journal of Biological Chemistry, 275*(8), 5626–5632. https://doi.org/10.1074/jbc.275.8.5626.

Wang, Q., Walsh, D. M., Rowan, M. J., Selkoe, D. J., & Anwyl, R. (2004). Block of long-term potentiation by naturally secreted and synthetic amyloid beta-peptide in hippocampal slices is mediated via activation of the kinases c-Jun N-terminal kinase, cyclin-dependent kinase 5, and p38 mitogen-activated protein kinase as well as metabotropic glutamate receptor type 5. *The Journal of Neuroscience, 24*(13), 3370–3378. https://doi.org/10.1523/JNEUROSCI.1633-03.2004.

Xie, L., Helmerhorst, E., Taddei, K., Plewright, B., Van Bronswijk, W., & Martins, R. (2002). Alzheimer's beta-amyloid peptides compete for insulin binding to the insulin receptor. *The Journal of Neuroscience, 22*(10). RC221. doi: 20026383. http://www.jneurosci.org/cgi/content/full/6383.

Xu, J., Zhu, Y., Contractor, A., & Heinemann, S. F. (2009). mGluR5 has a critical role in inhibitory learning. *The Journal of Neuroscience, 29*(12), 3676–3684. https://doi.org/10.1523/JNEUROSCI.5716-08.2009.

Yaar, M., Zhai, S., Pilch, P. F., Doyle, S. M., Eisenhauer, P. B., Fine, R. E., et al. (1997). Binding of beta-amyloid to the p75 neurotrophin receptor induces apoptosis. A possible mechanism for Alzheimer's disease. *Journal of Clinical Investigation, 100*(9), 2333–2340. https://doi.org/10.1172/JCI119772.

Yan, S. D., Chen, X., Fu, J., Chen, M., Zhu, H., Roher, A., et al. (1996). RAGE and amyloid-beta peptide neurotoxicity in Alzheimer's disease. *Nature, 382*(6593), 685–691. https://doi.org/10.1038/382685a0.

Yang, T., Hong, S., O'Malley, T., Sperling, R. A., Walsh, D. M., & Selkoe, D. J. (2013). New ELISAs with high specificity for soluble oligomers of amyloid beta-protein detect natural Abeta oligomers in human brain but not CSF. *Alzheimer's & Dementia, 9*(2), 99–112. https://doi.org/10.1016/j.jalz.2012.11.005.

Yang, T., Li, S., Xu, H., Walsh, D. M., & Selkoe, D. J. (2017). Large soluble oligomers of amyloid beta-protein from Alzheimer brain are far less neuroactive than the smaller oligomers to which they dissociate. *The Journal of Neuroscience, 37*(1), 152–163. https://doi.org/10.1523/JNEUROSCI.1698-16.2016.

Zempel, H., Thies, E., Mandelkow, E., & Mandelkow, E. M. (2010). Abeta oligomers cause localized Ca(2+) elevation, missorting of endogenous tau into dendrites, tau phosphorylation, and destruction of microtubules and spines. *The Journal of Neuroscience, 30*(36), 11938–11950. https://doi.org/10.1523/JNEUROSCI.2357-10.2010.

Zhang, D., Qi, Y., Klyubin, I., Ondrejcak, T., Sarell, C. J., Cuello, A. C., et al. (2017). Targeting glutamatergic and cellular prion protein mechanisms of amyloid beta-mediated persistent synaptic plasticity disruption: Longitudinal studies. *Neuropharmacology, 121*, 231–246. https://doi.org/10.1016/j.neuropharm.2017.03.036.

Zhang, Y., Venkitaramani, D. V., Gladding, C. M., Zhang, Y., Kurup, P., Molnar, E., et al. (2008). The tyrosine phosphatase STEP mediates AMPA receptor endocytosis after metabotropic glutamate receptor stimulation. *The Journal of Neuroscience, 28*(42), 10561–10566. https://doi.org/10.1523/JNEUROSCI.2666-08.2008.

Zhang, H., Wu, L., Pchitskaya, E., Zakharova, O., Saito, T., Saido, T., et al. (2015). Neuronal store-operated calcium entry and mushroom spine loss in amyloid precursor protein knock-in mouse model of Alzheimer's disease. *The Journal of Neuroscience, 35*(39), 13275–13286. https://doi.org/10.1523/JNEUROSCI.1034-15.2015.

CHAPTER FOURTEEN

The Neurobiology of D-Serine Signaling

Herman Wolosker[1]
Rappaport Faculty of Medicine and Research Institute, Technion—Israel Institute of Technology, Haifa, Israel
[1]Corresponding author: e-mail address: hwolosker@tx.technion.ac.il

Contents

Abstract

D-Serine is a physiological coagonist of NMDA receptors involved in synaptic plasticity, neurodevelopment, and neurodegeneration. D-Serine is synthesized by the enzyme serine racemase, which converts L- to D-serine. Recent studies indicate that the supply of L-serine by astroglia fuels the neuronal synthesis of D-serine. This pathway, named the serine shuttle, highlights the importance of the glia–neuron metabolic crosstalk for regulating NMDA receptor activity. Dysfunction of different components of the serine shuttle pathway leads to neurodevelopmental defects, neurodegeneration, and may be involved in psychiatric diseases. Serine racemase and other components of the serine shuttle are therefore promising targets for neuroprotective drugs. Here we review several aspects of the neurobiology of D-serine focusing on mechanisms regulating D-serine signaling in health and disease.

Advances in Pharmacology, Volume 82
ISSN 1054-3589
https://doi.org/10.1016/bs.apha.2017.08.010

ABBREVIATIONS

ALS amyotrophic lateral sclerosis
DAAO D-amino acid oxidase
LTP long-term potentiation
NMDA *N*-methyl D-aspartate
Phgdh 3-phosphoglycerate dehydrogenase
PIP_2 phosphatidylinositol 4,5-bisphosphate
SR serine racemase

1. INTRODUCTION

The NMDA type of glutamate receptors (NMDARs) plays a role in excitatory neurotransmission, synaptic plastic, and learning and memory (Traynelis et al., 2010). The activation of NMDARs requires the binding of a coagonist (D-serine or glycine) along with glutamate to its GluN1 and GluN2 subunits, respectively (Johnson & Ascher, 1987; Kleckner & Dingledine, 1988). D-Serine is considered the main NMDAR coagonist in the forebrain where it mediates several NMDAR-dependent processes ranging from normal neurotransmission to neurodegeneration (Billard, 2012; Boehning & Snyder, 2003; Wolosker, Dumin, Balan, & Foltyn, 2008).

D-Serine is synthesized by the enzyme serine racemase (SR), which converts L- to D-serine (Wolosker, Blackshaw, & Snyder, 1999; Wolosker, Sheth, et al., 1999). D-Serine was long considered a prototypical "gliotransmitter" (Henneberger, Papouin, Oliet, & Rusakov, 2010; Martineau, Baux, & Mothet, 2006b; Martineau et al., 2013; Mothet et al., 2005; Panatier et al., 2006; Schell, Molliver, & Snyder, 1995), but recent data from several laboratories indicate that D-serine and SR are predominantly localized to neurons in the normal brain (Balu, Takagi, Puhl, Benneyworth, & Coyle, 2014; Benneyworth, Li, Basu, Bolshakov, & Coyle, 2012; Ehmsen et al., 2013; Kartvelishvily, Shleper, Balan, Dumin, & Wolosker, 2006; Miya et al., 2008; Perez et al., 2017; Wolosker, Balu, & Coyle, 2016). Selective deletion of SR in neurons impairs NMDAR-dependent synaptic plasticity both in vitro (Benneyworth et al., 2012) and in vivo (Perez et al., 2017), establishing a physiological role of neuronal D-serine in the NMDAR regulation.

Astrocytes are key for the synthesis of D-serine by supplying L-serine to neurons, which is required for the activity of SR. This metabolic crosstalk, recently named the serine shuttle (Wolosker, 2011; Wolosker &

Radzishevsky, 2013) (Fig. 1), is critical for neuronal survival and neurodevelopment (de Koning et al., 2003; Furuya et al., 2000; Hirabayashi & Furuya, 2008). Astrocytic glycolytic activity generates 3-phosphoglycerate that is oxidized into 3-phosphohydroxypyruvate by the 3-phosphoglycerate dehydrogenase (Phgdh) enzyme (Fig. 1). Subsequent transamination and dephosphorylation reactions generate L-serine. The latter shuttles from astroglia to neurons to fuel the neuronal synthesis of D-serine. D-Serine is subsequently released from neurons to activate

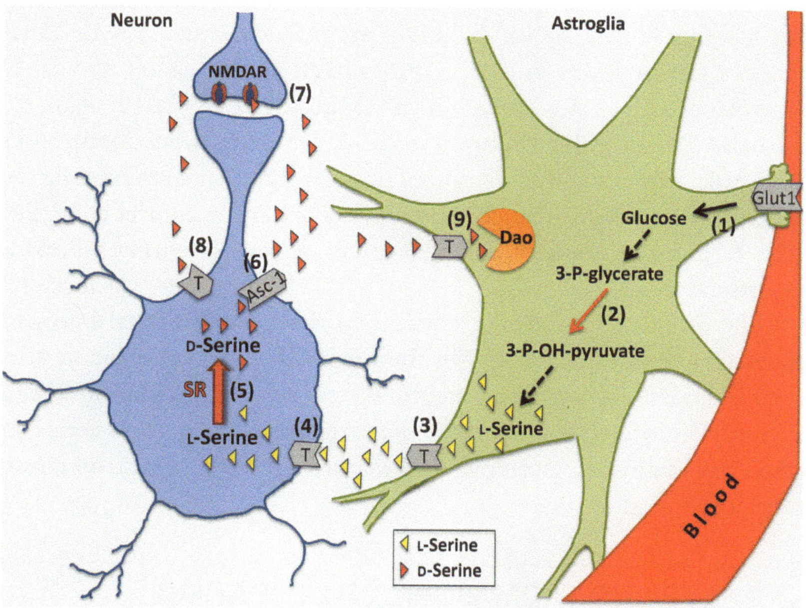

Fig. 1 Serine shuttle model of D-serine signaling. Astrocytes obtain glucose from blood vessels through glucose transporter 1 (GLUT1, step 1). Glucose is converted into L-serine in several steps, with the committed step catalyzed by the 3-phosphoglycerate dehydrogenase (Phgdh) enzyme (step 2). L-Serine exits the astrocytes by neutral amino acid exchangers, such as ASCT1 (Slc1a4) (T, step 3). Neurons take up L-serine by transport systems (T, step 4). Neuronal SR produces D-serine from L-serine (step 5). D-Serine is subsequently released from neurons through other transporters (step 6). Released D-serine allows synaptic NMDAR activation (step 7). D-Serine signaling may terminate through neuronal reuptake (step 8) or low-affinity astrocytic uptake and subsequent metabolism by the peroxisomal D-amino acid oxidase (step 9). *Dao*, D-amino acid oxidase; *glut1*, glucose transporter 1; *3-P-glycerate*, 3-phosphoglyceric acid; *3-P-OH-pyruvate*, 3-phosphohydroxypyruvate. *Adapted from Wolosker, H., Balu, D. T., & Coyle, J. T. (2016). The rise and fall of the D-serine-mediated gliotransmission hypothesis.* Trends in Neurosciences, *39(11), 712–721. https://doi.org/10.1016/j.tins.2016.09.007. S0166-2236(16)30118-7 [pii].*

NMDA receptors (Rosenberg et al., 2013, 2010; Sason et al., 2017). According to the serine shuttle hypothesis (Fig. 1), D-serine signaling is terminated by two mechanisms. The first is neuronal reuptake of D-serine, while the second mechanism consists of astrocytic uptake and subsequent metabolism by the D-serine catabolic enzyme, the peroxisomal D-amino acid oxidase (DAAO) (Fig. 1).

Dysfunction of several components of the serine shuttle is associated with pathological conditions. Mutations in enzymes specifically involved in the L-serine biosynthesis pathway cause severe neurodevelopmental problems and mental disability in infants (Acuna-Hidalgo et al., 2014; Hart et al., 2007; Klomp et al., 2000). In addition, missense mutation in DAAO increases D-serine levels in the cerebrospinal fluid and causes familial type of amyotrophic lateral sclerosis (ALS) (Mitchell et al., 2010; Paul & de Belleroche, 2014). Polymorphisms in SR locus are associated with schizophrenia risk, suggesting dysfunction of D-serine signaling in the disease (Balu et al., 2013; Bendikov et al., 2007; Labrie et al., 2009; Morita et al., 2007; Ripke & Schizophrenia Working Group of the Psychiatric Genomics Consortium, 2014).

While de novo synthesis of L-serine in the brain has been known for decades (Shank & Aprison, 1970), the significance of the serine shuttle to the production of D-serine in neurons was only recognized in the past few years. We will elaborate on the biochemical pathway for D-serine production and its physiological roles in the context of the glia–neuron crosstalk via the serine shuttle.

2. D-SERINE: FROM WORMS TO THE BRAIN

Unequivocal evidence for the presence of free D-serine in animals was first obtained in earthworms, where D-serine is required for the synthesis of lombricine, a phosphagen that buffers the ATP pool in annelids (Rosenberg & Ennor, 1961). D-Serine was subsequently described in silkworms, where millimolar concentrations of D-serine accumulate in the blood of the pupae, but rapidly decline at the end of the metamorphosis process (Srinivasan, Corrigan, & Meister, 1962, 1965). Injection of L-[^{14}C]serine into the pupae led to the accumulation of D-[^{14}C]serine, indicating a direct racemization reaction during pupation (Srinivasan et al., 1965). Several decades later, Esaki and colleagues detected racemization of L- into D-serine in partially purified silkworm extracts (Uo, Yoshimura, Shimizu, & Esaki, 1998), but a racemase has never been purified to homogeneity from silkworms.

Although the role of D-serine in the caterpillar remains a mystery, these early and mostly forgotten studies motivated our search for the mammalian SR and use it as a tool to unravel the physiological role of D-serine in the brain.

D-Serine is a high-affinity ligand of the coagonist site of NMDARs (Kleckner & Dingledine, 1988). Its natural occurrence in rodent brain was first reported by Hashimoto and Nishikawa when investigating the brain penetration of D-serine derivatives (Hashimoto et al., 1992). Levels of D-serine in the brain are a third of L-serine, reaching intracellular concentrations of about 0.3 mM in forebrain regions. By generating an antibody against D-serine, Snyder and coworkers found a close correlation between D-serine immunoreactivity and NMDAR localizations, suggesting D-serine as a potential endogenous modulator of the coagonist site (Schell et al., 1995).

3. SERINE RACEMASE: A MULTIFUNCTIONAL ENZYME

As a postdoctoral fellow at Sol Snyder's laboratory, I was greatly influenced by Sol's long-time pursuit of novel neurotransmitters and receptors. I became particularly interested in investigating the origin of brain D-serine, since the biosynthesis of D-amino acids was thought to be restricted to lower organisms. After failed attempts to raise enough silkworm pupae to confirm the existence of a serine racemase activity, I started to experiment with rat brains. Even though I could not detect any SR activity in crude brain extracts, I succeeded in detecting D-serine synthesis after carrying out a stepwise ammonium sulfate precipitation. Since the HPLC analysis of D-serine was tedious, Sol suggested that I develop an easy and sensitive method for detecting D-serine. Thus, I used a DAAO-based chemiluminescent assay, which greatly facilitated the determination of D-serine in the dozens of column eluates. Although the method was very tricky to work with, it allowed the complete purification and cloning of the SR from mammalian brain (Wolosker, Blackshaw, et al., 1999; Wolosker, Sheth, et al., 1999).

SR is a pyridoxal 5-phosphate (PLP)-dependent enzyme that directly converts L-serine to D-serine (Wolosker, Blackshaw, et al., 1999). Biochemical and crystallographic studies indicate that the production of D-serine is attained by the abstraction of a proton from the L-serine–PLP complex, leading to the formation of a planar carbanion intermediate, followed by reprotonation of the carbanion at the opposite side of the molecule in a so-called two-base mechanism (Foltyn et al., 2005; Goto et al., 2009; Ito et al., 2013).

Our lab subsequently found that SR also catalyzes the α,β elimination of water from L-serine generating aminoacrylate–PLP, an unstable intermediate that spontaneously decomposes into pyruvate and ammonia (De Miranda, Panizzutti, Foltyn, & Wolosker, 2002; Foltyn et al., 2005). This reaction is reminiscent of SR-limited homology to the serine/threonine dehydratase of *E. coli* (De Miranda, Santoro, Engelender, & Wolosker, 2000). The generation of pyruvate from L-serine is two to three times more efficient than the racemization under physiological-like conditions. SR-derived pyruvate was proposed to play a role in energy metabolism and protect cells from apoptosis (De Miranda et al., 2002; Talukdar et al., 2017). However, it is still unclear if the rate of pyruvate production by SR is fast enough to impact neuronal metabolism.

The ratio of the racemization and the α,β elimination reactions has physiological implications for the regulation of intracellular D-serine levels. D-Serine itself is a substrate for the α,β elimination, thereby limiting its physiological levels (Foltyn et al., 2005). It is possible that α,β elimination provides a catabolic route for D-serine in the forebrain areas devoid of endogenous DAAO expression. However, the elimination reaction with D-serine is about five times less efficient than the conversion of L-serine into D-serine (Strisovsky, Jiraskova, Mikulova, Rulisek, & Konvalinka, 2005), suggesting the preferential direction of SR is indeed the synthesis of D-serine.

In addition to use serine as substrate, SR catalyzes the α,β elimination of water from L-threonine generating α-ketobutyrate and ammonia, but without producing detectable levels of D-threonine (Foltyn et al., 2005; Strisovsky et al., 2005). This reaction has not been further explored, and it is not known whether it constitutes an important pathway for threonine degradation.

D-Aspartate is a D-amino acid that binds to the agonist site of NMDARs (Dunlop, Neidle, McHale, Dunlop, & Lajtha, 1986; Hashimoto & Oka, 1997). Like D-serine, D-aspartate is produced from its L-enantiomer in brain cultures (Long et al., 1998; Wolosker, D'Aniello, & Snyder, 2000). Recent studies indicate that SR-KO mice display a 50% decrease in brain levels of D-aspartate, indicating that SR may be responsible for half of the production of D-aspartate in the adult brain (Ito et al., 2016). The mammalian SR produces D-aspartate from L-aspartate at a rate 20-fold lower than for D-serine production (Uda et al., 2016). Therefore, SR is involved in the synthesis of five different products (D-serine, pyruvate, ammonia, α-ketobutyrate, and D-aspartate). Nevertheless, the role of SR-derived D-aspartate is unclear.

Postnatal levels of D-aspartate in the forebrain are about 40-fold lower than D-serine (Hashimoto & Oka, 1997), and there is no evidence that such low levels are sufficient to activate NMDARs (Ito et al., 2016).

4. NEURONAL VS ASTROGLIAL D-SERINE

D-Serine was originally proposed to be a glia-derived neuromodulator or gliotransmitter based on enrichment of D-serine (Schell et al., 1995) and SR (Wolosker, Blackshaw, et al., 1999) in astrocytes. Subsequent studies expanded this idea and suggested that vesicular D-serine release from astrocytes regulates several NMDAR-dependent processes (Bergersen et al., 2012; Martineau, Baux, & Mothet, 2006a; Martineau, Galli, Baux, & Mothet, 2008; Martineau et al., 2013; Oliet & Mothet, 2009; Oliet et al., 2008; Panatier et al., 2006; Papouin et al., 2012; Stevens et al., 2003; Williams, Diaz, Macnab, Sullivan, & Pow, 2006; Yang et al., 2003). As we recently reviewed (Wolosker et al., 2016), the methods used in these studies to specify gliotransmission by D-serine were prone to artifacts due to nonspecific antibody cross-reactivity, and recent studies using SR-KO mice as controls demonstrate that D-serine is mainly of neuronal origin.

By using more selective antibodies to SR and improved techniques to detect D-serine, we observed robust expression of SR and D-serine in glutamatergic neurons by immunohistochemistry (Kartvelishvily et al., 2006). These data led us to propose an alternative model whereby the neuronal D-serine plays a major role in NMDAR activation in an "autocrine" or "paracrine" manner (Wolosker, 2007; Wolosker et al., 2008).

Mori and coworkers reported preferential neuronal localizations of SR, with undetectable levels in astrocytes (Miya et al., 2008). They pioneered the use of SR-KO mice as negative controls to ensure the specificity of the antibodies. In collaboration with Sol Snyder group, we found that about 90% of forebrain neurons are positive for D-serine, while only a minority of astrocytes (10%) contain some D-serine (Ehmsen et al., 2013). The staining was abolished in SR-KO mice, confirming the specific detection of D-serine. Furthermore, we analyzed mice that expressed EGFP under the control of SR promoter, providing a highly sensitive assay to detect the cellular types that express SR (Ehmsen et al., 2013). EGFP localization was predominantly neuronal, confirming previous observations that neurons rather than glia are the main site of D-serine production.

Similar results demonstrating neuronal D-serine and SR were reported by Coyle group (Balu et al., 2014), who also demonstrated enrichment of

D-serine in GABAergic interneurons. Most importantly, cell-selective SR knockout revealed that only about 10% of SR is of glial origin (Balu et al., 2014; Benneyworth et al., 2012), indicating that D-serine is mostly produced in neurons.

5. PHYSIOLOGICAL ROLES OF THE NEURONAL AND NONNEURONAL D-SERINE

The investigation of the physiological roles of D-serine was made possible by the use of different strategies to knockdown D-serine levels. One strategy was to deplete D-serine in cell cultures or brain slices by adding enzymes that destroy D-serine, such as purified DAAO (Mothet et al., 2000) or D-serine deaminase (Shleper, Kartvelishvily, & Wolosker, 2005). Using the D-serine depletion strategy, Sol Snyder and coworkers demonstrated that D-serine is essential for NMDAR currents in primary cultures (Mothet et al., 2000). Subsequent studies demonstrated that D-serine is required for the NMDAR-dependent long-term potentiation (LTP) of the synaptic activity at the Schaffer collateral–CA1 synapse (Le Bail et al., 2015; Mothet, Le Bail, & Billard, 2015; Papouin et al., 2012; Yang et al., 2003) or amygdala (Li et al., 2013). Our lab demonstrated that depletion of endogenous D-serine by D-serine deaminase enzyme mostly abolished NMDAR-mediated neurotoxicity in hippocampal organotypic cultures (Shleper et al., 2005), indicating that D-serine is the dominant NMDAR coagonist for neurotoxicity. In the retina, degradation of D-serine by the D-serine deaminase enzyme demonstrates a role of D-serine in NMDAR-dependent light-evoked responses (Gustafson, Stevens, Wolosker, & Miller, 2007).

A more selective strategy was the use of SR-KO mice, which display a 90% decrease in brain D-serine (Basu et al., 2009; Miya et al., 2008). SR-KO mice exhibit a variety of phenotypes, including resistance to NMDAR-dependent neurotoxicity in vivo (Inoue, Hashimoto, Harai, & Mori, 2008), lower susceptibility to stroke damage (Mustafa et al., 2010), impairments in spatial (Basu et al., 2009; Labrie et al., 2009) and fear conditioning learning (Basu, Puhl, & Coyle, 2016), altered prepulse inhibition of the startle response (Labrie et al., 2009), and impairment of cocaine-induced conditioned place preference and locomotor sensitization (Puhl, Berg, Bechtholt, & Coyle, 2015).

Electrophysiological studies confirmed the impairment of the LTP in SR-KO mice under most experimental paradigms (Balu et al., 2013; Basu et al., 2009; Li et al., 2013; Rosenberg et al., 2013). However, in contrast to the severe phenotype of mutants of the coagonist site of the NMDARs (Kew et al., 2000), the SR-KO mice are viable, indicating that the synaptic activity of NMDARs is only partially mediated by D-serine in vivo. Other pathways (e.g., glycine release) are likely to overlap or compensate for the lack of D-serine. On the other hand, the remaining 10% of D-serine in SR-KO mice could be sufficient to partially saturate the NMDARs.

More recently, the role of neuronal D-serine was established by using cell-selective SR-KO mice. The LTP at the CA3–CA1 Schaffer collateral synapses in hippocampal slices was impaired when SR was deleted in glutamatergic neurons, but unaffected in astrocytic-selective SR-KO mice (Benneyworth et al., 2012). Deletion of SR in glutamatergic neurons also reduces the dendritic arborization and spine density, indicating a role in neurodevelopment (Balu & Coyle, 2012). Furthermore, deletion of SR in neurons using Thy1-mediated Cre recombination impairs hippocampal LTP in vivo, establishing a role of neuronal SR in synaptic plasticity (Perez et al., 2017).

Under normal conditions, astrocytes express little SR and do not significantly contribute to synaptic plasticity. However, reactive astrocytes, such as those present in primary cultures, overexpress SR (Kartvelishvily et al., 2006). A recent study demonstrates that traumatic brain injury causes reactive astrogliosis in the hippocampus and a switch of D-serine production from neurons to astrocytes. When SR is deleted from the reactive astrocytes, impairments in synaptic plasticity and learning were rescued, indicating that astrocytic D-serine plays a role in pathology, but not in the normal brain, where neuronal D-serine predominates (Perez et al., 2017).

The study of SR-KO mice revealed new roles of D-serine in peripheral tissues as well. Mori and coworkers demonstrated that skin SR is important for regulating keratinocytes development and the formation of the skin barrier (Inoue et al., 2014), suggesting that local D-serine production outside the brain also plays a physiological role and may be a target for therapies related to regeneration of skin cells.

6. THE SERINE SHUTTLE

Astrocytes are the main source of L-serine in the brain for they express the enzymes of the phosphorylated pathway that are involved in L-serine production from glucose (Yamasaki et al., 2001). Deletion of Phgdh enzyme, a committed step in L-serine biosynthesis, leads to a decrease in

D-serine and glycine levels in mice brain (Ehmsen et al., 2013; Yang et al., 2010) and the accumulation of cytotoxic deoxysphingolipids (Esaki et al., 2015). Patients with mutations in Phgdh or other enzymes of the phosphorylated pathway have severe neurodevelopmental problems, such as microcephaly, seizures, and mental disability (Acuna-Hidalgo et al., 2014; El-Hattab et al., 2016; Klomp et al., 2000).

The astrocytic source of L-serine inspired the formulation of two opposing hypotheses regarding the cellular origin of D-serine. The first was that higher levels of L-serine in astrocytes would be sufficient for astrocytic synthesis of D-serine and compensate for their lower SR levels. The alternative hypothesis was that astroglia would not synthesize much D-serine under normal conditions, but would export L-serine for the neuronal synthesis of D-serine by a glia–neuron crosstalk we called the serine shuttle (Wolosker, 2011; Wolosker & Radzishevsky, 2013). In order to investigate these possibilities, Jeff Ehmsen, an MD/PhD student from the Snyder lab, spent a couple of months in my laboratory at the Technion in Israel. By carefully titrating anti-D-serine antibodies using SR-KO mice as negative controls along with improved detection methods, Jeff found that D-serine was indeed predominantly neuronal. He carried out immunohistochemistry for D-serine in the brains of Phgdh-KO mice that have impaired L-serine synthesis in astroglia (Yang et al., 2010). Deletion of Phgdh in astroglia abolished D-serine immunoreactivity in neurons (Ehmsen et al., 2013). These data suggest that neuronal synthesis of D-serine depends on the astrocytic supply of L-serine, compatible with the serine shuttle hypothesis (Fig. 1).

A candidate to mediate L-serine release from astrocytes is the ASCT1 transporter (Arriza et al., 1993). Patients with mutations in ASCT1 (Slc1a4) have microcephaly and neurodevelopmental deficits that resemble those caused by mutations in the enzymes of the L-serine biosynthesis pathway (Damseh et al., 2015; Heimer et al., 2015). Although ASCT1 is capable of transporting L- and D-serine in transfected cells (Foster et al., 2016; Rosenberg et al., 2013), it is not known if it plays a role in serine homeostasis in vivo.

Asc-1 is a neutral amino acid transporter located at the plasma membrane that has relatively high affinity for D-serine and glycine and is present in neurons (Fukasawa et al., 2000; Helboe, Egebjerg, Moller, & Thomsen, 2003; Matsuo et al., 2004), though also proposed to be localized in astrocytes at the spinal cord (Ehmsen et al., 2016). Asc-1 works as an antiporter that exchanges D-serine for other neutral amino acids (Rosenberg et al., 2013; Sason et al., 2017). Surprisingly, we found that tonic release of endogenous

D-serine from cortical slices is lower in tissue from Asc-1-KO mice, suggesting that Asc-1 plays a role in D-serine release rather than uptake (Rosenberg et al., 2013; Sason et al., 2017). Moreover, blocking the Asc-1 transporter with a selective inhibitor decreases D-serine release, impairs the NMDAR-dependent LTP in the hippocampus, and decreases the NMDAR potentials (Sason et al., 2017).

Asc-1-KO mice also display lower synthesis of glycine in the brain and develop a fatal hyperekplexia phenotype due to glycinergic inhibitory transmission impairment (Safory et al., 2015). Even though Asc-1 plays a prominent role in the metabolism of glycine, in vivo experiments indicate that Asc-1 is also relevant for D-serine release. Administration of an Asc-1 inhibitor via brain microdialysis causes about 40% decrease in the extracellular levels of D-serine, confirming its role in a D-serine release pathway (Sakimura, Nakao, Yoshikawa, Suzuki, & Kimura, 2016; Sason et al., 2017).

Deletion of Asc-1 revealed that there is no other high-affinity transport system for D-serine (Rutter et al., 2007). As Asc-1 is involved in D-serine release, the absence of an efficient reuptake system for D-serine argues against the notion that D-serine is a fast-acting gliotransmitter released by exocytosis from astrocytes (Martineau et al., 2013; Mothet et al., 2005). In addition to the concerns regarding the low levels of D-serine in astroglia in vivo (Wolosker et al., 2016), it makes no sense to rapidly release D-serine if it cannot be efficiently removed from the synapse to terminate its signal. Indeed, we have shown that most D-serine is released from slices in a tonic fashion (Sason et al., 2017). Chelation of Ca^{2+} does not affect the kinetics of D-serine release from slices, while glutamate release under the same conditions is impaired (Rosenberg et al., 2010), suggesting that endogenous D-serine release from neurons is nonvesicular (Kartvelishvily et al., 2006; Rosenberg et al., 2013, 2010). In agreement with this notion, Bolshakov and coworkers found that D-serine is involved in the basal, but not activity-dependent, regulation of NMDARs at the amygdala (Li et al., 2013). Additional studies to clarify the roles and pathways mediating tonic and phasic D-serine release will be important to clarify the regulation of the serine shuttle and D-serine signaling.

7. REGULATION OF D-SERINE SIGNALING

Most of the known regulatory mechanisms of D-serine signaling focus on the activity of SR enzyme. SR is regulated by small ligands, protein interactors, posttranslational modifications, and subcellular localization (Table 1)

Table 1 Regulators of SR Activity and D-Serine Production

Modulators	Effects	References
Small ligands		
ATP, Mg^{2+}	Stimulates SR activity	De Miranda et al. (2002); Foltyn et al. (2005); Strisovsky et al. (2005)
NADH	Displaces ATP binding and inhibits SR	Bruno et al. (2016); Suzuki et al. (2015)
Protein interactors		
GRIP	Stimulates SR and targets it to the postsynapse	Kim et al. (2005)
Pick-1	Affects SR targeting	Fujii et al. (2006)
PSD-95	Affects SR targeting	Lin, Jacobi, Anderson, and Lynch (2016); Ma et al. (2014)
SAP102	Affects SR targeting	Ma et al. (2014)
Stargazin	Inhibits SR activity	Ma et al. (2014)
Golga3	Prevents SR degradation	Dumin et al. (2006)
Disc-1	Prevents SR degradation	Ma et al. (2013)
GAPDH	Decreases SR activity	Suzuki et al. (2015)
FBXO22	Decreases membrane binding of SR and increases its activity	Dikopoltsev et al. (2014)
Posttranslational modifications		
S-Nitrosylation	Decreases SR activity in an ATP-dependent manner	Mustafa et al. (2007)
O-Palmitoylation	Increases membrane association of SR	Balan et al. (2009)
PIP_2	Decreases SR activity	Mustafa et al. (2009)
Phosphorylation	Thr^{71}—major site, increases mouse SR activity Thr^{227}—increases membrane binding	Balan et al. (2009); Foltyn, Zehl, Dikopoltsev, Jensen, and Wolosker (2010)
Subcellular localization		
Membrane translocation	Inactivates SR	Balan et al. (2009)
Nuclear translocation	Inactivates SR	Kolodney et al. (2015)

(Wolosker & Mori, 2012). ATP and Mg^{2+} are the best characterized small ligand regulators (De Miranda et al., 2002). Both increase SR activity by severalfold. ATP is not hydrolyzed by the enzyme (De Miranda et al., 2002; Marchetti et al., 2013) but is required for stabilization of the SR dimer (Goto et al., 2009). Magnesium ion has a dual role: First, it increases the affinity of SR to ATP by complexing with the gamma and beta phosphates of ATP (De Miranda et al., 2002). Second, it directly stimulates the enzyme by binding to a cation binding site (Bruno et al., 2017; Cook, Galve-Roperh, Martinez Del Pozo, & Rodriguez-Crespo, 2002; De Miranda et al., 2002).

The second type of regulators are proteins interactors. The mouse SR displays a PDZ binding region consensus at its C-terminus and interacts with several postsynaptic proteins, including PSD-95, SAP102, Grip1, and Pick1 (Table 1). SR is present in dendrites and detergent-insoluble postsynaptic density fraction from the brain (Balan et al., 2009), supporting a model wherein neuronal SR regulates NMDARs in an "autocrine" or "paracrine" way (Kartvelishvily et al., 2006). Recent data demonstrating enrichment of SR in dendritic spines of cultured neurons and its interaction with PSD-95 are compatible with the postsynaptic production of D-serine (Lin et al., 2016; Ma et al., 2013). At the postsynapse, SR forms a ternary complex with PSD-95 and stargazin, which inhibits SR activity (Ma et al., 2014). AMPA receptor stimulation relieves SR inhibition by stargazing and increases D-serine synthesis, possibly increasing NMDAR activity (Ma et al., 2014).

SR interaction with Golga3 (Dumin et al., 2006; Ma et al., 2013) and Disc-1 (Ma et al., 2013) decreases SR ubiquitination and slows down its degradation by the ubiquitin-proteasome system. The ubiquitin ligase(s) responsible for SR ubiquitination is yet to be identified. SR interacts with the FBXO22 protein, which increases the synthesis of D-serine by preventing SR binding to intracellular membranes, but without affecting SR degradation rate or ubiquitination levels (Dikopoltsev et al., 2014).

Additional SR regulatory mechanisms encompass dynamic changes on its subcellular localization and posttranslational modifications. Stimulation of NMDARs in neuronal cultures leads to inactivation of SR by promoting its translocation from the cytosol (where SR normally resides) to the dendritic membrane (Balan et al., 2009). SR also interacts with lipids, especially phosphatidylinositol 4,5-bisphosphate (PIP_2), leading to inhibition of SR activity (Mustafa et al., 2009). Moreover, SR undergoes O-palmitoylation at serine or threonine residues, which may contribute to SR targeting to the membrane (Balan et al., 2009).

Upon apoptotic stimuli, SR accumulates in the nucleus of neurons, where the enzyme becomes inactive and strongly bound to the nuclear lamina (Kolodney et al., 2015). Mutations in the nuclear export sequences of SR also cause nuclear accumulation and inhibition of SR activity (Kolodney et al., 2015). It is proposed that SR translocation from the cytosol to other compartments (e.g., membranes and nuclear lamina) works as a fail-safe mechanisms to curb D-serine synthesis and prevent excitotoxicity of neighboring cells (Balan et al., 2009; Kolodney et al., 2015). SR translocation to the nucleus also reveals a nucleocytoplasmic shuttling mechanism that is disrupted early in apoptosis (Kolodney et al., 2015).

NO is an unconventional transmitter that is synthesized in the brain following NMDAR stimulation (Benhar, 2015; Boehning & Snyder, 2003). In addition to bind to heme-containing proteins, NO reacts with cysteine residues in a process called S-nitrosylation (Stamler, Lamas, & Fang, 2001). Snyder and coworkers were the first to demonstrate that numerous proteins are nitrosylated in vivo by nitric oxide following NMDAR stimulation (Jaffrey, Erdjument-Bromage, Ferris, Tempst, & Snyder, 2001). This was made possible by the development of the celebrated biotin-switch method, which allows selective purification of nitrosylated proteins (Jaffrey et al., 2001). Using this method, SR has been identified as an in vivo target of NO (Mustafa et al., 2007). NO nitrosylates Cys^{113} at the proximity of the ATP binding pocket of SR and inhibits the enzyme activity (Mustafa et al., 2007). NMDAR-dependent production of NO provides a feedback mechanism to decrease the synthesis of D-serine and the activity of NMDARs (Mustafa et al., 2007).

Mouse SR is phosphorylated at Thr^{71} and Thr^{227} (Foltyn et al., 2010). Thr^{71} is the main phosphorylation site of SR and this appears to increase D-serine production (Foltyn et al., 2010), while Thr^{227} phosphorylation takes place specifically at the membrane-bound enzyme and may facilitate SR association to membranes (Balan et al., 2009). However, none of these phosphorylation sites are conserved in human SR, suggesting species-specific regulatory processes.

8. D-SERINE AND PATHOLOGY

The resistance of SR-KO mice to NMDAR-mediated neurotoxicity and stroke damage (Inoue et al., 2008; Kolodney et al., 2015; Mustafa et al., 2010) suggests SR as a therapeutic target for neuroprotective drugs. Altered D-serine metabolism may also play a direct role in neurodegeneration.

A mutation in DAAO gene causes a familial form of ALS along with a large increase in the levels of D-serine in the spinal cord (Mitchell et al., 2010; Paul & de Belleroche, 2014). Mice expressing a catalytically inactive DAAO display motoneuron degeneration as well, indicating that increased D-serine levels may contribute to this neurodegenerative condition (Sasabe et al., 2012). However, cytotoxic effects caused by the formation of intracellular inclusions of aggregated DAAO might be also involved in this rare form of familial ALS. In any case, tissue samples from sporadic ALS cases have higher D-serine levels than controls (Sasabe et al., 2007, 2012), suggesting that the metabolism of D-serine is dysregulated in the disease.

Dysregulation of D-serine metabolism may also play a role in schizophrenia, where NMDARs are thought to have diminished activity (Balu & Coyle, 2014; Goff & Coyle, 2001; Javitt & Zukin, 1991; Krystal et al., 1994). In agreement, administration of D-serine ameliorates positive, negative, and cognitive symptoms of the disease when associated with conventional neuroleptics (Kantrowitz et al., 2010; Tsai, Yang, Chung, Lange, & Coyle, 1998). Schizophrenic subjects also display lower D-serine levels in the cerebrospinal fluid (Bendikov et al., 2007; Hashimoto et al., 2003), lower SR expression (Bendikov et al., 2007), and higher DAAO activity (Madeira, Freitas, Vargas-Lopes, Wolosker, & Panizzutti, 2008).

Genetic studies also implicate SR and DAAO variants in schizophrenia (Chumakov et al., 2002; Labrie et al., 2009; Morita et al., 2007; Schumacher et al., 2004). A large genome-wide association study with almost 37,000 patients and 110,000 controls identified SR as a schizophrenia risk gene, along with components of the glutamatergic pathway, such as GRIN2A and GRM3 (Ripke & Schizophrenia Working Group of the Psychiatric Genomics Consortium, 2014). The genetic data are compatible with the notion that schizophrenia is not limited to changes in the dopaminergic system but also involves glutamatergic dysfunction (Deutsch, Mastropaolo, Schwartz, Rosse, & Morihisa, 1989; Goff & Coyle, 2001). In agreement, SR-KO mice recapitulate several aspects of schizophrenia (Balu et al., 2013). Thus, enhancing SR activity or inhibiting its catabolism may provide a new therapeutic strategy for the disease.

9. CONCLUSION

D-Serine is now considered an important neuromodulator, which is required for NMDAR activity and is involved in several physiological and pathological processes. Studies from several laboratories now indicate that neurons rather than astrocytes are the main sources of D-serine. Dysregulation of the serine shuttle and brain D-serine metabolism is associated with neurodegeneration and schizophrenia risk, opening new therapeutic strategies to restore D-serine homeostasis in these conditions.

ACKNOWLEDGMENTS

I thank Sol Snyder for his continuous support throughout my career. My journey into this field was inspired by his iconoclastic pursuit of new transmitters and his unmatched originality and insight. I am indebted to my graduate students and research associates that dedicated their careers to study D-serine when the field was incipient and only a few labs believed on its importance. Work in my lab is funded by the Israel Science Foundation and the Allen and Jewel Prince Center for Neurodegenerative Disorders of the Brain.

CONFLICT OF INTERESTS

The author has no conflicts of interest to declare.

REFERENCES

Acuna-Hidalgo, R., Schanze, D., Kariminejad, A., Nordgren, A., Kariminejad, M. H., Conner, P., et al. (2014). Neu-Laxova syndrome is a heterogeneous metabolic disorder caused by defects in enzymes of the L-serine biosynthesis pathway. *American Journal of Human Genetics*, *95*(3), 285–293. https://doi.org/10.1016/j.ajhg.2014.07.012. S0002-9297(14)00321-8 [pii].

Arriza, J. L., Kavanaugh, M. P., Fairman, W. A., Wu, Y. N., Murdoch, G. H., North, R. A., et al. (1993). Cloning and expression of a human neutral amino acid transporter with structural similarity to the glutamate transporter gene family. *The Journal of Biological Chemistry*, *268*(21), 15329–15332.

Balan, L., Foltyn, V. N., Zehl, M., Dumin, E., Dikopoltsev, E., Knoh, D., et al. (2009). Feedback inactivation of D-serine synthesis by NMDA receptor-elicited translocation of serine racemase to the membrane. *Proceedings of the National Academy of Sciences of the United States of America*, *106*(18), 7589–7594.

Balu, D. T., & Coyle, J. T. (2012). Neuronal D-serine regulates dendritic architecture in the somatosensory cortex. *Neuroscience Letters*, *517*(2), 77–81.

Balu, D. T., & Coyle, J. T. (2014). The NMDA receptor 'glycine modulatory site' in schizophrenia: D-serine, glycine, and beyond. *Current Opinion in Pharmacology*, *20C*, 109–115. https://doi.org/10.1016/j.coph.2014.12.004.

Balu, D. T., Li, Y., Puhl, M. D., Benneyworth, M. A., Basu, A. C., Takagi, S., et al. (2013). Multiple risk pathways for schizophrenia converge in serine racemase knockout mice, a mouse model of NMDA receptor hypofunction. *Proceedings of the National Academy of Sciences of the United States of America*, *110*(26), E2400–E2409. https://doi.org/10.1073/pnas.1304308110.

Balu, D. T., Takagi, S., Puhl, M. D., Benneyworth, M. A., & Coyle, J. T. (2014). D-serine and serine racemase are localized to neurons in the adult mouse and human forebrain. *Cellular and Molecular Neurobiology*, *34*(3), 419–435. https://doi.org/10.1007/s10571-014-0027-z.

Basu, A. C., Puhl, M. D., & Coyle, J. T. (2016). Endogenous co-agonists of the NMDA receptor modulate contextual fear in trace conditioning. *Neurobiology of Learning and Memory*, *136*, 244–250. https://doi.org/10.1016/j.nlm.2016.09.006. S1074-7427(16)30181-2 [pii].

Basu, A. C., Tsai, G. E., Ma, C. L., Ehmsen, J. T., Mustafa, A. K., Han, L., et al. (2009). Targeted disruption of serine racemase affects glutamatergic neurotransmission and behavior. *Molecular Psychiatry, 14*(7), 719–727.

Bendikov, I., Nadri, C., Amar, S., Panizzutti, R., De Miranda, J., Wolosker, H., et al. (2007). A CSF and postmortem brain study of D-serine metabolic parameters in schizophrenia. *Schizophrenia Research, 90*(1–3), 41–51.

Benhar, M. (2015). Nitric oxide and the thioredoxin system: A complex interplay in redox regulation. *Biochimica et Biophysica Acta, 1850*(12), 2476–2484. https://doi.org/10.1016/j.bbagen.2015.09.010. S0304-4165(15)00242-1 [pii].

Benneyworth, M. A., Li, Y., Basu, A. C., Bolshakov, V. Y., & Coyle, J. T. (2012). Cell selective conditional null mutations of serine racemase demonstrate a predominate localization in cortical glutamatergic neurons. *Cellular and Molecular Neurobiology, 32*(4), 613–624. https://doi.org/10.1007/s10571-012-9808-4.

Bergersen, L. H., Morland, C., Ormel, L., Rinholm, J. E., Larsson, M., Wold, J. F., et al. (2012). Immunogold detection of L-glutamate and D-serine in small synaptic-like microvesicles in adult hippocampal astrocytes. *Cerebral Cortex, 22*(7), 1690–1697. https://doi.org/10.1093/cercor/bhr254.

Billard, J. M. (2012). D-amino acids in brain neurotransmission and synaptic plasticity. *Amino Acids, 43*(5), 1851–1860. https://doi.org/10.1007/s00726-012-1346-3.

Boehning, D., & Snyder, S. H. (2003). Novel neural modulators. *Annual Review of Neuroscience, 26*, 105–131.

Bruno, S., Marchesani, F., Dellafiora, L., Margiotta, M., Faggiano, S., Campanini, B., et al. (2016). Human serine racemase is allosterically modulated by NADH and reduced nicotinamide derivatives. *The Biochemical Journal, 473*(20), 3505–3516. https://doi.org/10.1042/BCJ20160566. BCJ20160566 [pii].

Bruno, S., Margiotta, M., Marchesani, F., Paredi, G., Orlandi, V., Faggiano, S., et al. (2017). Magnesium and calcium ions differentially affect human serine racemase activity and modulate its quaternary equilibrium toward a tetrameric form. *Biochimica et Biophysica Acta, 1865*(4), 381–387. https://doi.org/10.1016/j.bbapap.2017.01.001. S1570-9639(17)30001-8 [pii].

Chumakov, I., Blumenfeld, M., Guerassimenko, O., Cavarec, L., Palicio, M., Abderrahim, H., et al. (2002). Genetic and physiological data implicating the new human gene G72 and the gene for D-amino acid oxidase in schizophrenia. *Proceedings of the National Academy of Sciences of the United States of America, 99*(21), 13675–13680.

Cook, S. P., Galve-Roperh, I., Martinez Del Pozo, A., & Rodriguez-Crespo, I. (2002). Direct calcium binding results in activation of brain serine racemase. *The Journal of Biological Chemistry, 20*, 20.

Damseh, N., Simonin, A., Jalas, C., Picoraro, J. A., Shaag, A., Cho, M. T., et al. (2015). Mutations in SLC1A4, encoding the brain serine transporter, are associated with developmental delay, microcephaly and hypomyelination. *Journal of Medical Genetics, 52*(8), 541–547. https://doi.org/10.1136/jmedgenet-2015-103104. jmedgenet-2015-103104 [pii].

de Koning, T. J., Snell, K., Duran, M., Berger, R., Poll-The, B.-T., & Surtees, R. (2003). L-serine in disease and development. *The Biochemical Journal, 371*(3), 653–661. https://doi.org/10.1042/bj20021785.

De Miranda, J., Panizzutti, R., Foltyn, V. N., & Wolosker, H. (2002). Cofactors of serine racemase that physiologically stimulate the synthesis of the N-methyl-D-aspartate (NMDA) receptor coagonist D-serine. *Proceedings of the National Academy of Sciences of the United States of America, 99*(22), 14542–14547.

De Miranda, J., Santoro, A., Engelender, S., & Wolosker, H. (2000). Human serine racemase: Molecular cloning, genomic organization and functional analysis. *Gene, 256*(1–2), 183–188.

Deutsch, S. I., Mastropaolo, J., Schwartz, B. L., Rosse, R. B., & Morihisa, J. M. (1989). A "glutamatergic hypothesis" of schizophrenia: Rationale for pharmacotherapy with glycine. *Clinical Neuropharmacology*, *12*(1), 1–13.

Dikopoltsev, E., Foltyn, V. N., Zehl, M., Jensen, O. N., Mori, H., Radzishevsky, I., et al. (2014). FBXO22 protein is required for optimal synthesis of the N-methyl-D-aspartate (NMDA) receptor coagonist D-serine. *The Journal of Biological Chemistry*, *289*(49), 33904–33915. https://doi.org/10.1074/jbc.M114.618405. M114.618405 [pii].

Dumin, E., Bendikov, I., Foltyn, V. N., Misumi, Y., Ikehara, Y., Kartvelishvily, E., et al. (2006). Modulation of D-serine levels via ubiquitin-dependent proteasomal degradation of serine racemase. *The Journal of Biological Chemistry*, *281*(29), 20291–20302.

Dunlop, D. S., Neidle, A., McHale, D., Dunlop, D. M., & Lajtha, A. (1986). The presence of free D-aspartic acid in rodents and man. *Biochemical and Biophysical Research Communications*, *141*(1), 27–32.

Ehmsen, J. T., Liu, Y., Wang, Y., Paladugu, N., Johnson, A. E., Rothstein, J. D., et al. (2016). The astrocytic transporter SLC7A10 (Asc-1) mediates glycinergic inhibition of spinal cord motor neurons. *Scientific Reports*, *6*, 35592. https://doi.org/10.1038/srep35592. srep35592 [pii].

Ehmsen, J. T., Ma, T. M., Sason, H., Rosenberg, D., Ogo, T., Furuya, S., et al. (2013). D-serine in glia and neurons derives from 3-phosphoglycerate dehydrogenase. *The Journal of Neuroscience*, *33*(30), 12464–12469. https://doi.org/10.1523/JNEUROSCI.4914-12.2013.

El-Hattab, A. W., Shaheen, R., Hertecant, J., Galadari, H. I., Albaqawi, B. S., Nabil, A., et al. (2016). On the phenotypic spectrum of serine biosynthesis defects. *Journal of Inherited Metabolic Disease*, *39*(3), 373–381. https://doi.org/10.1007/s10545-016-9921-5. 10.1007/s10545-016-9921-5 [pii].

Esaki, K., Sayano, T., Sonoda, C., Akagi, T., Suzuki, T., Ogawa, T., et al. (2015). L-serine deficiency elicits intracellular accumulation of cytotoxic deoxysphingolipids and lipid body formation. *The Journal of Biological Chemistry*, *290*(23), 14595–14609. https://doi.org/10.1074/jbc.M114.603860. M114.603860 [pii].

Foltyn, V. N., Bendikov, I., De Miranda, J., Panizzutti, R., Dumin, E., Shleper, M., et al. (2005). Serine racemase modulates intracellular D-serine levels through an alpha,beta-elimination activity. *The Journal of Biological Chemistry*, *280*(3), 1754–1763.

Foltyn, V. N., Zehl, M., Dikopoltsev, E., Jensen, O. N., & Wolosker, H. (2010). Phosphorylation of mouse serine racemase regulates D-serine synthesis. *FEBS Letters*, *584*(13), 2937–2941. https://doi.org/10.1016/j.febslet.2010.05.022.

Foster, A. C., Farnsworth, J., Lind, G. E., Li, Y. X., Yang, J. Y., Dang, V., et al. (2016). D-serine is a substrate for neutral amino acid transporters ASCT1/SLC1A4 and ASCT2/SLC1A5, and is transported by both subtypes in rat hippocampal astrocyte cultures. *PLoS One*, *11*(6), e0156551. https://doi.org/10.1371/journal.pone.0156551. PONE-D-16-10510 [pii].

Fujii, K., Maeda, K., Hikida, T., Mustafa, A. K., Balkissoon, R., Xia, J., et al. (2006). Serine racemase binds to PICK1: Potential relevance to schizophrenia. *Molecular Psychiatry*, *11*(2), 150–157.

Fukasawa, Y., Segawa, H., Kim, J. Y., Chairoungdua, A., Kim, D. K., Matsuo, H., et al. (2000). Identification and characterization of a Na(+)-independent neutral amino acid transporter that associates with the 4F2 heavy chain and exhibits substrate selectivity for small neutral D- and L-amino acids. *The Journal of Biological Chemistry*, *275*(13), 9690–9698.

Furuya, S., Tabata, T., Mitoma, J., Yamada, K., Yamasaki, M., Makino, A., et al. (2000). L-serine and glycine serve as major astroglia-derived trophic factors for cerebellar Purkinje neurons. *Proceedings of the National Academy of Sciences of the United States of America*, *97*(21), 11528–11533. https://doi.org/10.1073/pnas.200364497.

Goff, D. C., & Coyle, J. T. (2001). The emerging role of glutamate in the pathophysiology and treatment of schizophrenia. *The American Journal of Psychiatry*, *158*(9), 1367–1377.

Goto, M., Yamauchi, T., Kamiya, N., Miyahara, I., Yoshimura, T., Mihara, H., et al. (2009). Crystal structure of a homolog of mammalian serine racemase from Schizosaccharomyces pombe. *The Journal of Biological Chemistry, 284*(38), 25944–25952.

Gustafson, E. C., Stevens, E. R., Wolosker, H., & Miller, R. F. (2007). Endogenous D-serine contributes to NMDA-receptor-mediated light-evoked responses in the vertebrate retina. *Journal of Neurophysiology, 98*(1), 122–130.

Hart, C. E., Race, V., Achouri, Y., Wiame, E., Sharrard, M., Olpin, S. E., et al. (2007). Phosphoserine aminotransferase deficiency: A novel disorder of the serine biosynthesis pathway. *American Journal of Human Genetics, 80*(5), 931–937. https://doi.org/10.1086/517888. S0002-9297(07)60948-3 [pii].

Hashimoto, K., Fukushima, T., Shimizu, E., Komatsu, N., Watanabe, H., Shinoda, N., et al. (2003). Decreased serum levels of D-serine in patients with schizophrenia: Evidence in support of the N-methyl-D-aspartate receptor hypofunction hypothesis of schizophrenia. *Archives of General Psychiatry, 60*(6), 572–576.

Hashimoto, A., Nishikawa, T., Hayashi, T., Fujii, N., Harada, K., Oka, T., et al. (1992). The presence of free D-serine in rat brain. *FEBS Letters, 296*(1), 33–36.

Hashimoto, A., & Oka, T. (1997). Free D-aspartate and D-serine in the mammalian brain and periphery. *Progress in Neurobiology, 52*(4), 325–353.

Heimer, G., Marek-Yagel, D., Eyal, E., Barel, O., Oz Levi, D., Hoffmann, C., et al. (2015). SLC1A4 mutations cause a novel disorder of intellectual disability, progressive microcephaly, spasticity and thin corpus callosum. *Clinical Genetics, 88*(4), 327–335. https://doi.org/10.1111/cge.12637.

Helboe, L., Egebjerg, J., Moller, M., & Thomsen, C. (2003). Distribution and pharmacology of alanine-serine-cysteine transporter 1 (asc-1) in rodent brain. *The European Journal of Neuroscience, 18*(8), 2227–2238.

Henneberger, C., Papouin, T., Oliet, S. H., & Rusakov, D. A. (2010). Long-term potentiation depends on release of D-serine from astrocytes. *Nature, 463*(7278), 232–236.

Hirabayashi, Y., & Furuya, S. (2008). Roles of L-serine and sphingolipid synthesis in brain development and neuronal survival. *Progress in Lipid Research, 47*(3), 188–203.

Inoue, R., Hashimoto, K., Harai, T., & Mori, H. (2008). NMDA- and beta-amyloid1-42-induced neurotoxicity is attenuated in serine racemase knock-out mice. *The Journal of Neuroscience, 28*(53), 14486–14491.

Inoue, R., Yoshihisa, Y., Tojo, Y., Okamura, C., Yoshida, Y., Kishimoto, J., et al. (2014). Localization of serine racemase and its role in the skin. *The Journal of Investigative Dermatology, 134*(6), 1618–1626. https://doi.org/10.1038/jid.2014.22. S0022-202X(15)36857-3 [pii].

Ito, T., Hayashida, M., Kobayashi, S., Muto, N., Hayashi, A., Yoshimura, T., et al. (2016). Serine racemase is involved in D-aspartate biosynthesis. *Journal of Biochemistry, 160*(6), 345–353. https://doi.org/10.1093/jb/mvw043. mvw043 [pii].

Ito, T., Maekawa, M., Hayashi, S., Goto, M., Hemmi, H., & Yoshimura, T. (2013). Catalytic mechanism of serine racemase from Dictyostelium discoideum. *Amino Acids, 44*(3), 1073–1084. https://doi.org/10.1007/s00726-012-1442-4.

Jaffrey, S. R., Erdjument-Bromage, H., Ferris, C. D., Tempst, P., & Snyder, S. H. (2001). Protein S-nitrosylation: A physiological signal for neuronal nitric oxide. *Nature Cell Biology, 3*(2), 193–197. https://doi.org/10.1038/35055104.

Javitt, D. C., & Zukin, S. R. (1991). Recent advances in the phencyclidine model of schizophrenia. *The American Journal of Psychiatry, 148*(10), 1301–1308.

Johnson, J. W., & Ascher, P. (1987). Glycine potentiates the NMDA response in cultured mouse brain neurons. *Nature, 325*(6104), 529–531.

Kantrowitz, J. T., Malhotra, A. K., Cornblatt, B., Silipo, G., Balla, A., Suckow, R. F., et al. (2010). High dose D-serine in the treatment of schizophrenia. *Schizophrenia Research, 121*(1–3), 125–130. https://doi.org/10.1016/j.schres.2010.05.012.

Kartvelishvily, E., Shleper, M., Balan, L., Dumin, E., & Wolosker, H. (2006). Neuron-derived D-serine release provides a novel means to activate N-methyl-D-aspartate receptors. *The Journal of Biological Chemistry*, *281*(20), 14151–14162.

Kew, J. N. C., Koester, A., Moreau, J.-L., Jenck, F., Ouagazzal, A.-M., Mutel, V., et al. (2000). Functional consequences of reduction in NMDA receptor glycine affinity in mice carrying targeted point mutations in the glycine binding site. *The Journal of Neuroscience*, *20*(11), 4037–4049.

Kim, P. M., Aizawa, H., Kim, P. S., Huang, A. S., Wickramasinghe, S. R., Kashani, A. H., et al. (2005). Serine racemase: Activation by glutamate neurotransmission via glutamate receptor interacting protein and mediation of neuronal migration. *Proceedings of the National Academy of Sciences of the United States of America*, *102*(6), 2105–2110.

Kleckner, N. W., & Dingledine, R. (1988). Requirement for glycine in activation of NMDA-receptors expressed in Xenopus oocytes. *Science*, *241*(4867), 835–837.

Klomp, L. W., de Koning, T. J., Malingre, H. E., van Beurden, E. A., Brink, M., Opdam, F. L., et al. (2000). Molecular characterization of 3-phosphoglycerate dehydrogenase deficiency—A neurometabolic disorder associated with reduced L-serine biosynthesis. *American Journal of Human Genetics*, *67*(6), 1389–1399. https://doi.org/10.1086/316886.

Kolodney, G., Dumin, E., Safory, H., Rosenberg, D., Mori, H., Radzishevisky, I., et al. (2015). Nuclear compartmentalization of serine racemase regulates D-serine production: Implications for N-methyl-D-aspartate (NMDA) receptor activation. *The Journal of Biological Chemistry*, *290*(52), 31037–31050. https://doi.org/10.1074/jbc.M115.699496. M115.699496 [pii].

Krystal, J. H., Karper, L. P., Seibyl, J. P., Freeman, G. K., Delaney, R., Bremner, J. D., et al. (1994). Subanesthetic effects of the noncompetitive NMDA antagonist, ketamine, in humans. Psychotomimetic, perceptual, cognitive, and neuroendocrine responses. *Archives of General Psychiatry*, *51*(3), 199–214.

Labrie, V., Fukumura, R., Rastogi, A., Fick, L. J., Wang, W., Boutros, P. C., et al. (2009). Serine racemase is associated with schizophrenia susceptibility in humans and in a mouse model. *Human Molecular Genetics*, *18*(17), 3227–3243.

Le Bail, M., Martineau, M., Sacchi, S., Yatsenko, N., Radzishevsky, I., Conrod, S., et al. (2015). Identity of the NMDA receptor coagonist is synapse specific and developmentally regulated in the hippocampus. *Proceedings of the National Academy of Sciences of the United States of America*, *112*(2), E204–E213. https://doi.org/10.1073/pnas.1416668112. 1416668112 [pii].

Li, Y., Sacchi, S., Pollegioni, L., Basu, A. C., Coyle, J. T., & Bolshakov, V. Y. (2013). Identity of endogenous NMDAR glycine site agonist in amygdala is determined by synaptic activity level. *Nature Communications*, *4*, 1760. https://doi.org/10.1038/ncomms2779.

Lin, H., Jacobi, A. A., Anderson, S. A., & Lynch, D. R. (2016). D-serine and serine racemase are associated with PSD-95 and glutamatergic synapse stability. *Frontiers in Cellular Neuroscience*, *10*, 34. https://doi.org/10.3389/fncel.2016.00034.

Long, Z., Homma, H., Lee, J. A., Fukushima, T., Santa, T., Iwatsubo, T., et al. (1998). Biosynthesis of D-aspartate in mammalian cells. *FEBS Letters*, *434*(3), 231–235.

Ma, T. M., Abazyan, S., Abazyan, B., Nomura, J., Yang, C., Seshadri, S., et al. (2013). Pathogenic disruption of DISC1-serine racemase binding elicits schizophrenia-like behavior via D-serine depletion. *Molecular Psychiatry*, *18*(5), 557–567. https://doi.org/10.1038/mp.2012.97.

Ma, T. M., Paul, B. D., Fu, C., Hu, S., Zhu, H., Blackshaw, S., et al. (2014). Serine racemase regulated by binding to stargazin and PSD-95: Potential N-methyl-D-aspartate-alpha-amino-3-hydroxy-5-methyl-4-isoxazolepropionic acid (NMDA-AMPA) glutamate neurotransmission cross-talk. *The Journal of Biological Chemistry*, *289*(43), 29631–29641. https://doi.org/10.1074/jbc.M114.571604.

Madeira, C., Freitas, M. E., Vargas-Lopes, C., Wolosker, H., & Panizzutti, R. (2008). Increased brain D-amino acid oxidase (DAAO) activity in schizophrenia. *Schizophrenia Research*, *101*(1–3), 76–83.

Marchetti, M., Bruno, S., Campanini, B., Peracchi, A., Mai, N., & Mozzarelli, A. (2013). ATP binding to human serine racemase is cooperative and modulated by glycine. *The FEBS Journal*, *280*(22), 5853–5863. https://doi.org/10.1111/febs.12510.

Martineau, M., Baux, G., & Mothet, J. P. (2006a). D-serine signalling in the brain: Friend and foe. *Trends in Neurosciences*, *29*(8), 481–491. https://doi.org/10.1016/j.tins.2006.06.008.

Martineau, M., Baux, G., & Mothet, J. P. (2006b). Gliotransmission at central glutamatergic synapses: D-serine on stage. *Journal of Physiology, Paris*, *99*(2–3), 103–110. https://doi.org/10.1016/j.jphysparis.2005.12.011.

Martineau, M., Galli, T., Baux, G., & Mothet, J. P. (2008). Confocal imaging and tracking of the exocytotic routes for D-serine-mediated gliotransmission. *Glia*, *56*(12), 1271–1284. https://doi.org/10.1002/glia.20696.

Martineau, M., Shi, T., Puyal, J., Knolhoff, A. M., Dulong, J., Gasnier, B., et al. (2013). Storage and uptake of D-serine into astrocytic synaptic-like vesicles specify gliotransmission. *The Journal of Neuroscience*, *33*(8), 3413–3423. https://doi.org/10.1523/JNEUROSCI.3497-12.2013.

Matsuo, H., Kanai, Y., Tokunaga, M., Nakata, T., Chairoungdua, A., Ishimine, H., et al. (2004). High affinity D- and L-serine transporter Asc-1: Cloning and dendritic localization in the rat cerebral and cerebellar cortices. *Neuroscience Letters*, *358*(2), 123–126.

Mitchell, J., Paul, P., Chen, H. J., Morris, A., Payling, M., Falchi, M., et al. (2010). Familial amyotrophic lateral sclerosis is associated with a mutation in D-amino acid oxidase. *Proceedings of the National Academy of Sciences of the United States of America*, *107*(16), 7556–7561. https://doi.org/10.1073/pnas.0914128107.

Miya, K., Inoue, R., Takata, Y., Abe, M., Natsume, R., Sakimura, K., et al. (2008). Serine racemase is predominantly localized in neurons in mouse brain. *The Journal of Comparative Neurology*, *510*(6), 641–654.

Morita, Y., Ujike, H., Tanaka, Y., Otani, K., Kishimoto, M., Morio, A., et al. (2007). A genetic variant of the serine racemase gene is associated with schizophrenia. *Biological Psychiatry*, *61*(10), 1200–1203.

Mothet, J. P., Le Bail, M., & Billard, J. M. (2015). Time and space profiling of NMDA receptor co-agonist functions. *Journal of Neurochemistry*, *135*(2), 210–225. https://doi.org/10.1111/jnc.13204.

Mothet, J. P., Parent, A. T., Wolosker, H., Brady, R. O., Jr., Linden, D. J., Ferris, C. D., et al. (2000). D-serine is an endogenous ligand for the glycine site of the N-methyl-D-aspartate receptor. *Proceedings of the National Academy of Sciences of the United States of America*, *97*(9), 4926–4931.

Mothet, J. P., Pollegioni, L., Ouanounou, G., Martineau, M., Fossier, P., & Baux, G. (2005). Glutamate receptor activation triggers a calcium-dependent and SNARE protein-dependent release of the gliotransmitter D-serine. *Proceedings of the National Academy of Sciences of the United States of America*, *102*(15), 5606–5611. https://doi.org/10.1073/pnas.0408483102.

Mustafa, A. K., Ahmad, A. S., Zeynalov, E., Gazi, S. K., Sikka, G., Ehmsen, J. T., et al. (2010). Serine racemase deletion protects against cerebral ischemia and excitotoxicity. *The Journal of Neuroscience*, *30*(4), 1413–1416. https://doi.org/10.1523/JNEUROSCI.4297-09.2010.

Mustafa, A. K., Kumar, M., Selvakumar, B., Ho, G. P., Ehmsen, J. T., Barrow, R. K., et al. (2007). Nitric oxide S-nitrosylates serine racemase, mediating feedback inhibition of D-serine formation. *Proceedings of the National Academy of Sciences of the United States of America*, *104*(8), 2950–2955.

Mustafa, A. K., van Rossum, D. B., Patterson, R. L., Maag, D., Ehmsen, J. T., Gazi, S. K., et al. (2009). Glutamatergic regulation of serine racemase via reversal of PIP2 inhibition. *Proceedings of the National Academy of Sciences of the United States of America*, *106*(8), 2921–2926.

Oliet, S. H., & Mothet, J. P. (2009). Regulation of N-methyl-D-aspartate receptors by astrocytic D-serine. *Neuroscience*, *158*(1), 275–283. https://doi.org/10.1016/j.neuroscience.2008.01.071. S0306-4522(08)00166-8 [pii].

Oliet, S. H., Panatier, A., Piet, R., Mothet, J. P., Poulain, D. A., & Theodosis, D. T. (2008). Neuron-glia interactions in the rat supraoptic nucleus. *Progress in Brain Research*, *170*, 109–117. https://doi.org/10.1016/S0079-6123(08)00410-X. S0079-6123(08)00410-X [pii].

Panatier, A., Theodosis, D. T., Mothet, J. P., Touquet, B., Pollegioni, L., Poulain, D. A., et al. (2006). Glia-derived D-serine controls NMDA receptor activity and synaptic memory. *Cell*, *125*(4), 775–784. https://doi.org/10.1016/j.cell.2006.02.051. S0092-8674(06)00506-X [pii].

Papouin, T., Ladepeche, L., Ruel, J., Sacchi, S., Labasque, M., Hanini, M., et al. (2012). Synaptic and extrasynaptic NMDA receptors are gated by different endogenous coagonists. *Cell*, *150*(3), 633–646. https://doi.org/10.1016/j.cell.2012.06.029. S0092-8674(12)00786-6 [pii].

Paul, P., & de Belleroche, J. (2014). The role of D-serine and glycine as co-agonists of NMDA receptors in motor neuron degeneration and amyotrophic lateral sclerosis (ALS). *Frontiers in Synaptic Neuroscience*, *6*, 10. https://doi.org/10.3389/fnsyn.2014.00010.

Perez, E. J., Tapanes, S. A., Loris, Z. B., Balu, D. T., Sick, T. J., Coyle, J. T., et al. (2017). Enhanced astrocytic D-serine underlies synaptic damage after traumatic brain injury. *The Journal of Clinical Investigation*, *127*, 3114–3125. https://doi.org/10.1172/JCI92300. 92300 [pii].

Puhl, M. D., Berg, A. R., Bechtholt, A. J., & Coyle, J. T. (2015). Availability of N-methyl'D-aspartate receptor coagonists affects cocaine-induced conditioned place preference and locomotor sensitization: Implications for comorbid schizophrenia and substance abuse. *The Journal of Pharmacology and Experimental Therapeutics*, *353*(3), 465–470. https://doi.org/10.1124/jpet.115.223099. jpet.115.223099 [pii].

Ripke, S., & Schizophrenia Working Group of the Psychiatric Genomics Consortium (2014). Biological insights from 108 schizophrenia-associated genetic loci. *Nature*, *511*(7510), 421–427. https://doi.org/10.1038/nature13595nature13595 [pii].

Rosenberg, D., Artoul, S., Segal, A. C., Kolodney, G., Radzishevsky, I., Dikopoltsev, E., et al. (2013). Neuronal D-serine and glycine release via the Asc-1 transporter regulates NMDA receptor-dependent synaptic activity. *The Journal of Neuroscience*, *33*(8), 3533–3544. https://doi.org/10.1523/JNEUROSCI.3836-12.2013.

Rosenberg, H., & Ennor, A. H. (1961). The occurrence of free D-serine in the earthworm. *The Biochemical Journal*, *79*, 424–428.

Rosenberg, D., Kartvelishvily, E., Shleper, M., Klinker, C. M., Bowser, M. T., & Wolosker, H. (2010). Neuronal release of D-serine: A physiological pathway controlling extracellular D-serine concentration. *FASEB Journal*, *24*(8), 2951–2961. https://doi.org/10.1096/fj.09-147967.

Rutter, A. R., Fradley, R. L., Garrett, E. M., Chapman, K. L., Lawrence, J. M., Rosahl, T. W., et al. (2007). Evidence from gene knockout studies implicates Asc-1 as the primary transporter mediating D-serine reuptake in the mouse CNS. *The European Journal of Neuroscience*, *25*(6), 1757–1766. https://doi.org/10.1111/j.1460-9568.2007.05446.x.

Safory, H., Neame, S., Shulman, Y., Zubedat, S., Radzishevsky, I., Rosenberg, D., et al. (2015). The alanine-serine-cysteine-1 (Asc-1) transporter controls glycine levels in

the brain and is required for glycinergic inhibitory transmission. *EMBO Reports*, *16*(5), 590–598. https://doi.org/10.15252/Embr.201439561. embr.201439561 [pii].
Sakimura, K., Nakao, K., Yoshikawa, M., Suzuki, M., & Kimura, H. (2016). A novel Na(+)-independent alanine-serine-cysteine transporter 1 inhibitor inhibits both influx and efflux of D-serine. *Journal of Neuroscience Research*, *94*(10), 888–895. https://doi.org/10.1002/jnr.23772.
Sasabe, J., Chiba, T., Yamada, M., Okamoto, K., Nishimoto, I., Matsuoka, M., et al. (2007). D-serine is a key determinant of glutamate toxicity in amyotrophic lateral sclerosis. *The EMBO Journal*, *26*(18), 4149–4159.
Sasabe, J., Miyoshi, Y., Suzuki, M., Mita, M., Konno, R., Matsuoka, M., et al. (2012). D-amino acid oxidase controls motoneuron degeneration through D-serine. *Proceedings of the National Academy of Sciences of the United States of America*, *109*(2), 627–632. https://doi.org/10.1073/pnas.1114639109.
Sason, H., Billard, J. M., Smith, G. P., Safory, H., Neame, S., Kaplan, E., et al. (2017). Asc-1 transporter regulation of synaptic activity via the tonic release of D-serine in the forebrain. *Cerebral Cortex*, *27*(2), 1573–1587. https://doi.org/10.1093/cercor/bhv350. bhv350 [pii].
Schell, M. J., Molliver, M. E., & Snyder, S. H. (1995). D-serine, an endogenous synaptic modulator: Localization to astrocytes and glutamate-stimulated release. *Proceedings of the National Academy of Sciences of the United States of America*, *92*(9), 3948–3952.
Schumacher, J., Jamra, R. A., Freudenberg, J., Becker, T., Ohlraun, S., Otte, A. C., et al. (2004). Examination of G72 and D-amino-acid oxidase as genetic risk factors for schizophrenia and bipolar affective disorder. *Molecular Psychiatry*, *9*(2), 203–207.
Shank, R. P., & Aprison, M. (1970). The metabolism in vivo of glycine and serine in eight areas of the rat central nervous system. *Journal of Neurochemistry*, *17*(10), 1461–1475.
Shleper, M., Kartvelishvily, E., & Wolosker, H. (2005). D-serine is the dominant endogenous coagonist for NMDA receptor neurotoxicity in organotypic hippocampal slices. *The Journal of Neuroscience*, *25*(41), 9413–9417.
Srinivasan, N. G., Corrigan, J. J., & Meister, A. (1962). D-serine in the blood of the silkworm Bombyx mori and other lepidoptera. *The Journal of Biological Chemistry*, *237*, 3844–3845.
Srinivasan, N. G., Corrigan, J. J., & Meister, A. (1965). Biosynthesis of D-serine in the silkworm, Bombyx mori. *The Journal of Biological Chemistry*, *240*, 796–800.
Stamler, J. S., Lamas, S., & Fang, F. C. (2001). Nitrosylation. The prototypic redox-based signaling mechanism. *Cell*, *106*(6), 675–683. doi:S0092-8674(01)00495-0 [pii].
Stevens, E. R., Esguerra, M., Kim, P. M., Newman, E. A., Snyder, S. H., Zahs, K. R., et al. (2003). D-serine and serine racemase are present in the vertebrate retina and contribute to the physiological activation of NMDA receptors. *Proceedings of the National Academy of Sciences of the United States of America*, *100*(11), 6789–6794.
Strisovsky, K., Jiraskova, J., Mikulova, A., Rulisek, L., & Konvalinka, J. (2005). Dual substrate and reaction specificity in mouse serine racemase: Identification of high-affinity dicarboxylate substrate and inhibitors and analysis of the beta-eliminase activity. *Biochemistry*, *44*(39), 13091–13100.
Suzuki, M., Sasabe, J., Miyoshi, Y., Kuwasako, K., Muto, Y., Hamase, K., et al. (2015). Glycolytic flux controls D-serine synthesis through glyceraldehyde-3-phosphate dehydrogenase in astrocytes. *Proceedings of the National Academy of Sciences of the United States of America*, *112*(17), E2217–E2224. https://doi.org/10.1073/pnas.1416117112. 1416117112 [pii].
Talukdar, G., Inoue, R., Yoshida, T., Ishimoto, T., Yaku, K., Nakagawa, T., et al. (2017). Novel role of serine racemase in anti-apoptosis and metabolism. *Biochimica et Biophysica Acta*, *1861*(1 Pt. A), 3378–3387. https://doi.org/10.1016/j.bbagen.2016.08.020. S0304-4165(16)30320-8 [pii].
Traynelis, S. F., Wollmuth, L. P., McBain, C. J., Menniti, F. S., Vance, K. M., Ogden, K. K., et al. (2010). Glutamate receptor ion channels: Structure, regulation, and function. *Pharmacological Reviews*, *62*(3), 405–496.

Tsai, G., Yang, P., Chung, L. C., Lange, N., & Coyle, J. T. (1998). D-serine added to antipsychotics for the treatment of schizophrenia. *Biological Psychiatry*, *44*(11), 1081–1089.

Uda, K., Abe, K., Dehara, Y., Mizobata, K., Sogawa, N., Akagi, Y., et al. (2016). Distribution and evolution of the serine/aspartate racemase family in invertebrates. *Amino Acids*, *48*(2), 387–402. https://doi.org/10.1007/s00726-015-2092-0. 10.1007/s00726-015-2092-0 [pii].

Uo, T., Yoshimura, T., Shimizu, S., & Esaki, N. (1998). Occurrence of pyridoxal 5′-phosphate-dependent serine racemase in silkworm, Bombyx mori. *Biochemical and Biophysical Research Communications*, *246*(1), 31–34.

Williams, S. M., Diaz, C. M., Macnab, L. T., Sullivan, R. K., & Pow, D. V. (2006). Immunocytochemical analysis of D-serine distribution in the mammalian brain reveals novel anatomical compartmentalizations in glia and neurons. *Glia*, *53*(4), 401–411.

Wolosker, H. (2007). NMDA receptor regulation by D-serine: New findings and perspectives. *Molecular Neurobiology*, *36*(2), 152–164.

Wolosker, H. (2011). Serine racemase and the serine shuttle between neurons and astrocytes. *Biochimica et Biophysica Acta*, *1814*(11), 1558–1566. https://doi.org/10.1016/j.bbapap.2011.01.001.

Wolosker, H., Balu, D. T., & Coyle, J. T. (2016). The rise and fall of the D-serine-mediated gliotransmission hypothesis. *Trends in Neurosciences*, *39*(11), 712–721. https://doi.org/10.1016/j.tins.2016.09.007. S0166-2236(16)30118-7 [pii].

Wolosker, H., Blackshaw, S., & Snyder, S. H. (1999). Serine racemase: A glial enzyme synthesizing D-serine to regulate glutamate-N-methyl-D-aspartate neurotransmission. *Proceedings of the National Academy of Sciences of the United States of America*, *96*(23), 13409–13414.

Wolosker, H., D'Aniello, A., & Snyder, S. H. (2000). D-aspartate disposition in neuronal and endocrine tissues: Ontogeny, biosynthesis and release. *Neuroscience*, *100*(1), 183–189.

Wolosker, H., Dumin, E., Balan, L., & Foltyn, V. N. (2008). D-amino acids in the brain: D-serine in neurotransmission and neurodegeneration. *The FEBS Journal*, *275*(14), 3514–3526.

Wolosker, H., & Mori, H. (2012). Serine racemase: An unconventional enzyme for an unconventional transmitter. *Amino Acids*, *43*(5), 1895–1904. https://doi.org/10.1007/s00726-012-1370-3.

Wolosker, H., & Radzishevsky, I. (2013). The serine shuttle between glia and neurons: Implications for neurotransmission and neurodegeneration. *Biochemical Society Transactions*, *41*(6), 1546–1550.

Wolosker, H., Sheth, K. N., Takahashi, M., Mothet, J. P., Brady, R. O., Jr., Ferris, C. D., et al. (1999). Purification of serine racemase: Biosynthesis of the neuromodulator D-serine. *Proceedings of the National Academy of Sciences of the United States of America*, *96*(2), 721–725.

Yamasaki, M., Yamada, K., Furuya, S., Mitoma, J., Hirabayashi, Y., & Watanabe, M. (2001). 3-Phosphoglycerate dehydrogenase, a key enzyme for L-serine biosynthesis, is preferentially expressed in the radial glia/astrocyte lineage and olfactory ensheathing glia in the mouse brain. *The Journal of Neuroscience*, *21*(19), 7691–7704.

Yang, Y., Ge, W., Chen, Y., Zhang, Z., Shen, W., Wu, C., et al. (2003). Contribution of astrocytes to hippocampal long-term potentiation through release of D-serine. *Proceedings of the National Academy of Sciences of the United States of America*, *100*(25), 15194–15199.

Yang, J. H., Wada, A., Yoshida, K., Miyoshi, Y., Sayano, T., Esaki, K., et al. (2010). Brain-specific Phgdh deletion reveals a pivotal role for L-serine biosynthesis in controlling the level of D-serine, an N-methyl-D-aspartate receptor co-agonist, in adult brain. *The Journal of Biological Chemistry*, *285*(53), 41380–41390. https://doi.org/10.1074/jbc.M110.187443.

Kolibri 360 GmbH
Ferdinand-Jühlke-Straße 7
99095 Erfurt, Deutschland
produktsicherheit@kolibri360.de